Ollie

Stephen Venables is best known as the mountaineer who in 1988 became the first Briton to climb Everest without oxygen – one of many pioneering expeditions around the world. He began climbing while at New College, Oxford, in the early seventies, and has written eight books about his mountain travels, winning the Boardman Tasker Prize, the King Albert Medal and the Grand Award at Banff International Mountain Literature Festival. He has also appeared in several television documentaries and the IMAX movie, *Shackleton's Antarctic Adventure*. He lives in Bath with his wife Rosie and Ollie's brother Edmond.

'An uplifting tribute to a remarkable child' *Daily Express*

'Venables celebrates his son's "gigantic, quirky, enigmatic, defiant personality", and describes their twelve years together as an adventure that enriched his life . . . A testament not only to a brave boy, but to an exceptional marriage' *New Statesman*

'Extraordinary and inspirational . . . Mischievous and playful, Ollie's determination and zest for life brought joy and laughter into the lives of those around him, leaving a legacy of love and endurance' *Good Book Guide*

Ollie

STEPHEN VENABLES

arrow books

Published by Arrow Books in 2007

1 3 5 7 9 10 8 6 4 2

Copyright © Stephen Venables 2006

The right of Stephen Venables to be identified as the author
of this work has been asserted by him in accordance with
the Copyright, Designs and Patents Act, 1988

This book is a work of non-fiction based on the life, experiences and
recollections of the author. In some limited cases names of people have
been changed solely to protect the privacy of others. The author has stated
to the publishers that, except in such minor respects not affecting the
substantial accuracy of the work, the contents of this book are true

First published in the United Kingdom by Hutchinson in 2006

Arrow Books
The Random House Group Limited
20 Vauxhall Bridge Road, London SW1V 2SA

www.randomhouse.co.uk

Addresses for companies within The Random House Group Limited
can be found at: www.randomhouse.co.uk/offices.htm

The Random House Group Limited Reg. No. 954009

A CIP catalogue record for this book is available from the British Library

ISBN 9780099478799

The Random House Group Limited makes every effort to ensure that the
papers used in its books are made from trees that have been legally sourced
from well-managed and credibly certified forests. Our paper procurement
policy can be found at: www.randomhouse.co.uk/paper.htm

Typeset by Palimpsest Book Production Limited, Grangemouth, Stirlingshire
Printed and bound in the United Kingdom by Bookmarque Ltd, Croydon, Surrey

Acknowledgements

When Ollie became autistic our family embarked on an extraordinary journey into the unknown. During that journey, complicated by leukaemia, we encountered many wonderful people whom we would otherwise never have met. Only some of the several hundred people who touched Ollie's life are mentioned by name in this book, some by first name only; others – in the interests of privacy or to avoid a confusing surfeit of names – are mentioned only anonymously; many do not appear at all. But all of you – friends, relatives, neighbours, teachers, social workers, psychologists, doctors, surgeons, radiographers, nurses, carers, therapists, cooks, cleaners, gardeners, shoppers, shopkeepers, drivers, administrators, technicians – I thank you for all you did to help us and our son.

Special thanks are due to the Margaret Coates Unit, Option Institute, Prior's Court School and Sunfield; and to the Royal United Hospital Bath, Bristol Children's Hospital, Bristol Eye Hospital, Frenchay Hospital and Royal Free Hospital London.

And to the charities and trusts who helped pay for Ollie's care and home education: Lizzie Bingley Trust, CLIC, Family Fund Trust, R.J. Harris Trust, Jessie's Fund, Mead Nursery, Oldham Foundation, Malcolm Sargent Fund, Sharon Spratt Trust, Thompson Charitable Trust, St John's Hospital, Wessex Cancer Trust and S.D. Whitehead Trust; and the many individuals – too many to list here – who also donated money, both towards Ollie's education and for setting up Peach.

I would also like to thank the people who helped me in the writing of this book: Hamish Hamilton for permission to quote from Elfrida Vipont's *The Elephant and the Bad Baby*, Donna Williams for allowing me to quote from her film *Inside Out*, and Mosby – Yearbook Inc. for permission to use passages from *Mosby's Medical Dictionary*; Tom and Alice Craigmyle for providing a peaceful sanctuary at St Catherine's; Avery Cunliffe, *Bath Evening Chronicle*, Sam Farr, Simon Prentice, Southwest News and Ed Webster for allowing me to use their photographs; Dr Charles Clarke, Dr David Rushton and Professor Seth Love for checking relevant medical sections of the manuscript; my agents Euan Thorneycroft and Vivienne Schuster at Curtis Brown; James Nightingale, Neil Bradford, Emma Mitchell and my ever encouraging editor Tony Whittome at Hutchinson; and of course my wife Rosie, the best mother Ollie could possibly have had, for all her vital suggestions, corrections and enormous encouragement.

Stephen Venables
January 2006

For Rosie

Chapter One

We buried him on the last day of October, a day of low clouds scudding through a sodden sky. The matting draped over the excavated mound of stony earth was luminous green, like the artificial seaweed in an old-fashioned fishmonger. The real grass underfoot was cold and dank where Edmond, Rosie and I – brother, mother, father – stood closest to the grave, flinching at the terrible finality of those ancient words, 'Earth to earth, ashes to ashes, dust to dust'. Echoing their elemental truth, the coffin settled with a hollow groan in its hard bed, oak reverberating on rock.

The service ended and the others stood back slightly in a hushed semicircle while we three stooped to admire the flowers. Then Rosie began suddenly to laugh. Uncles, aunts, godparents and grandparents shuffled uncomfortably behind us: oh no, she's finally cracked! Another peal of laughter rang brightly through the silent cemetery and she pointed at the puzzling floral arrangement of brilliant banded colours which I had taken for some kind of funerary urn. 'Look,' she giggled, 'it's a *watering can*! That's what it is: see – it's even got a sprinkler rose.' And I looked closer and laughed too at the cheerful sunflower spout from which sprinkled a threaded arc of pale slender grass seeds. It was the perfect tribute from his special school to the boy called Ollie, whose obsessive baffling passion for watering cans seemed emblematic of his whole gigantic, quirky, funny, beautiful, enigmatic, defiant personality.

Like the swallows he arrived in the spring and left in the autumn. In between, we joined him on a journey which lasted twelve years and four months. At first we never called him Ollie, preferring his full name, Oliver. I liked the unhurried resonance of those three soft syllables and it was only after something happened in his brain, upsetting the whole subtle balance of sensory perceptions to the point where language became almost impossible for him to process, that we changed to the simpler 'Ollie', so much easier to hear and to say.

Now that perky staccato seems inseparable from the boy we loved, synonymous with the laughter he brought to our lives. But also inseparable from a kind of radiance – an innate joyfulness which was never quashed, despite the huge challenges he had to face. So, as I try to tell the story of how he grappled with those challenges, I shall call him Ollie, right from the beginning. But what was the beginning? How did it start – this extraordinary journey, this adventure which so totally changed and enriched our lives?

I suppose that it really began in a country churchyard, another graveyard, on a hot June afternoon in 1986 – a sudden meeting of strangers' eyes over the headstones as Rosie and I wandered out independently from the wedding of two mutual friends. At the reception afterwards she was bubbling and flirtatious. She was thirty, had just finished studying aesthetics at Goldsmiths' College in London, and was about to start teaching at a rumbustious inner-city primary school. She was brave and beautiful and she was married to someone else.

I managed to forget about her and was soon gone – away to the Alps to climb mountains, because climbing mountains was what I did. That summer's glorious odyssey culminated in success on a climb I had dreamed about for fifteen years – the magnificent, awesome, irresistible North Face of the Eiger. In October I returned, elated but penniless, to London and, with no other jobs on the immediate horizon, started working at my Eiger companion Luke's furniture-making business in Covent Garden. My first book, about mountain explorations in Kashmir, had just been published and one lunchtime I had to go over to the BBC for a radio interview. I was on my way back to the workshop from Broadcasting House, threading the jostling crowds, anonymous in a city of eight million people, when I suddenly saw her – emerging from a wine bar in a burst of golden laughter. I shouted across the street 'Rosie!' There was a moment of startled incomprehension, then sudden recall and a hurried exchange of phone numbers before she rushed off to catch up with her sister who asked, 'Who was that strange man?'

Another three years passed before the strange man was taken to meet Rosie's parents. During those three years she left an unsatisfactory marriage and enjoyed a brief spell of manless contentment before I began to see more of her. Meanwhile I had given up carpentry and committed myself to the vagaries of freelance writing and lecturing, based around my expeditions. It was a momentous time, making epic journeys through the Karakoram, climbing a spectacular new route up Mount Everest and, back in London, falling in love with Rosie. Then one summer's evening in 1989, in a friend's Shropshire garden, she told me to propose to her. So I did; and the following day we went to tell her parents.

Her mother, Kay, was admirably direct: 'We think you're a splendid chap, Stephen; we just wish you had a bit of money.' Robin was more tolerant of my wayward life, attributing romantic and completely unrealistic notions of courage and heroism to my rather self-indulgent Everest climb of the previous year. He seemed confident that, somehow, I would support his youngest daughter, and his only real concern was that she should have babies. 'She has a very strong maternal instinct, you know. She always wanted to have children and I think she really needs that fulfilment.'

I mumbled agreement, hoping privately to defer fatherhood for a little longer. In any case, we had first to sort out somewhere to live. Rosie wanted to stay in London. I wanted a little more space, with a garden, close to the country. She agreed reluctantly to move a hundred miles west to Larkhall, on the edge of Bath. My parents had lived for twelve years on the other side of the city, so I knew the area quite well and had grown fond of its steep hills, winding valleys and villages built of mellow, golden, oolitic limestone. Of course it is a landscape which can seem cloyingly pretty, verging even on the twee, and in the city itself, for all its gracious beauty, I still yearn for some outrageous brash modernism to challenge the relentless Georgian respectability; but Larkhall, on the edge of town, is less obviously bourgeois. There we took out a mortgage on a small Victorian terrace house with bedroom and study upstairs, and downstairs, adjoining the kitchen, a single long room with space for the Broadwood grand piano I had just inherited from my godfather. We moved in September 1989, ten weeks before I was due to depart on an expedition to the sub-Antarctic island of South Georgia. It was an oddly turbulent time. Rosie missed London and hated the temporary job she had taken at the local infants' school; and we still had to adjust to our strange new shared life, knowing that any progress was soon going to be disrupted by four months' separation.

I disappeared to South Georgia. Rosie spent the winter working in the French Alps and it was only when we both returned the following spring, in 1990, that we began to achieve some kind of equilibrium. We pottered contentedly in our tiny garden, digging, planting, watering, nurturing, discussing endlessly the possibilities of colour and texture as the summer days lengthened languorously. We drove over the Severn Bridge to spend evenings rock climbing in the Wye Valley. Friends came to stay. I started work on a new book about the South Georgia expedition, often stealing guiltily downstairs to play the piano, relishing the novelty of domestic stability. Babies were mentioned again, but as part of a future plan, to be scheduled contraceptively around my expeditions and Rosie's horticultural enthusiasms. Every morning that summer she got up at sunrise to rattle up the Fosse Way in her open-top Deux Chevaux to the plant nursery where she spent the day potting, propagating and weeding, returning in the late afternoon, sometimes with a few precious green sweepings from the potting-room floor, to be nurtured in our own garden. It was the happiest summer she had spent since her childhood in East Africa. In the autumn she was starting a horticultural course at the local agricultural college; the following year she hoped to study landscape design.

In September I was invited to Switzerland, as a special guest of the mountain film festival at Les Diablerets. It was a chance to do some climbing, enjoy faultless Swiss hospitality and rub shoulders with some of the great legends of the mountain world, such as Anderl Heckmair, the Bavarian who had led the very first ascent of the Eiger North Face in 1938. My head was still buzzing with tales of heroic deeds when I returned to Larkhall on a Monday evening. Rosie was in the sitting room, having a drink with our acupuncturist friend Lizzie Bingley. After a quick hello kiss I went upstairs to dump luggage and check my answer machine, then came back down to rejoin Rosie and Lizzie.

The two women looked rather edgy. 'Have you looked in the study?' asked Rosie. 'Didn't you notice anything?'

'Er . . .'

'Right in the middle of your desk, staring you in the face! What *is* it about men that makes them incapable of seeing things?' I ran obediently back upstairs to have another look. And there it was – the overlooked white plastic stick, a bit like a pen, with a little window and a blue line, indicating . . . ? I tried unsuccessfully to make sense of the instructions – another disability of the chromosomally challenged male sex. Was it positive or negative?

'What do you think it means?' she laughed, as I returned downstairs to pour myself some wine.

'So . . . you *are* –'

'Oh dear . . . are you angry? You look rather shell-shocked. That's why I asked Lizzie to be here, for some moral support.'

'Of course I'm not angry. Am I such an ogre? No . . . yes . . . no, it's wonderful . . . yes – wonderful news.' Which of course it was. I just felt a little dazed. Departure on the great journey into the unknown, scheduled for some future, still unspecified date, had suddenly, without warning, been brought forward. I felt nervous about being ready in time, anxious about this sudden awesome responsibility for a new life.

But as the winter drew in I began to share Rosie's unqualified joy. Christmas came, Rosie's delayed divorce papers finally arrived and, after just one week as an officially unattached woman, she retied the knot on 29th December. We married at the register office – I in a sober grey morning suit, Rosie in dazzling crimson velvet, with some hasty last-minute letting out of seams to accommodate the bulge. We both wore buttonholes of blue iris. Thirty or so friends and family came to lunch at my parents' house; then the two of us left in pouring rain for Cornwall, to spend a brief honeymoon amongst the winter gales battering the Atlantic coast.

Back in Bath Rosie grew bigger and bigger, struggling now to get into her boiler suit for tractor-maintenance classes at the agricultural college. At home, I spent mornings wrestling with my South Georgia book, before coming downstairs each lunchtime to follow the progress of the Gulf War on the radio. It was strange to listen to the civilised, measured voices of the 'Defence' experts analysing the bombardment of Saddam Hussein's army, neglecting to mention that this consisted of human beings – thousands of young men, being pulverised, atomised, eviscerated, obliterated in the desert sand, while we, at a safe distance from all that horror, were preparing to nurture and protect new life.

We went through all the prescribed rituals, attending ante-natal classes, looking at the little pulsing heart on the CTS monitor, decorating the house, buying and borrowing baby equipment. Rosie's Siamese cats, Coco and Chai, snuggled proprietorially into the white lace of the beautiful cradle now standing expectantly in the sitting room, and the pale yellow fragrance of spring seemed imbued with new meaning. Then quickly the colours and scents deepened. Rosie was due at the end of May but by 3rd June nothing had happened. Restless and uncomfortable, she suggested a walk, so we lumbered across the roaring London Road and headed for the calm of the canal. The yellow irises were out and a swan glided past with six downy grey cygnets. Everything was singing with new life but still we were having to wait.

It was the week of the Bath Festival, and the following day, Tuesday, we went to a concert in the Guildhall with Lizzie Bingley. There were anxious glances all around as Lizzie and I manoeuvred Rosie into her seat, assessing emergency escape routes. The concert was a cello recital by Steven Isserlis, pouring all his Slavic flamboyance into a gloriously romantic programme, including both the Chopin *and* Rachmaninov sonatas. And it did the trick. Soon after we got home Rosie felt the first little warning stabs of pain and we drove over to the Royal United Hospital.

The midwife on duty told her to stay but thought that things were going to be quite slow. So I slept at home and bicycled back to the hospital the next morning to find Rosie sitting cross-legged on a bed, bent forward and groaning. When I asked superfluously how she was feeling, she snapped, 'Bloody awful. And this TENS machine is a complete waste of time.' She had followed the ante-natal tutors' advice and hired the special battery pack and electrodes which emit a gentle pain-numbing pulse when attached to your back. Or that was the theory. In reality, they hardly impinged on waves of previously unimaginable pain. Nor did the gas and air seem to make a huge difference. The pain just surged in ever bigger rollers, hour after hour after hour. The garden courtyard outside the window was bathed in rainy, grey-green light. A little finch pecked chirpily at the gravel, mocking the misery inside. Then darkness fell and the hospital drew in on its own bleak fluores-cent light. Doctors and midwives came and went, and eventually announced at about midnight that it was time to go down to the delivery room.

As Rosie sprawled on the bed under a stark flood-light, surrounded by medical equipment, I couldn't banish inappropriate cinematic images of the Gestapo at work. 'Why does it have to be so horrific?' I kept asking myself angrily. 'Why must life be initiated by such hideous torture?' In desperation, Rosie agreed eventually to have an epidural injection. It gave some relief but still no baby appeared. The young midwife seemed out of her depth. The obstetrician looked worried. A student on an obstetrics placement sat in the corner practising delivery with a foetal doll inside a plastic pelvis. He just looked bemused, wiggling and twisting the doll's head backwards and forwards, failing dismally to extricate it. Then Rosie started screaming with a new, different, stabbing pain, so intense that she was convinced she was about to die. Only afterwards did we discover that her catheter had fallen out, unnoticed, causing her drip-fed bladder to inflate agonisingly.

She was given another epidural, which reduced but didn't eliminate this new mystery pain. I asked whether she should have a Caesarean. The doctor agreed that that might be the best thing, but there was no anaesthetist available – too many road accidents to deal with. So we had to stay put in the torture chamber. Then, at about three in the morning an older, highly experienced midwife came on duty. She was a large authoritative woman and she rolled up her sleeves with an air of capable determination, announcing firmly that it was time to get this baby out. Numb, drugged and exhausted, Rosie had to make one final huge effort. All I could do was whisper encouragement in her ear as she clutched me, sinking fingernails into my wrists. Then at last, after thirty hours' relentless struggle, a slippery blue-grey bundle was pulled from between her legs. The cord was cut and the bundle was whisked over to a special reviving machine, where a doctor did a quick check that the prolonged traumatic birth had done no damage. The bundle cried and someone announced, 'It's a boy and he's fine.' They brought him back, laid him on Rosie's breast and for the first time we met Ollie.

After nine months' waiting both of us had imagined that we knew him already, but this person was a complete stranger. He peered uncomprehendingly at us and we stared back at the wobbly, banana-shaped head, with its crumpled brow, unsmiling eyes and large squashed nose. 'Hello, little man,' Rosie said; then laughed, 'he's not very beautiful, *is* he?' Somehow she – and I – had expected an instant flood of loving recognition. But nothing had prepared us for the trauma of the birth. Rosie was completely exhausted and all she wanted was to sleep; I was just dazed and it was only as I bicycled home through the still dark streets that I began to feel excited. I was a father! I had a son! A whole new life – an unwritten, unknown story stretching ahead for seventy . . . eighty . . . (who knew – ninety ?!) years – had just started, right now on this very Thursday morning, June the sixth, D-Day, the sixth day of the sixth month . . . and I – we – would be there, right at the heart of the story, observing and shaping every moment of its first few chapters.

Ollie weighed 6lb 5oz at birth – a touch thin, but nothing to be alarmed about. There was some concern about the difficult delivery so the doctors kept a check on him at first, pricking his tiny bony heels to determine glucose levels in his blood, but after three days they announced that he was perfectly healthy and could go home.

He was fine. Rosie, however, was still very sore. More seriously, she was also suffering psychologically from the trauma of the birth, reliving the pain and terror. She was also finding breastfeeding extremely painful: her voluptuous bosom, source of delight to adult men, seemed less well suited to its primary purpose of feeding a tiny baby mouth. Two years later, when Edmond was born, a friend told her about Rotasept – a magic numbing spray for sore nipples; with Ollie no-one mentioned this simple solution to a problem which was souring the mother–child relationship. So, reluctantly, she gave up breastfeeding and switched to bottle-feeding with a formula based on cow's milk.

Later, much later, when it became clear that Ollie had an intolerance to dairy products – and was having increasing problems with his immune system – we would wonder whether things might have worked out differently if Rosie had known about Rotasept and been able to continue breastfeeding. But at the time, in June 1991, it was just a relief to escape the pain which had come between her and her baby. With bottles, feeding became a pleasure. And the love, which had at first surprised us with its hesitancy, like a bud furled protectively against a late frost, now burst into flower, intoxicating with its heady scent and luminescence. Like billions of parents before us, convinced that we alone were privileged to experience a unique miracle, we watched the eyes brighten and focus, look, stare, question and, best of all, *smile*.

With Ollie the smile seemed to have a special intensity. Experts are unable to agree whether that manipulation of facial muscles by the six-week-old baby is simply a physical skill learned by copying the mother, or whether it is an innate expression of joy; but, whatever the mechanism, with Ollie, once that first thrilling contact was made, there was never, ever, anything passive about his smile. It was a smile which engaged robustly with the world. And soon the smile became a laugh. For him the world was a funny place, full of delight. And the more he delighted in the world, the more we delighted in him.

Rosie's burgeoning enchantment with her baby soon banished the demons of post-natal depression. She had looked forward to having a baby ever since she was a teenager, and now she had that gift she simply adored him. I was at first more ambivalent about fatherhood. Of course I was proud to have been through this rite of passage – in fact, I had been so elated, the Sunday after Ollie was born, that I had driven over to Bristol to lead a friend up the soaring wall of 'Yellow Edge', the greatest rock climb in the Avon Gorge, on a surge of confidence – but as the summer ripened and deepened, I was surprised by the way that facile pride was supplanted by a new, deeper contentment, a sense of life having a whole new dimension.

In the meantime I had to earn a living. The South Georgia book advance was all spent. Summer tends to be a thin time for freelancers so I was very grateful when a seasoned journalist friend gave me a lead to Will Ellsworth-Jones, then editor of the Weekend section at the *Daily Telegraph*. Once the frighteningly inscrutable replies to my telephone overture were over, Will proved to be that rarest of creatures – a friendly approachable Fleet Street editor. He warned me that his boss, Max Hastings, demanded a full quota of hearty blood sports in the 'Outdoors' pages, but he promised to try and squeeze in some additional mountainous and environmental stories from me, starting with four articles on my own forthcoming trip to Nepal.

The expedition was still six weeks away, and Rosie needed a holiday. How to pay? I suddenly remembered Catherine Destivelle – the brilliant French climber who had just soloed a new route up the mirror-smooth monolith of the Petit Dru, above Chamonix. At home in Paris she was now more famous than the French prime minister, but there hadn't been a single column inch in the British press. 'What's so special about her?' Will asked warily. I waxed enthusiastic, detected a flicker of interest on the other end of the telephone, then explained that I would need to go to Paris to interview her: there would be a return fare and a hotel night to pay on top of the fee. This was a bit of cheek, coming from an untried freelance who had not yet produced a single word for the paper, but occasionally you have to be bold. Will asked a few more questions then muttered resignedly, 'Oh, all right – you'd better go.'

In those pre-budget-flight days the boat ferry cost no more than an air ticket, so I could justify taking the car and including the whole family. We sailed from Portsmouth on a warm September night, drove lazily through Normandy the next day and reached Paris with plenty of time for me to prepare for the interview. Catherine was her usual ebullient self – giggling and enthusing about the eight days she had spent alone on the thousand-metre-high vertical sheet of granite, giving me total concentration for two hours before leaving to prepare for that evening's television chat show. For the whole of the next morning I sweated at a table in the hotel courtyard, ripping sheet after abortive sheet from the Olivetti. By lunchtime I still hadn't managed the first sentence. By tea time I had one sketchy paragraph to show for my labours. Rosie came to see how I was getting on and I snapped at her to go away. So she wheeled Ollie back to the Jardins de Luxembourg to while away the rest of the afternoon. An hour before the deadline I finally galvanised my brain into action, racing to a blotchy, Tipp-Exed finish and despatching the agreed 800 words with one minute to spare. Two days later I spoke on the phone to Will who queried a couple of minor ambiguities then added lugubriously, 'You'll be pleased to hear I liked the piece.'

Phew! What a blessed relief! Now we were free, the three of us, to enjoy our little holiday which, for me, was a return to old haunts. Like Ollie, I had first come to Paris as a baby – in my case to stay with my grandparents who had lived here. Later, at sixteen, I had stayed here with our friends the Potiers. The parents, Marion and Jean-Pierre, were now in their sixties and retired, but they and their apartment on the Boulevard St Germain seemed unchanged. While Rosie and I joined them for dinner at the familiar round table by the tall elegant window overlooking Rue du Bac, one of their grandchildren played with Ollie who was chuckling contentedly in his reclining rocker chair.

In just three months our ugly duckling, maligned so uncharitably at birth, had metamorphosed into a beautiful baby who seemed to delight everyone with his radiant good humour. At the gardens of Vaux le Vicomte near Fontainebleau next day an extended family of Italians – fellow holidaymakers – went wild with excitement, summoning nephews, nieces, grandchildren, aunts and uncles, shouting to them to ignore the grandiose artifice of Le Nôtre's fabulous landscape and gather instead around our pushchair, to cluck and coo over the *bello bambino*. At restaurants each night Ollie gurgled contentedly in his carry basket, resting on a chair beside our table. At Chartres, crammed into the tiny bedroom of a grimy hotel, he transformed our seedy garret into a theatre of laughter. Amongst the ancient sandstone boulders of the Fontainebleau forest, where I had first climbed with the Potiers twenty-one years earlier and where we now met Catherine for a morning's play, Ollie seemed to share Rosie's wry amusement at my futile efforts to emulate the rock-climbing superstar. He seemed both to absorb our contentment and to enrich it, reflecting it back to us, adding a glow of enchantment to what would otherwise have been merely a pleasant holiday.

A few days after returning home I set off again, this time alone. The Mountain Club of South Africa had invited me to be principal guest at their centenary dinner in Cape Town, offering also to organise some paid lectures, justifying my trip as 'work' and allowing me to escape nappy duty with a clear conscience. It was a thrilling whirlwind tour, filled with dazzling sensations: the canyons of the Magaliesberg mountains near Johannesburg; the towering Sentinel in the Drakensberg, redolent with memories of Michael Caine and Stanley Baker sweating it out in *Zulu*; the tropical lushness of Durban; the Garden Route; the vineyards of Stellenbosch, serried beneath red mountains; the foghorn booming over the blasted heath at the Cape of Good Hope; and Table Mountain, where on my last morning, a little jaded from the previous night's dinner, we swung up the giddy, vertiginous, sandstone rungs of 'Jacob's Ladder', banishing centennial hangovers with buckets of sweet spring air.

Packed into just ten days, the South African tour hardly impinged on family life in Larkhall. But only two weeks after my return we had to face a longer, harder separation as Rosie and Ollie waved me onto the flight to Nepal. I would not be returning for seven weeks. This was my first Himalayan expedition since the Everest climb three years earlier. The objective – a beautiful peak called Kusum Kanguru, about twenty miles south of Everest – was my own project and it was I who had chosen the team. My two partners for the climb, Dick Renshaw and Brian Davison, were totally dependable;

Henry and Sarah Day were wonderful company on the long trek to base camp; Pasang Norbu, our Sherpa cook from the Everest expedition, was one of the kindest, most cheerful people I knew. This venture was entirely my own idea and I ought to have enjoyed it unequivocally. Most of the time I *did* enjoy myself and the final climb to the summit, completing a new route up the mountain, was intensely satisfying. But I was surprised by how much I missed Ollie, particularly in the evenings, when the autumn mist rolled up from the valley. Pondering fatherhood before it actually happened, I had always assumed that I would stick firmly to my schizophrenic way of life – switching effortlessly between domestic security and wilderness adventure, settler and nomad – but now, confronted with the reality of that dislocating wrench, I realised that it was not going to be quite so easy.

One evening, in a fit of egotism, I took my cassette recorder over to a hollow behind a boulder, out of earshot from the others – who might think I had gone barking mad – and talked to Ollie, telling him all about what I was doing on Kusum Kanguru, anxious that he should not forget the sound of my voice. I even sang his bedtime song: 'Go to sleep my baby, close your pretty eyes. Angels will be watching; peeping at you from the skies. Great big moon is shining; stars begin to peep. Time for little Ollie Venables; to go to sleep.' The tape was sent home the next day, along with the latest despatch to the *Telegraph*.

Afterwards Rosie said, 'We did listen to the tape for a while, but I'm afraid we got a bit bored with it.' It certainly seemed to have little effect on Ollie, who looked very unimpressed when a strange man returned to Heathrow airport and started kissing his mother. He became even more alarmed when the stranger got into the back of the car. Every time I raised my head above the level of the front seat he screamed. Talking drew the same response. So I had to huddle silently, head down, all the way back to Bath.

It took a few days for both Ollie and Rosie to adjust to the man who had intruded on their domestic routine. I was large and loud and clumsy and, until things settled down, superfluous. But we soon got over the awkward transition. Ollie either retrieved subconscious images of the pre-departure me, or just accepted the new me. Whatever the mechanism, the bond was re-established. At the airport I had also hardly recognised *him*. There was a new luminosity in his dark brown eyes, and a bloom to his skin; his nose was straighter and finer, his forehead broader, his chin more defined. He was starting to crawl and soon after I returned I hung a bouncer from the beam between the kitchen and sitting-dining room. At night he settled happily in his cot, chuckling and smiling through the bars; in the morning the same contentment greeted us.

At times it seemed that he was *too* easy. Surely there ought to be more struggle and angst in this child-rearing business? Shouldn't he throw more tantrums? Afterwards, when the contentment of those enchanted times was shattered, we wondered what signs there had been of impending catastrophe; but even now, years later, we can find few clues. Despite his traumatic birth, he was a very healthy baby. Rosie was slightly concerned that he was not very cuddly; but apart from that he was extremely sociable. He loved to be with us, but didn't cling; he had a self-contained serenity.

His weight gain was on target and he was passing all his developmental milestones. However, Rosie did worry about the cow's-milk formula which was still the mainstay of his diet. During the first weeks of bottle-feeding, he had sometimes arched his back, as if in pain. At times he also seemed unduly windy and snuffly. A couple of times, after visiting the GP, he was treated with anti-biotics. Back in July, Rosie had queried the bottle formula, but the doctors felt that Ollie had no serious intolerance to cow's milk, one GP, as we later discovered in the notes, dismissing Rosie rather patronisingly as an 'anxious mother'. The only other slight worry, early in 1992, was his strange crawling, with one hip apparently not abducting properly. However, the orthopaedic specialist found no serious abnormality and Rosie subsequently saw a cine film of herself as a baby doing exactly the same lopsided crawl, with one leg stretched straight behind her.

Soon after Ollie was born an old climbing friend, Phil Bartlett, had said what a relief it must be that 'there was nothing wrong with him'. It had never occurred to me that our baby would be anything other than 'normal', and as the months passed that assumption seemed to be confirmed. He was strong, healthy and full of promise. And if I sometimes resented the drudgery of changing nappies and the relentless routine of sterilising bottles, boiling water, measuring formula powder – 'No, you bumbling dolt: it has to be *exactly* seven measures and you *must* level off the powder with a knife and *don't forget* to sterilise the knife: you're not on a mountain now' – even if those domestic trivia seemed irksome, the object of all this attention repaid us with more and more pleasure as the days passed.

Winter melted and for the third time Rosie and I watched the glaucous daffodil spears pierce the little plot of land we called home. Her professional horticultural ambitions were still on hold, especially as we hoped to have another child soon, but even at our microcosmic amateur level, this whole business of painting pictures with plants was a huge shared pleasure compatible with child-rearing. And for inspiration we had the great set-piece gardens of southern England. That spring we visited Margery Fish's magical hellebore 'ditch' at East Lambrook. We wheeled the pushchair through Sissinghurst and continued the next day to Great Dixter. On Easter Monday we drove north through the Cotswolds to the sublime garden rooms of Hidcote Manor. It was a gorgeous spring afternoon and Ollie thrilled to the wide gracious space of the Great Walk, relishing the huge velvet expanse of lawn, crawling, climbing, laughing, playing to the crowd and, for the first time in his life, getting to his feet and standing upright.

These idylls were interspersed with reminders of a harsher world: interviews with the cave diver Martin Farr and the polar traveller Ran Fiennes, about to start his epic walk across Antarctica with Mike Stroud. There was a new book on Himalayan climbing to get started, meetings of the British Mountaineering Council to yawn through and, looming more urgently, a new expedition. Just six months after returning from Kusum Kanguru, I was leaving again for the Himalaya. It was a joint Indian-British venture co-led by my old Mumbai friend, Harish Kapadia, and the public face of British mountaineering, Chris Bonington. We planned to explore the Panch Chuli – the five sacred cooking hearths of the mythic Pandava brothers, four of them unclimbed, rising to over 6,000 metres in Kumaon, on the India–Nepal border. I was looking forward to seeing Harish and the Mumbai-wallahs again. I was excited by the prospect of unknown, untouched summits. I was even more excited by the deep forested river gorges we would explore to reach those summits. But I was also dreading the separation from Rosie and Ollie. I was going to miss my son's first birthday and, even though I was departing with an incredibly strong, experienced team, there was, as always, the lurking, unspoken fear that I might not come back.

Chapter Two

The accident happened on the summer solstice, just before dawn. Late the previous afternoon we had reached the summit of Panch Chuli V – the first human beings ever to touch this elusive dome of snow 6,456 metres above sea level. It had been the culmination of a strenuous last-minute dash up a completely unexplored glacier system, right at the head of a remote uninhabited valley, and now, after descending wearily through the night, Dick Renshaw, Victor Saunders, Stephen Sustad and I were nearly back down at the tent, where Chris Bonington waited, perched on a metre-wide ledge. It was the last day of the expedition and, thirty miles away in the village of Munsiari, Harish Kapadia and the rest of the Indian team were preparing for our return to the plains.

We were descending in a series of abseils, taking turns each time to slide fifty metres down the double ropes, before pulling one end to bring them down for the next abseil. Sometimes the knot joining the two ropes jammed behind a rock, forcing one of us to climb back up in the dark to free it. It was cold, exhausting work and we had had virtually nothing to eat or drink for twenty-four hours. However, we had all dealt with countless similar situations in the past and by dawn we would be back at the tent. After a quick breakfast we would then continue down to the valley, reaching base camp that evening. From there everything would be easy, and in just a few days' time I would be back home with Rosie and Ollie.

It was on the penultimate abseil, soon after I lowered myself over the edge, committing my life to the ropes, that the anchor failed. I had only gone a few metres, feet braced wide against the rock, when I heard the bright, mocking ring of a steel peg ripping from granite and felt a sudden backward lurch into space. The understanding seemed only to come gradually, in slow motion, out of sync with the violent, strident battering, as my body was flung down the mountain, bouncing from rock to rock, flung headlong into the dark void, and I realised with resigned regret that this was death. And somewhere, in the middle of all that hideous tumbling cacophony, hurtling towards the final moment of annihilation, I glimpsed blurred images of the wife and son I would never see again.

I awoke to desolate grey silence, amazed at being alive, terrified of the damage I might find. But I was lucky: neither my skull nor my spine had been damaged during the eighty-metre plunge down the cliff. And my brave companions, watching the body cartwheel through the darkness, had managed incredibly to grab the ends of the ropes and stop me falling a further 300 metres down a huge ice face. That instant, instinctive reaction probably saved my life. However, the battering had still done considerable damage. My left ankle was fractured and my right knee was gashed open. The whole right leg had seized up and the slightest movement was excruciatingly painful. As I hacked out a ledge with my ice axe and heaved my body into some kind of stable position, waves of fear and nausea swept over me. But then I thought of the people who had survived similar disasters. And I thought of Rosie in the labour room – the hours of searing pain and struggle – and I realised that this couldn't be as bad as that. For the first time in my life I was just going to have to try to be brave.

Nevertheless, as the grey dawn brightened and I saw the blood oozing into the snow, and as I stared down the plunging snowfield – and, below it, the tortured labyrinthine cataracts of ice which we had fought our way up two days earlier – my courage wavered. When Victor reached me with the first-aid kit, I croaked, 'If I don't manage to get out of this alive, will you tell Rosie I'm sorry.' He brushed aside the melodrama, assuring me that there was going to be no dying, and from that moment I never doubted that, somehow, I would get home to my wife and son.

I was lucky to be with four of the world's best Himalayan climbers. While Dick and Victor lowered me, ropelength by weary ropelength, down the long ice face, Stephen Sustad rejoined Chris to carry tents, stoves and sleeping bags from Chris's perch down to the comparatively flat basin below, where we eventually established camp, thirty-six hours after setting out on the summit push. There I waited four days with Dick and Victor, while the other two descended to the valley to alert Harish Kapadia and try to organise a rescue.

We got very, very hungry in our tent, but we had a stove to melt snow, so there was enough to drink. With my swollen battered right leg immobilised in a splint, the pain subsided to a dull ache and it was only when the helicopter arrived, on the fourth day, that I had again to be brave. It was an Indian Air Force Lama on its third attempt to find a way through gathering monsoon clouds to our remote camp, nearly 6,000 metres above sea level. With no flat landing spot, the pilot had to hover with one skid resting against the slope and the rotor blades scything inches from the mountain, while Victor dragged my inert body across to the side door. The whole world was reduced to a violent, deafening, pulsating maelstrom of flung snow and exhaust fumes.

As Victor said afterwards, 'One mistake by the pilots and we would all have been turned into salami.' Cowering beneath the thrumming blades, I had to drag my aching torso upwards and backwards into the helicopter doorway, arms reaching out behind me, cracked left ankle bracing in front, right leg flapping loose in a torment of grating gristle and bone. Victor gave my leg one final grinding shove. I shrieked with agonised exultation and collapsed inside the warm haven of the helicopter cockpit.

The pilots had risked their lives to pick me up, and moments later we were fleeing the dangerous mountain cauldron, speeding back to Munsiari, where we touched down for a brief emotional reunion with Chris and Harish. As we took off again to head south for a military hospital in the plains, Harish handed me a bundle of letters. I had been writing home regularly during the last seven weeks, but no return mail had got through to our base camp. Now, luxuriating in the warm comfortable safety of the helicopter, a solipsist immersed in the miracle of my own survival, I discovered for the first time what had been going on in my absence.

In the first letter Rosie was pregnant. In the second she had had a miscarriage; she felt lousy and was devastated by the loss of a new life. In between, her brother Jake, who ran a travel company, had given her, a friend called Elaine and Ollie a free holiday near Mombasa. Later I saw the photos of Ollie there and at home that early summer – face and hair golden brown, eyes sparkling – paddling, playing in the oak sandpit I had made just before I left for Panch Chuli, standing up proudly with his first birthday card, looking at his first picture book, playing with Nana and Grandpop's bathtime present and saying his first word, 'duck', followed a few days later by his second word 'shoe' . . . a whole succession of special unrepeatable events I had missed. What I had also missed was his sudden attack of diarrhoea on the return from Kenya – the wrenching pain and screaming, so inconsolable one night at Rosie's parents' house that she had left at midnight to drive Ollie home over the dark empty expanse of Salisbury Plain. A stool test had revealed salmonella, contracted either in Kenya or during the hideous charter flight home, and after several days of agony the infection finally subsided.

It was a mark of Ollie's robust health that he recovered quickly and totally from that debilitating attack. By the time I was speeding south over the Himalayan foothills to the military hospital at Bareilly, he had regained all his weight and the agonised screaming was just a bad memory. But Rosie had had a hard time in my absence, and the last thing she needed was a battered, shrivelled husk of a husband to nurse back to health. When I arrived back in England eight days after the accident, anger was the predominant emotion as she drove me from Heathrow to Larkhall, telling me that I could spend one night at home but that after that I was to stay in hospital until I was properly mended.

Neighbours helped to manoeuvre my wheelchair through the front door. Then Rosie left me parked in the sitting room while she went to collect Ollie from our friends at the end of the terrace. She returned with him a few minutes later. 'Look who's here: it's Daddy.'

This time he didn't scream. There *was* a moment's hesitation, but then he moved forward, holding a chair for balance. He stopped just short of me, as if to make sure who this really was, stared hard then broke into a huge, giggling smile.

In the morning Rosie delivered me to the men's trauma ward at the Royal United Hospital, where I stayed for the next five weeks. Apart from a quick patching up of another knee injury nineteen years earlier, some brief frostbite amputations after Everest and the more recent visit to the maternity ward with Rosie, I had no experience of hospitals, none of serious illness. This was a whole new world and I never completely accepted its rituals and hierarchies. I resented the delegation of personal control, the subjugation to some unknown authority, and the delays while other more urgent cases took precedence.

I had two operations: one to repair the fractured left ankle and to insert special beads of antibiotic onto the infected bone of my right knee; then, once the infection had gone, a second operation to repair the right knee with wire, steel screws and a slice of my hip grafted onto the tibial plateau. I emerged from anaesthesia in a filthy temper, cursing everyone in sight. Then I lay inert for several days, watching enviously as Ollie took his first unaided steps across the ward, laughing each time he wobbled and fell to the floor.

Rosie brought him to see me most days, then, if she could find a babysitter, returned on her own in the evening. She was working flat out to keep the Venables family functioning on a dwindling budget, and the strain of the situation was not helped by some vindictive apparatchik from the Customs and Excise sending the bailiffs round on an exploratory snoop just because I was slightly late with the VAT. We badly needed money and I could not afford to cancel two corporate speaking engagements which had been booked long before the accident. So, ignoring the dire warnings about post-operative infections, Rosie decided to spring me from hospital six days after the big operation. Just as she was about to leave home the car broke down. Desperate, she banged on the door at Number One. Yes – Mick and

Sue could spare their car for the evening. It was a venerable old Peugeot, a piebald creature of infinite variety, all dents and blotches and moulting decrepitude, and it caused quite a stir as it rattled to a halt amongst the fat, sleek executive saloons parked outside the British Gas training centre. The trainees were even more astonished to see their evening's motivational speaker wife-handled from the old banger and trundled in, plastered leg first, on a squeaking Red Cross wheelchair.

A strange way to earn a living, but that and another engagement at Henley Management College kept us afloat during the healing process. At first it was painful and depressing and I got absolutely nowhere with the first essential step to recovery – a 'straight leg raise'. Time after time I stared at the lifeless foreign object stretched in front of me, focusing all my attention, willing it to lift. Then, suddenly, three weeks after the operation, sitting on the grass at my parent's home on a day out from hospital, the neurological signal got through, nerves connected with muscles, and I shouted triumphantly as the object came alive and lifted from the ground.

It was a shimmeringly beautiful summer afternoon and Ollie was playing beside me in the garden. I was incredibly lucky to be alive, I was mending, and the future looked good. Over the next few days, although I was not officially discharged, hospital became a mere formality. I had been separated from Rosie for three months and she was keen to get pregnant again as quickly as possible, so I spent most nights at home, checking back into the RUH for the morning ward round. And then, five weeks after admission, I was finally sent home for good. Little did we know how often we would be returning to hospital in the years to come.

★

Ollie was a picture of robust health. At the Abbey, where we went to the family communion service most Sundays, he would stand up on the pew and join heartily and tunelessly in the hymns. On an afternoon trip to The Courts gardens, a few miles outside Bath, he first developed his passion for escape, playing hide-and-seek amongst the columns of a neo-classical temple, threatening to jump into the lily pond, running across the lawn, tempting and teasing me, as I raced after him on my crutches, then curling up in fits of laughter when I caught him.

He was christened one Sunday morning at the end of September, at the untraditionally mature age of fifteen months, dressed in navy blue cords and a red jumper. Our acupuncturist friend, Lizzie Bingley, was godmother, along with Rosie's ex-sister-in-law Fiona Close, a nurse by profession. Both lived nearby and had known Ollie since he was born. For godfathers he had my second cousin, Lucius Cary, engineer, entrepreneur, tree-house builder and professional optimist; and Henry Noltie, a taxonomist and art historian at the Royal Botanic Gardens Edinburgh, who had a pet rabbit running loose under the harpsichord in his exquisite Georgian drawing room. They were a wise, kind, eclectic group to watch over his life, and after the service they came back to Larkhall, along with seven children, Rosie's parents, my parents and one of my sisters. The adults filled all the available space, so we fed the children, rabbit fashion, under the piano.

Ollie was bright and cheerful that Sunday, 29th September, but for the previous three nights he had been feverish with nightmares. At the time, still obsessed with my own recovery from the accident, I was hardly aware of these problems. A heavy sleeper, I never heard the anguished screams, nor Rosie's attempts to soothe and sing him back to sleep. Nor, on Thursday the 24th, had I been particularly aware that while I went to the hospital for physiotherapy, Rosie had been taking Ollie to the local clinic for his vaccination against measles, mumps and rubella.

Later I would learn much more about MMR. At the time of Ollie's injection I was hardly aware of its existence. It had never occurred to me that anyone would want to vaccinate children against the common childhood illnesses I, my brothers and sisters and all our friends had experienced without any problems. Of course I knew that mumps could be extremely unpleasant after puberty, and that rubella in pregnant women could damage their unborn children. Hence the importance we had attached to being exposed to these illnesses at an early age – a natural process which happened once we started to mix with other children at school, at an age when we were robust enough to tolerate the illnesses and gain lifelong immunity. Measles I remembered particularly well: my two younger brothers and I incarcerated in our bedroom for a week during the hot summer of 1959 . . . wet flannels and calamine lotion soothing our itchy irritability . . . Mrs Armstrong bringing us speckled brown eggs from her hens . . . the longing to join the adult voices in the garden outside . . .

It had been irksome at the time, but never once, during the thirty-three years between my childhood measles and Ollie's MMR vaccination, did I know anyone – or anyone who knew anyone else – who had been damaged by measles. That may be a reflection on my comfortable middle-class upbringing – measles *can* be very risky for malnourished children living in crowded, insanitary conditions – but that just seems to reinforce the argument for fighting disease by improving people's overall health and living conditions, rather than trying to vaccinate the disease away.

The line put to Rosie when she delayed making an appointment for Ollie's MMR was rather different. Measles was extremely dangerous and if she did not vaccinate him she would be playing with fire. How would she feel if he became blind or suffered brain damage? And what about her responsibility to the community – her son's part in the 'herd immunity' which was designed to ensure against outbreaks? And what about mumps, where there was a very tiny risk of encephalitis? And how would she feel if he were to pass rubella to a pregnant woman with no immunity?

The health visitor was just doing her job, relaying Department of Health policy. However, looking later at the wording of official pronouncements on childhood diseases, it seemed that the whole perception of risk had been changed, as if to justify the blanket MMR coverage introduced to Britain in 1988. For instance, the *Macmillan Guide to Family Health* 1982 describes mumps as 'generally a mild disease' where 'the usual outcome is complete recovery'; in 1995, the same editor, this time in the British Medical Association publication *Family Health*, has mumps described as 'a highly uncomfortable illness' before emphasising its many potential, admittedly rare, side effects. With measles the change in tone is more dramatic: the 1982 *Macmillan Guide* states that 'in the vast majority of children who catch measles the disease disappears within 10 days and the only after-effect is life-long immunity to another attack'. The BMA 1995 guide, on the other hand, labels measles 'a potentially dangerous viral illness', describes the potential complications (including a 1 in 1,000 chance of encephalitis) and goes on to stress the importance of prevention through immunisation, reassuring the reader that 'side effects are generally mild'. A Department of Health booklet sent to families in 1994 warned any parent wavering over immunisation that 'unfortunately, measles can be much more serious than most people think. School-age children who get it are likely to be very ill.' The goalpost hadn't just been shifted; it had been moved to the other end of the pitch. When questioned on the wisdom of combining three live vaccines so conveniently and economically into one single shot, the Chief Medical Officer could reply that this greatly improved the chances of getting irresponsible feckless mothers to deliver their children for vaccination: they couldn't be trusted to come in for three separate injections, but with just one shot to worry about they ought to be able to cope.

For an intelligent, responsible, educated mother like Rosie, this assumption that she should bow to standardised policy and, against all her instincts, inject three live viruses simultaneously into her precious fifteen-month-old child was hard to stomach. He had only recovered recently from a vicious attack of salmonella and although he now seemed robustly healthy, his whole metabolism could still be vulnerable. But the scare tactics wore down her resistance and she dutifully took Ollie to the clinic for his injection. The first night after the jab he ran a temperature and had nightmares. For a fortnight he remained intermittently ill and the night terrors continued. He also began to develop a slight tremor in his right hand. Over the next few months his medical notes recorded a continuing saga of unspecific but worrying 'malaise'.

16.10.92
'Screaming for hours at night – inconsolable. Feeds well, OK during the day. Mum concerned re recur-

rence of Salmonella − same symptoms as in late May.'
[No salmonella was found.]
16.11.92
'Frantic crying in cot − lying on back − bouts of
crying then cheerful . . . Refused to let me examine
him but has red drums.'
Augmentin
4.12.92
Malaise . . .
22.12.92
Off colour . . .
3.2.93
In pain suddenly . . .
5.2.93
Unhappy babe since seen two days ago . . . occasional
screaming bouts
6.2.93
6.45 am restless night in pain
10.2.93
Discharge note from RUH. Reason for admission −
crying. On examination − distressed. Red dull left
TM. Final diagnosis − Otitis Media. Discharge
prescriptions − Amoxil

Otitis − inflammation of the ear drum − is common
in young children and may have been completely
unconnected, but it seemed to be part of an overall
pattern of reduced health. Rosie's fear of a return of
salmonella was prompted by Ollie's diarrhoea, which,
alternating with constipation, was to be a problem for
the rest of his life. Whatever was wrong with him, it
seemed to be centred in his gut. It is possible that cow's
milk did something to unbalance the natural gut flora.
Perhaps salmonella played a part. Perhaps antibiotics,
such as Augmentin and Amoxil exacerbated the problem.

And perhaps – on the basis of what we later learned about other children with similar histories – the combined vaccine at fifteen months did lasting damage. At the time, during the winter of 1992–3, all Rosie knew was that Ollie was not the same healthy child he had been before MMR. His digestive system was erratic, his sleep was often disturbed and he suffered increasingly from non-specific viral infections.

At the time I was only dimly aware of these problems. Illness had never been a part of my landscape and I didn't want to know about it. Pathologically optimistic, I assumed that these bouts of malaise were just minor kinks in the ascending graph of Ollie's development. Most of the time he was fine – more than fine: he was a bright, alert, adventurous, loving, laughing, blossoming personality who filled our lives with pleasure, so that now, in my mental scrapbook of images, it is the pleasurable daily rituals which shine most vividly in the memory. The steamy warmth of bath-time. Saying his night-time prayers, then lingering to stare through his cot bars – the two of us smiling at each other in mutual admiration, pleasure erupting into bursts of laughter. Christmas Eve carols at the Abbey, with Ollie singing loudly through the prayers, drowning out the Rector in his pulpit. Story time – no, story times – all through the day, sitting together on the pink candy-striped 'frequent use' sofa bed which Rosie had brought from her London flat. His first picture dictionary which my parents, 'Granny and Granchie', gave him for his first birthday. *Mr Gumpy's Outing* with its satisfying repetition, animal noises and mounting drama, culminating in the big 'Splash' as Mr Gumpy's boat overturns and all the animals fall into the river – Ollie tipping onto the floor between my legs – before going home to a huge restorative tea at the idyllic house beside the river. The same ritual anticipation in Ollie's favourite story of all, *The Elephant and the Bad Baby*: Ollie pointing to the pictures and later to the words, then holding my hands to his head to act out the final chaotic denouement as 'The elephant went BUMP, the old lady went BUMP, the butcher went BUMP, the barrow boy went BUMP etc. etc.' . . . followed by chastisement of the bad baby who 'never once said PLEASE!' but who, like Mr Gumpy's friends, is treated to a final redemptive tea party. Then Ollie might climb onto the crimson damask stool at the piano, mimicking my hands on the keyboard, swivelling index finger over thumb, experimenting with incipient melodies; or go outside to play on the swing strung from the pergola, shrieking with pleasure as I held him high by the feet then let him go in a swooping arc.

More snapshots, from early spring 1993. Ollie barefoot in the rain, striding purposefully up the garden path, mouth pursed in concentration. A courtyard café in Bath; two tweedy old ladies at the next table, grey heads thrust together over weighty handbags, mouths puckered in disapproval as they share some scandalous secret; beside them Ollie's face smooth and serene, with an enigmatic smile hovering about the mouth. Ollie exploring a strange house in Cumbria, looking puckish as he starts to rifle through the irreplaceable slide collection of the world-famous mountaineer Doug Scott. A bright Saturday morning two weeks later, back at home, Ollie comes downstairs to find Harish Kapadia, leader of the Panch Chuli expedition, asleep on the sofa bed; instant rapport as Harish tickles him and chats to him in a bubbling torrent of English and Gujarati.

Harish was in Britain to speak at a mountaineering conference. I had met him and Chris Bonington at the gathering in Buxton the previous weekend and followed

Chris up a short rehabilitative rock climb. It was 21st March, nine months exactly from my midsummer nightmare on Panch Chuli. Rosie's own nine months was also nearly at an end, and she was now rotund with our second child.

Edmond was born on the fifth day of the fifth month. Again Rosie had an exhausting struggle. But this time she managed without an epidural, there were no cockups with dropped catheters, and, despite the unspeakable pain, the whole experience was much less traumatic. Keen to prepare Ollie for the new arrival, she had bought him a life-size baby doll, but he never really saw the point of the ugly, bald, plastic bath companion. Far more interesting was the huge toy car Rosie instructed me to give him on the day Edmond was born. He was clutching it proprietorially when we brought his baby brother home two days later.

It soon became obvious that we had been spoiled with Ollie, the easy baby. Edmond was much more demanding and prepared to scream loudly if thwarted. Thanks to the magic Rotasept spray, Rosie was able to breastfeed him successfully and he loved to guzzle, long and often, so that for a year she never had more than two or three consecutive hours' sleep. While she nursed Edmond through the first weeks of his life, I took Ollie out on long bike rides. It was the best possible therapy for my recently mended knee and Ollie loved to sit up on the child seat, shouting gleefully along the narrow lanes brimming with cow parsley and May blossom, laughing at my motorbike noises as we careered down the steep winding lanes past Woolley, Langridge, Little Solsbury, Bailbrook, Swainswick and St Catherine . . . or bounced along the canal towpath, alarming those pedestrians who didn't notice the toddler on the back and saw only a demented thirty-nine-year-old racing towards them making loud brrumm-brrumm noises.

One year on from Panch Chuli, I felt very blessed to be alive and was in no hurry to return to the mountains. A good run of lectures on the back of the fortieth anniversary of Everest's first ascent was keeping us solvent but still leaving me plenty of time at home. Edmond, for all his stroppiness, was a gorgeous smiling baby, much more cuddly than Ollie had ever been. But in his own way Ollie was equally affectionate and was rewarding us with the thrill of fantastically fast learning.

He was fascinated by cars and loved to categorise them according to their owners – a Ford Escort was a 'Mick car', while a Volvo saloon was a 'Nana-Gwanpop car'. By the autumn, at twenty-seven months, he was experimenting with his first sentences and showing an impressive memory. Several weeks after visiting his godfather Henry in Edinburgh he pointed excitedly to a Volkswagen Golf, shouting, 'There's a Henry car'; examining a dolphin picture in a new book, he recalled the carved wooden fish he had seen next to the harpsichord and observed, 'Henry's got dolphins.' And the categorising continued. When we woke in the mornings we would hear him in his cot, chatting to himself: 'Mummy's a woman; Daddy's a man; Emmun's a boy; Coco's a cat. Mummy's called Rosie; Daddy's called Stephen.' But there was also poetry in his ordering of the world: stringy fronds on a tree were 'bit like an octopus'. And, perhaps even more than with most two-year-olds, he was full of delighted curiosity: 'What *is* it? What *is* it? It's *cheesepie*!' – pointing to the oven as Rosie pulled out an exquisite quiche, filling the house with golden cream and Gruyère aromas.

By November Ollie was counting to two. I was not particularly impressed, but his nursery-teacher mother assured me that this was a big conceptual leap into numeracy for a two-and-a-half-year-old. He was also beginning to recognise words on the page, and we felt that he would soon be reading. He also seemed quite musical, prompting us to wonder whether he might go to choir school in a few years' time. There was just a slight niggling worry about his occasional aloofness from other children. At the pre-school gym class where I took him every Thursday morning, he did well at the balancing, jumping and bouncing but seemed indifferent to the communal 'circle time' with the other children. In his intellectual development he seemed also, occasionally, to be taking time out – even regressing slightly – after his too-frequent viral illnesses. In August, sharing a large house in the country with my step-cousin Anna Black and her two young children, Ollie had seemed disconnected, either not comprehending what we were all up to, or wilfully going his own way. Having always had a deep mistrust of team games and all things pandering to the herd instinct, I rather admired Ollie's anarchic tendencies, but Rosie was uneasy about his moments of disconnectedness.

In August she had also noticed the tremor in his hand increase after a viral infection. As autumn progressed, she became more alarmed by increasing bouts of trembling and thirst, and alternating lethargy and hyperactivity; she noticed that his speech diminished during these episodes. She wondered whether he was diabetic, but a urine test on 15th November proved negative. Nevertheless the problems – along with the familiar bouts of diarrhoea – persisted. And, as 1993 came to an end, his whole metabolism seemed to respond to a growing sense of angst, as our family was suddenly engulfed in a series of crises.

★

It started late on the night of 23rd November. I was driving back from a lecture when the second-hand gearbox packed up. The old Ford just managed to limp home before grinding to a permanent halt outside the terrace, leaving us carless on the very day I was going into hospital to have the wire, plates and screws removed from my legs. With my right leg once more sliced open to the bone, I had to stay in hospital for observation. After a couple of days the leg began to feel hot and tight beneath its bandage. I asked the houseman under whose care I had been put to have a look, but he insisted it wasn't necessary. The next day the leg burned hotter and tighter and I felt as though I were getting flu. Still the young man insisted that the blood pressure and pulse readings on my chart indicated no serious infection – no need to interfere with the bandages. I continued to sweat and shiver. The skin beneath the bandages stretched drum-taut, pulling at the eighteen-inch stapled wound seam. Rosie became extremely anxious, but still the youth stuck to the statistics on his chart and refused to look at the actual wound.

At last, sprawled feverishly, trying to get to sleep after lights out one evening, I felt a gush of warm liquid soak my bed. A nurse unwrapped the sodden bandages to reveal that, sure enough, the leg had erupted in a Vesuvius of pus. I was put immediately on antibiotics but the next few days were frightening for Rosie, tormented by visions of being lumbered with a one-legged husband. The antibiotics worked, thank God. My temperature subsided, the leg stabilised and after ten days in the trauma ward I came home on crutches, just in time to set off on a vital overdraft-busting lecture tour, chauffeured by one of the many kind friends helping to keep the Venables family functional.

We were getting ready for Christmas when another

crisis struck. Rosie's mother, who had been becoming increasingly frail from what transpired to be Parkinson's disease, fell down the stairs and broke her hip. *She* was now in hospital; her husband Robin was all alone at home and needed help. Neither Rosie's sister nor brother could get over to Alresford, in Hampshire, so we would have to go. My parents had kindly rented for us a temporary replacement car, into which Rosie now packed presents, clothes, bedding, travel cot, nappies, dummies, medicine, wine, champagne, goose, Christmas pudding, brandy butter, husband, crutches, baby and toddler – the latter, Ollie, ill again with a temperature of 102° Fahrenheit, which his GP ascribed to another virus.

As we headed south-east on the familiar trail – along the Avon, across the river Frome, round Warminster, over the huge bleak spaces of Salisbury Plain, on past Stonehenge and then down into a softer landscape of chalk streams meandering past thatched cottages – I wondered what our hastily convened ad hoc Christmas was going to be like, never guessing that this Christmas of 1993 would be the fulcrum around which our life was bent and changed for ever.

Chapter Three

We tried hard to be jolly, starting with Rosie's traditional Buck's Fizz for breakfast. At Winchester
Cathedral Robin smiled approvingly at his two grandchildren sitting so serenely through Matins, apparently
as moved as he by the transcendent music of the choir-
boys soaring out over the longest nave in Europe. For
a moment nothing in Ollie's demeanour suggested
internal turmoil, but back at the house he grew tired
and went to bed. While Rosie and Robin visited Kay
in hospital, I tried to get Ollie to unwrap some of his
presents, but he was bored, indifferent, listless. And silent.
Speech seemed to require too much effort.

The flu-like viral infection passed and by New Year,
when we were back home, he was looking a bit better.
However, it was a new, changed Ollie who came down
to breakfast each morning during the first days of 1994.
The bubbling, questing, creative eagerness was stifled by
a new rigidity of purpose. With unvarying routine he
now took out his toy cars and arranged them meticulously on the upholstered arm of the sofa bed, aligning
them with the piping, precisely perpendicular to the
pink stripes. And unless cajoled into some alternative
activity, after breakfast he would return to his work-
station and continue lining cars, head leaning sideways,
sighting out of the corner of his eye, mouth slightly
open, occasionally dribbling.

The only other toys which really seemed to interest
him were the Duplo bricks, with which he had once

made such flamboyant structures. Now they too were reduced to predictable, unvarying two-dimensional lines. His books were neglected and when Rosie tried to read his familiar stories he pulled away, as if frightened by language. His own speech, which had until recently, despite the intermittent setbacks, been flowering so colourfully, began to wither. First it was just the pronunciation which went, so that 'duck', for instance, became 'dawk', 'darling' distorted to 'dorning'. But soon the actual vocabulary began to dwindle. Alone with his cars, he whispered to himself. With us, words were replaced increasingly by primal grunts and bleats. Our own requests to him were met by incomprehension or by confused echolalia – repeating the same words back to us, as if in a foreign language. Something seemed to be short-circuiting the intricate wiring of his neural pathways and all we could do was watch helplessly as learning and language evaporated, like files vanishing from the screen of a corrupted computer.

Fear made Rosie angry. She grew impatient with Ollie's apparently obtuse behaviour, on one occasion even shouting in desperation, 'What's wrong with you?' I, for once, was the calm one, insisting ostrich-like that this could not really be anything serious – just another kink, albeit a bigger one, in the graph – a temporary computing problem which would soon fix itself. I could not countenance the idea of anything being wrong with my son. For a while I even admired the purposefulness of his car-marshalling sessions – his determined getting down to 'work' in the morning. His GP gave the impression this was probably just some temporary developmental glitch, though he did ask for a hearing assessment. However, by March I was having to admit to myself that something really was drastically wrong. The bright little boy who had engaged so eagerly with the world had become withdrawn and timid and the light had gone out of his eyes.

He was enslaved by distressing phobias. The vacuum cleaner reduced him to screaming terror. Repair work on the house had to wait until he was out of doors because he could not bear the sound of the electric drill. 'Uncle Hike', with whom he had recently enjoyed such boisterous rapport, was devastated by the total change in his nephew. Out of doors Ollie was also fearful, incomprehensibly terrified by the field at the end of the terrace where he had played since he was a baby. Several weeks passed before Rosie realised that his terror was induced by the remaining winter leaves on the Lombardy poplars, rustling in the breeze. Some of his phobias seemed very astute: he found the twin portraits on the spine of Alan Bullock's *Hitler and Stalin – Parallel Lives* so upsetting that he turned the book round on the shelf, spine to the wall. As well as phobias, there were baffling new obsessions. Some – such as a compulsion to poke his finger into the exhaust pipes of parked cars or his fascination with light switches – were short-lived; others, in particular a passion for running water and liquids of all kinds, would remain with him for the rest of his life.

Later, much later, we – and he – would be able to laugh about these things; but as the winter days of 1994 lengthened into a fraught spring there was little laughter. While Edmond grew and flourished, a cheerful, healthy, affectionate baby, Ollie was drifting away into a parallel inaccessible world. It was as though we had been given some unimaginably precious gift, to which we had become ever more attached, only to have it snatched suddenly away from us.

★

On 29th March Ollie was finally referred to a hearing specialist. After exhaustive tests the consultant assured Rosie that Ollie's hearing was perfect – or at least he was detecting sounds at the correct volume. But as for his understanding and processing of those sounds . . . something seemed to be not quite right. The letter despatched to Ollie's GP on 5th April commented:

'Many thanks for referring Oliver for hearing assessment. I enclose a copy of our clinic notes. As you can see we eventually got a normal hearing test off him. However, he does seem to have problems with social communications, rigidity of thought etc. I have therefore taken the liberty of referring him on for a full developmental assessment, and speech therapy assessment.'

Rosie, meanwhile, had become desperate. Three months had passed since the devastating viral infection at Christmas. Now that the simple explanation of deafness had been ruled out, she knew that something was seriously wrong with Ollie's mental processes and she was frantic to find out what on earth was happening. There was no time to wait for laborious internal referrals. On Good Friday, 1st April, she persuaded me to telephone Charlie Clarke, a well-known expedition medic and consultant neurologist at St Bartholomew's Hospital in London, nearly always available to talk on the phone to fellow mountaineers about anything from frostbitten toes to brain tumours and pull strings on their behalf. His wife Ruth Seifert, a consultant psychiatrist by trade, answered the phone and was wonderful. 'Yes, of course you're worried. *Of course* he must see someone immediately. Charlie's away, but I'll get him to phone you when he returns on Monday.' Which he did, promising to speak to our GP in Bath first thing on Tuesday morning, 5th April. By Tuesday afternoon the GP had made an appointment for Ollie to see the Consultant Community Paediatrician at the first available clinic on 11th April.

We arrived punctually at four forty-five, noticing that the car parked in the consultant's space was an old Deux Chevaux. The owner, who met us in the waiting room, wore saggy trousers and a jersey, and had his long dark hair gathered in a ponytail. Simon Lenton may not have presented like a typical consultant, but the superficially hippyish impression was actually rather encouraging. He was quiet, direct and good at listening to parents. Despite the gentle demeanour, as a consultant he had serious clout and over the years he was to become a powerful and sympathetic ally. At that first meeting he observed Ollie briefly in the waiting-room play area, then took Rosie into the consulting room, leaving me to watch our son. After about twenty-five minutes Rosie came out and we swapped places. With me he was more brief, repeating without delay what he had just confirmed to Rosie – that, as far as he could tell, Ollie was autistic.

So they were right. Several friends had tentatively uttered the dreaded A word. Rosie herself, when interviewed by Simon Lenton, had said that she wondered whether Ollie might have become autistic. In a sense the paediatrician was just giving professional confirmation of her fears. That provisional diagnosis had to be reconfirmed later that month by a specialist psychologist's assessment, but much of what Rosie had told him about Ollie fitted the label. Our unique, precious, clever, beautiful son, so rich in promise, was in fact autistic.

Simon – he used first-name terms from the beginning – asked me what I knew about the condition. Very little, I replied. I had never knowingly met an autistic person. I was barely even aware of the word. I could only recall hearing it once, quite recently, on television, in a programme about the famous prodigy artist Stephen Wiltshire, and even then I hadn't really understood what it meant. Simon gave a very brief explanation about impaired social interaction and language skills. He told me that he had encouraged Rosie to contact the National Autistic Society and order some of their information booklets. I asked him how all of this might affect our lives. How able would Ollie be? Would he be capable, for instance, of attending a normal school? 'Well – possibly not,' he replied.

He accompanied me back to the waiting room where Rosie was watching gloomily as Ollie lined up toy cars. Simon told her that he would arrange various tests and an appointment with the psychotherapist, then left to see his next patient. We walked out into the bright blossom-scented afternoon, strapped Ollie into his child seat, and drove slowly back down the hill to Larkhall to start our new life in a foreign country called Autism.

In 1911 a psychiatrist called Eugen Bleiler coined the term autism – from the Greek *autos*, meaning 'self' – to describe an aspect of schizophrenia where the individual withdraws totally from the outside world and retreats inside himself. But the modern definition of childhood autism really dates from 1943 when Dr Leo Kanner, an Austrian psychiatrist working at Johns Hopkins University in America, published his response to four developmentally impaired children in whom he observed five common characteristics:

1. The inability to relate to and interact with people from the beginning of life.
2. The inability to communicate with others through language.
3. An obsession with maintaining sameness and resisting change.
4. A preoccupation with objects rather than people.
5. The occasional evidence of good potential for intelligence.

Reading that bleak, damning assessment fifty-one years later, it was immediately obvious to Rosie and me that this narrow definition of 'classical autism' did not fit our son. He *was* having problems relating to and interacting with other people, he *was* having trouble with language and he *was* becoming a creature of obsessive habit, but these were emphatically *new* problems. Right from the start, we were punctilious in telling people that Ollie had *become* autistic, or that he *had autism*. This was something which had happened to him; it was not some innate quality he had been born with. And as for good potential for intelligence, he had actually seemed unusually bright until his central nervous system began to unravel.

The National Autistic Society provided a less damning summary of current thinking on the subject, setting out four simplified diagnostic criteria:

1. Difficulty with social relationships.
2. Difficulty with verbal and non-verbal communication.
3. Difficulty in the development of play and imagination.
4. Resistance to change in routine.

One of their booklets also recorded the current 'triad of impairments' as defined by the American Psychiatric Association:

1. Qualitative impairment in reciprocal interaction.
2. Qualitative impairment in verbal and non-verbal communications and imaginative activity.
3. Markedly restricted repertoire of activities and interests.

With many autistic children that 'restricted repertoire' is reduced to bizarre, obsessive activities such as spinning, rocking, moaning or flicking hands in front of the eyes — self-stimulating rituals designed perhaps to exclude the outside world. It is the kind of extreme behaviour seen recently, for instance, in traumatised children at some Romanian state orphanages. Bruno Bettelheim observed a similar extreme withdrawal in some of his fellow inmates at a concentration camp during the Second World War. He managed to escape to America where he became director of the Sonia Shankham Orthogenic School for children with developmental problems. Observing in his autistic charges some of the same obsessive, ritualistic behaviours he had seen in the camp, he deduced that these children were similarly protecting themselves from trauma — trauma which he attributed to their parents. In his seminal 1969 book *The Empty Fortress* he suggested that autistic children were emotionally deprived, filled with anxiety and suppressed hatred as a result of inadequate parenting.

By the Nineties Bettelheim's theories had been discredited — it transpired that he had had no medical training and had treated parents with disdain, barring them from visiting the children whom, according to some sources, he beat and terrorised – but there were still lingering pockets of expert opinion which attributed autism to early trauma and poor bonding, causing us to pick again over the possible clues in Ollie's early life. What about those first few days when the breast-feeding didn't go well? What about the time we had to leave him overnight, while we went to London? What about the arrival of Edmond, which seemed to leave Ollie subdued, resorting to comfort from his dummy and snuggly – the piece of towelling he still carried everywhere with him? What about the recent Christmas crisis, when the car disappeared, I went into hospital and we then moved camp to Alresford? They were all upsetting disruptions for a sensitive child, perhaps, but hardly the stuff of extreme trauma. As for parental bonding, I had been away for four months during the first year of his life, but my absences had been more than compensated for by Rosie's intense, joyful devotion; she and Ollie had been a model of mutual adoration.

The more we read around the subject, and the more we re-examined the clues in Ollie's specific case, the more clear it seemed that the causes of his autism were physical, organic, chemical. Something was happening to the metabolism which affected his neural pathways, skewing his whole sensory and intellectual perception to the point where the world around him – and the people around him – seemed frighteningly incomprehensible.

What was also clear was that there was no standard, typical autistic person. As Simon Lenton stressed at our very first meeting, there was an 'autistic spectrum' ranging from Kanner's 'classically autistic' severely impaired child to the person with 'Asperger's syndrome' who is highly intelligent but whose intelligence may be highly specific, to the detriment of imaginative and social development. (Independently of Kanner, and researching in Vienna, Hans Asperger also used the term 'autism' to describe a group of higher-functioning, but socially impaired, children in 1944; it was the British researcher, Lorna Wing, who coined the term 'Asperger's syndrome' in 1981, shortly after Asperger himself had died.) Autism was a 'continuum', and trying to define Ollie's position on that continuum was the job of the psychotherapist who saw him on 11th May.

All four of us went to the family counselling department at the hospital, so that the psychotherapist could observe us together. She watched Ollie playing, noted the differences between him and his younger brother, then took a long history from Rosie. In her subsequent letter to Simon Lenton she noted all the medical incidents, including the apparent problems with cow's milk, the salmonella attack and the adverse reaction to the MMR vaccination. Summing up her assessment, she wrote:

'Oliver presented as a calm, contented child whose language delay, restricted social use of language, very limited play skills, lack of imaginative play and very limited social interaction are consistent with a diagnosis of autism. However, the pattern of Oliver's development with the acquisition and subsequent loss of interpersonal, language and play skills and interest in his environment is unusual and not consistent with the pattern most usually seen in autistic children of the failure of the normal development of these skills. It is possible that Oliver comes into the small category of children with a Heller type of pervasive disintegrative disorder. These children may eventually present as indistinguishable from autistic children who show the more familiar developmental pattern and whose prognosis is less uncertain. Another significant aspect of Oliver's development is the coincidence of regression and viral infections. I wonder if further neurological investigations are indicated? I look forward to discussing Oliver with you and Mr and Mrs Venables on 24th May at 1.30 pm.'

We duly arrived for the meeting on the 24th. Simon was inscrutable. The psychotherapist looked gloomily sympathetic as she talked us through the letter. She had no explanation for Ollie's drastic regression, nor did she offer any great hope for the future. Autism was a life-long condition. There were systems in place to help children with 'special needs', although there was no statutory requirement for specific educational help until Ollie became five. He was now just coming up to his third birthday. 'But surely there must be something *I* can do, *now* – some kind of therapy, some kind of intensive treatment – some way of retrieving that learning?' Rosie asked.

The psychotherapist mentioned a few 'management strategies', then added, 'You should be glad when he is sitting around lining up his cars; at least it'll give you a chance to get on with some housework.'

'Well – I don't think much of *that*,' Rosie announced as we got into the car to drive home. From the very first day of Ollie's provisional diagnosis six weeks earlier, she had set to work, determined to tackle autism head-on, researching, studying, exploring – trying to understand the enemy which had stolen away our son so that she could then fight back at that enemy. She began to make contact with a network of researchers, all following interconnected parallel paths. Over the years ahead it became obvious that these paths, like sheep trails contouring a mountainside, crossing and merging tantalisingly, often petered out or sidetracked towards new destinations. Just as there was no single, standard type of autism, there was no single obvious cause or cure. But that was no reason not to do everything possible to fight Ollie's autism and, at the very least, ameliorate his condition, working on two fronts — metabolic and educational — trying both to remove the biochemical causes of his condition and to salvage his lost cognitive skills.

Rosie led the way while I followed, reluctantly at first, shamed by her defiant energy. For both of us it was a schizophrenic process because, however much we wanted to fight Ollie's condition, we had at the same time to live with it — had to learn to love the new Ollie and his bizarre ways, whilst cherishing the affectionate, funny, sensitive, mischievous soul of the old Ollie which continued to shine through the distorting fog of autism.

Friends and neighbours were sympathetic, but sometimes the sympathy seemed to be directed exclusively towards Rosie, Edmond and me, as if Ollie were somehow to blame. Or, because he had virtually stopped talking, they might assume that he was also deaf or unable to understand what they were saying. When someone asked brusquely, 'Will he *always* be like this?' a wounded shadow seemed to pass over Ollie's face. Lying in bed that night, exhausted by another long day of care, Rosie said, 'Sometimes I think I see a faraway look of sadness in his eyes, as though he is remembering how he used to be.' Perhaps, like an elderly person in the early stages of Alzheimer's disease, Ollie really was aware of slipping over the edge, losing his grasp on reality — or at least the familiar, comfortable, neurotypical reality he had until recently shared with us.

That reality included holidays and we were determined that the autism which had taken over our lives
should not thwart previously made plans to visit
France. After years of shoestring expeditionary
vagabondage, I had decided it was time for a proper
family holiday in that most predictable middle-class
destination – the Dordogne. With my cousins the
Blacks and some other friends we had booked a chateau
near Périgueux and, three days after the final consultation with the psychologist, we packed the car and
headed south.

The Channel ferry was a potential sensory nightmare of
metallic booms, vibrations, strange smells and bewildering crowds, so we took the precaution of booking a
cabin. But Ollie screamed frantically, apparently frightened by the dark confinement. So I took him to the
upper deck, where he laughed and shouted, enthralled
by the wind and the sky, and tried repeatedly to climb
out of my arms and hurl himself into the sea.

Once in France, we drove slowly south. The dead Ford
had been replaced by a decidedly 'compact' Fiat, its roof
piled high with bicycles, clothes, cot, nappies and a bucketful of rose blooms we couldn't bear to leave rotting
unloved on the pergola at home. Edmond and Ollie sat
contentedly in their child seats in the back; in the front
I drove, ranting occasionally at Rosie's woeful map-
reading. Dusk arrived and the children had to be put to
bed. We drove forlornly through a wilderness of tiny
hamlets devoid of hotels, until at last we found a seedy
bar with a bedroom upstairs. Drunken voices, stale
smoke and old greasy food smells wafted up through
the floorboards, and the sheets were so filthy we slept
with our clothes on to avoid contamination.

'Do you think this is suitable for a woman of my age

and class?' Rosie demanded shrilly. 'God knows what germs the children will pick up.'

'I'm sorry, this is all there is. Anyway, at least there are no fleas.'

'Why didn't you organise something in advance?'

'Where's your sense of adventure?'

We escaped at dawn, and the following night in Limoges found a hotel more suitable to a woman of Rosie's station. Then on the third day we arrived at our chateau, where David and Anna had kept us the north wing. The following afternoon Leah arrived with her daughter Tashi, along with Jenny (at whose wedding I had first met Rosie) and her sons Luke and Ryan (father John was prospecting for their new home in Australia). For two weeks we lived in a gentle, unhurried, sun-baked limbo. In the evenings we drank copious Bergerac wine in a gorgeously gracious dining room, living in the style to which I wished I were accustomed. By day we ate long lunches under an avenue of lime trees, or sprawled amongst the giant hay bales on the meadow below the chateau. I rigged one of my climbing ropes to make a swing for the children (well, really for myself). Rosie and I drove off to different restaurants with the boys, or put them on the bike seats for long rides through forests of coppiced chestnut. Edmond spent hours playing content-edly in the dust with fellow one-year-old, Matthew Black.

In the normal order of events, Matthew's older sister Alice would have played with Ollie, but she found him unpredictable, even slightly frightening – or merely indifferent, quietly getting on with his own pursuits. Time after time, when I forgot to lock the car, he would rush out and play with all the switches, turning lights on and off and removing the indicator arm. Our greatest fear was the big drop at the end of the chateau's court-yard – a sort of Gallic super ha-ha – which we had to patrol relentlessly, now that Ollie's spatial awareness was distorted to the point where he had no conventional sense of danger. During the daytime he was generally content, but at night he took ages to settle. Rosie and I took turns to sit and sing to him, trying to soothe his troubled spirit. Occasionally he would let us rub his back gently; at other times he preferred not to be touched. Then eventually he would fall asleep, on his side, knees drawn up slightly, hands still clasped to his snuggly, dummy in his mouth. It was only later, after discovering to what extent Ollie's problems originated in his gut, that Rosie realised he was probably suffering horrible stomach spasms during those long summer evenings.

We celebrated his third birthday with a huge picnic lunch under the lime avenue. Briefly, tentatively, smiling conspiratorially at Rosie's words of praise, he explored his main present – an enormous set of interconnecting plastic wheels and cogs. Then he ran off to play alone on the infinitely more exciting dumper truck belonging to the builders renovating the south wing.

On the way home we stopped at a hotel near the Loire where we had stayed so happily three years earlier when Ollie was a baby. This time, after a long day's drive, it was laborious getting *two* boys bathed, changed and ready for bed, before plugging in the baby alarm and going over to the dining room for supper and a vital restorative drink. We had just started the first course when the alarm piped up. Ollie was inconsolable, so we brought him over to the dining room. That did no good, so I carried him to the one place where he felt really safe – the car – and left him strapped in his baby seat while we continued with dinner. Next day, slightly early for the ferry, we made a detour into Rouen to see the great west front of the cathedral which had so entranced Monet. But instead of misty, shimmery pastel tones, we

found harsh light and jangling crowds. In the middle of
the large square in front of the cathedral something filled
Ollie with terror (or was it a spasm in his gut?) and he
began to scream, struggling to escape from the scene.
We beat a hasty retreat through the crowds, and heads
turned to stare disapprovingly at the tall angular man
wrestling a shrieking three-year-old back to his car. Late
that night we drove onto the ferry and headed home
to Larkhall, ending what would prove to be our last
proper family holiday for many years.

David Black commented afterwards on how shell-
shocked Rosie and I had seemed in the Dordogne. I
actually remember it – apart from the obvious crises –
as a period of warm tranquillity. But there was also a
sense of being in limbo – of trying to adjust to an aching
sense of grief at the loss of the old Ollie – whilst
preparing, in my case rather reluctantly, to embark on a
new, arduous journey, not quite sure that I shared Rosie's
energy and selfless determination to do everything
possible for our son.

　She had already started work before we left for France;
back at home she renewed the task with increased
vigour. On the metabolic front, she discovered a whole
network of researchers trying desperately to find out
what biochemical processes were causing such catastrophic damage to children like Ollie. What soon
became apparent was that autism was a very poor rela-
tion to the big players like cancer and heart disease when
it came to funding for medical research. Much of the
work on autism was being done by parents of autistic
children, such as Brenda O'Reilly, founder of Allergy
Induced Autism, Dr Paul Shattock, head of Sunderland
University's Autism Research Unit and Dr Bernard
Rimland, founder of the Autism Society of America, all

of them operating on shoestring budgets, co-opting other professionals − such as Dr Rosemary Waring at Birmingham University (and later the gastroenterologist, Dr Andrew Wakefield, at the Royal Free Hospital) − as best they could. There was talk of heavy metal contamination, of enzyme deficiencies, of inadequate oxidation of sulphur, of opioid peptides, of candida, of gluten and casein intolerance, of vitamin B12 deficiency . . . a whole melting pot of interconnected hypotheses on the furthest frontiers of advanced microbiology.

For a layman like me, with virtually no scientific training, it was bewildering. Rosie, always more rational and methodical, was more assiduous in following the leads and pointing out that all the research revolved round one central hypothesis − that children like Ollie had difficulty both in absorbing nutrients and excluding toxins. So she put him on special vitamin supplements recommended by Bernard Rimland. Then in Oxford she met a physician who had stopped work to care full-time for her autistic daughter. She put Rosie onto Brenda O'Reilly, who had said she knew of a child who recovered from autism after vitamin B12 injections.

When Rosie came back to me with the news of B12 salvation my eyes lit up. 'So you *do* care,' she said. 'You seemed almost indifferent, while I've been so grief-stricken.'

'Well perhaps men are just less good at showing it, and . . . well . . . I suppose we still have to try and enjoy life somehow.' Of course I was distressed, devastated by the loss of our former son, but also selfishly resentful at the way we were having to sacrifice normal pleasures to the endless search for therapies.

Rosie tracked down the information on B12 injections. Ollie would need to have a blood test and for a clear result he would first have to stop all his regular vitamin supplements. So she removed the supplements and Ollie started eating stones and sucking pieces of metals – a condition called pica. Then the two of them had to endure the trauma of the blood test, only to hear three weeks later that the lab had not found any significant B12 deficiency.

End of that little spark of hope.

The research continued. Apart from possible damage from heavy metals such as mercury, one of the most convincing hypotheses for a cause of (or contributor to) autism was opioid peptides – long chains of harmful proteins which are normally broken down by digestive enzymes, but in the case of children like Ollie pass through the damaged gut wall into the bloodstream, and thence to the central nervous system. As their name indicates, they can mimic the hallucinatory effects of opiates. They derive in particular from gluten (a protein in wheat and other grains) and casein (found in dairy products). Paul Shattock had found that many autistic children, along with quite a few hyperactive children – the two seem to be interrelated – improved on a gluten- and casein-free diet.

So, grumbling conservatively at the wrench from culinary normality, I agreed to abandon cream and yoghurt and cheesepie and buttered toast and tagliatelli con pesto and milk chocolate and Bath Olivers and all the other things we loved, at least during meals with Ollie. It seemed to help and he became markedly calmer. Over the following years we stuck to the diet whenever possible and usually when it did lapse – particularly the gluten exclusion – Ollie became immediately, obviously distraught, uncomfortable, sometimes violent.

Some medics were – and often still are – sceptical about the whole notion of mental processes being affected by what is happening in the gut. Given the immediate and obvious mental effects of alcohol – or the countless drugs which are also absorbed through the alimentary canal – this seems surprising. The scepticism about diet treatments seems doubly surprising when a well-known developmental defect – PKU, short for polyketonuria, now tested for routinely at birth – is treated successfully with a special diet. Perhaps scepticism about the metabolic origins of autism also stems from the traditional view of autism as a condition which children are born with and which belongs purely in the province of the shrinks. Which is why it was so refreshing, that summer of 1994, to visit Dr John Richer, a consultant psychologist at the John Radcliffe Hospital in Oxford, who took a thoroughly holistic view of autism.

On the face of it, his pedigree was off-putting: he had studied with the ethologists Niko and Elisabeth Tinbergen, whose work with autistic children had explored perceived failures of mother–child bonding – shades of Bettelheim's *Silent Fortress*, albeit expressed in infinitely less damning terms. However, Rosie's search for answers and treatments was exhaustively eclectic, so off we went to Oxford. John Richer had no instant cure on offer, but he did offer constructive hope. He confirmed the importance of play, praise and rewards. He told us how he prescribed special diets for autistic children in his care, and he stressed that his policy as autism advisor to his Local Education Authority was to aim for eventual integration of autistic children in mainstream schools.

We wanted to try mainstream straight away and Rosie had already made the first moves for a nursery place back in May, before Ollie's autism diagnosis was even confirmed. Now, in July, we took him to the school in question. The head teacher was bright-eyed and surprisingly enthusiastic – overzealous even – to have Ollie in her nursery class. Uncharitable thought, perhaps, but I did wonder whether she wanted to add the words 'integration of Special Needs child' to her CV. Rosie was herself a trained and highly experienced nursery teacher, who had run a class of sixty children. She had also done a huge amount of research into autism and, more to the point, she knew Ollie better than anyone else in the world. She had very clear ideas about what he needed and at the very least she expected to be consulted closely; so she was somewhat alarmed when the attendant educational psychologist announced rather patronisingly that she and the head would sit down together to prepare an educational plan for Ollie. Still, it was encouraging to think that, once he had his 'Statement of Special Educational Needs' and special assistant in place, Ollie could join 'normal' children in a small unthreatening nursery, whose introductory booklet stated emphatically:

'To start with we would like you to stay with your child in the nursery. Some children may find a whole session too long at first. When the child is ready (and it will vary greatly from child to child) you will be able to leave your child . . . Please don't get anxious or impatient if the settling-in period takes a while. Our experience has shown that it is vital not to rush this stage.'

I, far more than Rosie, had an innate wariness of all public institutions, national and local, but I warmed to this apparent promise of teacher–parent co-operation. Meanwhile, for the time being Ollie was still with us at home, all day, every day. As well as modifying his diet, we were trying to protect his new sensory sensitivities by limiting exposure to crowds, noise and confusion. The supermarket, for instance, was now a no-go area. Later we saw a film made by Donna Williams, an autistic woman who has the language to write and speak eloquently about how she perceives the world. One scene (with her former boyfriend, also autistic) shows her in a supermarket, struggling to stay on track because of 'the sounds of the people's shoes on the ground and all the pinging of the trolley metal and the jumble of all . . . and all their intertwined blah-blah and the different intoned hum of all the refrigerators competing with what's being seen'. I tried to think of my own idea of sensory hell, and imagined a strident strobe-lit disco, where I am drunk and everyone is shouting in Japanese.

So we tried to keep Ollie's routine calm and predictable. We limited speech to simple sentences devoid of sub-clauses. Rather than 'What do you think about stopping what you're doing and going for a walk now, Ollie?' we would cut to the chase with '*Ollie, we're going for a walk.*' His own speech was recovering a bit, particularly at home, where he felt secure. He even felt confident enough to try an occasional sentence, once asking a visiting child to 'come and look at my cars'. With Edmond, he enjoyed playing on the see-saw and swinging side by side at the local park. When two visiting older boys demonstrated their affection for Rosie's Siamese cats, he briefly emulated them, stroking instead of chasing Coco and Chai.

Our front door was separated from the garden by a communal path which led straight up to a one-way street with dangerous traffic. Because Ollie had no sense of danger he had to be watched constantly, and I made a temporary gate to put across the path. At first this infuriated one of the older residents of the terrace, until a sympathetic neighbour gave him a severe telling-off, explaining that the poor child was 'artistic'. There were no more complaints after that from the elder of the terrace, even when Ollie rushed uninvited into his house and helped himself to a bowl of strawberries, and from that day he and his family became staunch allies.

The social boundaries and conventions which begin normally to structure the life of a three-year-old hardly applied with Ollie. When my two brothers dropped in that summer, perhaps too boisterously for Ollie at that particular moment, he went up to the older one, Mark, looked him steadily in the eye, took him by the hand and saw him to the door. He then did the same with Philip, who paused for a moment on the threshold, wondering whether he really had to go through with this indignity, until Ollie gave him a firm shove and shut the door in his face. Our conversation had to be continued with the two of them standing outside and talking through the window.

The world had to accept Ollie on his terms, but equally his acute sensitivity to every mood and nuance of the people around him, contrary to stereotypical assumptions about the alienating effects of autism, seemed to have become even more finely tuned by his new condition. His godmother Lizzie, who lived in the next street, remained a loyal friend to Rosie and was a frequent visitor. Ollie had known her all his life and was comfortable with her, but he seemed to detect an underlying sadness. Lizzie had recently split up with a disastrously uncommitted boyfriend and was longing desperately to find a satisfactory man and have a baby before it was too late. One evening, as we were sitting with a drink, Ollie picked up the baby doll bought a year earlier when Edmond was born, walked across the room and, with uncanny prescience, handed it silently to Lizzie.

Perhaps the hardest – and bravest – thing for Ollie was to accept all the Local Authority professionals who now entered our lives – the speech therapist, the psychotherapist, the social worker and the expert we called the 'Wee and Pooh Man' who came to advise us on getting Ollie out of nappies. His strategies were highly successful and, autism notwithstanding, Ollie had soon got the hang of using a lavatory. This acquisition of new skills coincided with some building work on one of the other houses in the terrace. Caught short whilst exploring that particular garden one afternoon, Ollie defecated proudly in the lavatory he found abandoned, unplumbed, on the lawn. We had to admire his faultless logic.

Throughout his life, Ollie would have problems with irritable unpredictability, so that he would often have to relieve himself in the wrong place – usually without an abandoned lavatory to hand – resulting in a compulsive need to disperse the turds. 'Smearing', we discovered, is a common trait in children with autism, whose sensory perceptions are often very different from ours, so that the stench of faeces is not necessarily offensive to them. Often that summer, collapsing with a drink after a hard day, our guard would slip and, too late, we would discover Ollie, usually on the inappropriately carpeted stairs, plastering treads, risers, banister and walls with a comprehensive skim of fresh excrement. With a resigned groan we would abandon our drinks and set to work, one of us cleaning up Ollie while the other started the long process of scrubbing and disinfecting the staircase. We were just starting to clear up after one of Ollie's most creative faecal graffiti sessions one fine summer evening, when there was a knock at the door and Siri arrived to meet us.

Siri had been suggested by the Social Services as a possible Family Link worker to help look after Ollie and the last thing we wanted was to put her off, so I opened the door just wide enough to stick my head out, explain that we had a little crisis and ask could she come back in an hour's time? We scraped and scrubbed manically. Then out came the concentrated lavender oil. And the joss sticks. And the scented candles. I was just emerging from the garden with a handful of fresh mint when Siri returned and I asked her if she would like to join us for a glass of Pimm's.

She was a little older than us, had until recently run a hotel in North Wales, was now living in Bath and had just started part-time work on the Family Link scheme, providing respite care for several families with Special Needs children. She came from Australia, which partly explained, perhaps, her firm, plain-speaking, efficient manner. But she also had a calm reserve which was imme-diately appealing, both to us and, when he met her a few days later, to Ollie. She had other children to look after, and in any case our care entitlement was limited, but for two or three sessions a week, lasting two hours each, she would now have total charge over Ollie, usually taking him off to run and play in one of the city's parks – or to her house if it were raining – giving Rosie a complete break from his demanding presence. Of all the myriad people who were to touch Ollie's life over the next few years, she was one of the kindest and most dependable.

In August we moved for two weeks to Henley, house-sitting for the family of Ollie's godfather, Lucius, while they had their annual holiday in France. For us the space and silence of the large house, with its lawns and fields and beech wood, was a great treat. It was also littered with potential dangers for a three-year-old with damaged spatial awareness. The first morning I neglected to lock one of the upstairs bedroom windows which opened onto the curved sloping roof of the kitchen window bay. I was in the bathroom cleaning my teeth when Ollie slipped into the bedroom to do some exploring. Rosie was downstairs in the kitchen, looking out through the French window, when the fragile little body dropped through the air, limbs flailing, and landed with a hard thud. She rushed out to find him sprawled, still and silent, on the brick terrace; then after an agonising delay he opened his eyes and she carried him into the house.

I spent the rest of the morning in Lucius's workshop improvising a temporary door to block off the staircase and keeping an eye on Edmond, while Rosie endured hours of anxiety in the hospital at Reading. By the time Edmond and I got there in the evening, the 'bouncing baby' had had every bone in his body X-rayed and was running riot in the children's ward. Apart from a hair-line fracture in his collarbone he was fine and we brought him back that night. For the rest of the fort-night we kept windows and the stair door firmly locked and there were no more dramas.

Edmond was starting to talk. And to enjoy the stories which Ollie had now abandoned, observing religiously the same unvarying rituals with *The Elephant and the Bad Baby*, *Mr Gumpy's Outing* and all the other books which Rosie chose so unerringly. From the start he had always been plumper and more robust than Ollie, more conven-tionally affectionate. And more prone to tantrums. At one stage that summer, deprived increasingly of his mother's attention, he started banging his head on the floor when frustrated, and occasionally flapping his hands, filling us with dread that he too was going to flip over the edge into autism. Whatever metabolic insult sparked off Ollie's transformation, we knew that the *susceptibility* to autism had a strong genetic component. As a precaution, we declined the invitation to take Edmond to the clinic for an MMR vaccination; more proactively, Rosie decided that he needed individual supervision. She was working flat out to cope with Ollie's problems and I had to devote at least some time to earning a living; we needed someone else to look after Edmond. And somehow he or she would have to be paid.

Right from the start Rosie had been determined to find imaginative ways of extracting maximum benefit from the system: we paid our taxes and now we were going to reap the rewards. 'Resources' might be limited but there *was* potential help available, if you were prepared to go and find it. It was she who asked the local childcare college if they could find a school leaver to look after Edmond as work experience; she who then made sure we got Ollie's statutory Disability Living Allowance to pay the helper's wages. And so, as the rustling poplars (now less troubling to Ollie) turned gold and the starlings heralded winter with their autumnal chatter, Tanya arrived one fine morning to meet her sixteen-month-old charge, Edmond. For Rosie the extra help was a huge relief, but also confirmation of what autism had stolen from her: the chance with her second son to witness and enjoy all those first experiences – those uniquely precious little epiphanies – which she had shared so joyfully with Ollie. For years afterwards she would regret that day as the start of her severance from the most formative period of Edmond's young life.

I remember Tanya's first day, 21st September, for different reasons. The previous night we had been taken out to dinner by a couple from Seattle, Jim and Mary-Lou Wickwire, who were to become special friends. Jim I knew by repute, as the mountaineer who had, amongst many other achievements, made the third ascent of K2, running out of oxygen on the summit and, rather like me on Everest, bivouacking alone, with no tent or sleeping bag, at 27,000 feet above sea level. Now, many years later, he had invited me to join a trip to Monte Sarmiento, a peak rising above the Straits of Magellan, in Tierra del Fuego. The expedition was planned for spring 1995 and would be my first serious climb since the Panch Chuli accident of 1992.

Jim and I talked business and studied maps upstairs while Mary-Lou – seeing that Rosie was busy introducing a rather shy Tanya to Venables mayhem and was unavailable for chat – rolled up her sleeves and started sweeping the back garden. What a star! For me, the Sarmiento plans were a reminder of my ostensible job of being a mountaineer. After Jim and Mary-Lou left, I drove up to Birmingham where I was giving the keynote motivational presentation at an insurance company's annual conference. Then home via Wiltshire, where I had an environmental piece to research for the *Telegraph*. Then, two weeks later, a run of four lectures in three days, returning late each night, by day only sporadically helping Rosie with the children. Then, after a day's break for manic preparations, the drive to Heathrow to catch a flight to South Africa for a three-week lecture tour.

'Lecture tour' is perhaps too grandiose a term for what was really a glorious holiday, with some magical days returning to the kloofs of the Magaliesberg, driving to the far northern Transvaal to climb up the huge quartzite walls of a great monolith called the Blouberg, thrilling to the endless mountains, flowers and wine of the Western Cape and the shimmering granite cone of the Spitzkoppe piercing the Namibian desert. But as well as playing hard, I worked hard, with eleven engagements, on several topics, in six different cities, earning another vital wodge of cash to keep the Venables family functioning. It was Philip Weinberg's entrepreneurial flair

which made the tour happen; Paul Fatti and other South
African climbers who shared with me some of their
country's most magical wilderness; Janet Fatti who gave
up a whole day to drive me to the remote city of
Bloemfontein. As we were driving back across the veld,
she started to talk about Ollie, about the inexplicable
metamorphosis which had stolen a part of him away
from us, about the turmoil which had disrupted our
family. Then, with the directness which I always found
quite startling, she announced suddenly, 'I pray for him
every night.' It was only later I discovered that she had
then already suffered the first bout of the cancer which
would eventually kill her.

Janet was the foundation rock of the Fatti family,
nurturing four children while Paul supported the whole
edifice through his professorship at De Wits University.
Most of the other climbers who hosted me in South
Africa also had solid, well-paid professional positions.
And here was I, freewheeling frivolously through the
mountains while my wife stayed at home fighting the
cause of our disabled son. Of course I felt pangs of guilt.
Of course I wondered endlessly whether I should pack
it all in and get a 'proper job'. But at forty, with no
serious track record in any corporate or academic institution, I wasn't sure that a job would actually be that
easy to find. And there was also the question of pride.
Having invested so much time and emotional energy,
staking my whole identity to this freelance career, I felt
determined to stick it out and continue down that
awkward path. And I persuaded myself disingenuously
that at least when I *was* at home I had the time and
flexibility to help with the children.

While I was away, Tanya settled into her new job tending
Edmond, while Rosie took Ollie on his first weekly

visits to the nursery class. At first he was extremely nervous and could hardly bear to look at the other children, but with his mother at his side, he played cautiously with the school toys. After a couple of sessions he began to give surreptitious sidelong glances at the other pupils and by December he managed a whole forty-five-minute session, playing happily and even joining in tentatively with the other children. However, his total time at the nursery, spread over several weeks, had only amounted to five hours.

The Special Needs statement arrived finally at Christmas and in January Ollie was enrolled officially as a pupil in the nursery class, with a young woman employed to help him. Our naïve assumption was that Rosie and Ollie would have several meetings with the assistant, giving Ollie ample time to get to know her and Rosie a chance to pass on everything she knew about her son.

Not a bit of it. On the first day, 9th January 1995, Rosie was asked to go after five minutes, leaving her very sensitive autistic child for one and a half hours in the care of a complete stranger, apparently with no specific training in Special Needs education. When Rosie brought Ollie in for his second morning, the 11th, she was asked to leave immediately. The head had drawn up a rigorously detailed plan for Ollie, bristling with unrealistic 'targets' and language far beyond Ollie's current comprehension and based, as far as we could tell, on some hypothetical off-the-shelf autistic child. When Rosie objected to her exclusion from the classroom she was told that this was the best thing for Ollie – that autistic children need a firm routine and that in any case Ollie was coping fine.

His way of coping was in fact to retreat from the world. When Rosie arrived to collect him on 11th January she found him staring sadly out of the window, clutching his

snuggly and her own jersey, which she had left for additional comfort. As she approached, he turned away and
withdrew. Over the next week he became increasingly
remote. By day he developed new quirky behaviours; at
night-time the old terrors returned. From the 17th to the
20th I was away in the Alps on a photo shoot. I returned
to find a very gloomy Rosie and a silent Ollie. On
Monday, the 23rd, she took him in reluctantly and, despite
her agonised concern, was asked to leave after five
minutes. On his seventh day, the 24th, we were just sitting
down to lunch with a friend, Rosie telling her how
worried she was, when the phone rang. Ollie was very
distraught. We had better come and fetch him.

He was standing alone in the playground, staring at
the red door of a store shed, screaming in terror. When
Rosie arrived, the head told her she wished that Ollie
could have stayed to 'work it through'; but Rosie wasn't
taking any more chances. Ollie came straight home and
we never took him back to the school. He had suffered
quite enough trauma and the remnants of his speech,
which had survived falteringly up to this moment, had
now disappeared completely.

It was only in the spring that we made a formal
complaint, recording the whole saga in detail, correcting
point by point the head's very different interpretation
of events. In our letter to the Child Health and
Educational Special Needs departments Rosie blazed:

'I feel extremely angry at the way Ollie's induction has been mishandled and believe that this has
caused distress and some damage to my son and
wasted the LEA's money. I do not feel that the
school has complied with Ollie's Statement,
particularly the paragraph which reads "Every effort
should be made to ensure parental involvement in

the delivery of a structured curriculum or behaviour management programme within the home,"
nor do I think it has complied with Clause 2.28
of the Code of Practice on Special Educational
Needs which states "School based arrangements
should ensure that assessment reflects a sound and
comprehensive knowledge of a child and his or her
responses to a variety of carefully planned and
recorded actions which take account of the wishes,
feelings and knowledge of parents at all stages.'"

At a special meeting in May I represented Rosie,
placing myself deliberately at the head of the table, opposite the Senior Educational Psychologist, who chaired
the proceedings. I noted with satisfaction the taut neck
and awkward squirming of our ambitious head teacher,
then chided myself for being vindictive and considered
backing down, then thought, 'No, her wounded pride is
her problem; my sole job here is to represent the interests
of my son.' So I went through all the points I had
rehearsed at home with Rosie. The head refuted several
of those points, maintaining that she had tried hard to
cooperate with Rosie. I reiterated my points, insisting
politely that the head had made mistakes and expressing
the sincere desire that in future we would have a harmo-
nious partnership with the Local Education Authority.
The Senior Ed. Psych. seemed sympathetic and I sensed
that he could become a very useful ally.

We had no idea where our journey with Ollie was
taking us but, whatever happened, we were going to
need lots of help from our LEA in the years to come.
At some stage Ollie would have to return to some kind
of school. For the time being, though, we were busy
following a different, parallel path, educating him
ourselves, on our own terms, in our own home.

Chapter Four

No-one knows exactly what mechanisms alter the minds of autistic children. There is no indication, for instance, of the dramatic, degenerative shrinking which ravages so cruelly the brains of Alzheimer's patients. The problem, as far as Rosie and I could gather from our researches, seemed to lie more in the intricate circuitry, with several experts suggesting that with children like Ollie toxins damage the myelin sheaths protecting and insulating the axons – the microscopic tails which transmit signals between neurons. But even that very plausible short-circuiting explanation was only a hypothesis and as yet there has been no definitive proof of extensive demyelination in autistic people. The more we read around the subject the more obvious it became that the human brain was the last great frontier of exploration – an immense uncharted continent, teeming with baffling, wondrous phenomena. Most wondrous and encouraging of all was the brain's ability to repair itself, to make new connections, to restructure its compartments to compensate for traumatic damage. If this could happen in the brains of middle-aged stroke victims, surely there was hope for the young, flexible, still-growing brain, which would not normally be fully developed until the age of about sixteen.

Rosie was convinced that, in addition to addressing what seemed to be a metabolic disorder, we should also try to repair connections with some kind of intensive educational programme. Nothing was on offer in Britain, and it seemed that all the really dynamic ideas were coming from America, including the Option Institute's special programme for autistic children. We read *Son Rise*, by the institute's founder Barry Kaufman, which describes the journey he and his wife made to engage their profoundly autistic son to the point where he emerged from his silent autistic world, began to speak and became a perfectly socialised, communicative 'normal' person. Their methodology started from a position of total acceptance – entering their son's world, copying every bizarre nuance of his behaviour to create the bond which allowed them eventually to entice him, step by patient step, into their neurotypical world.

Rosie was so impressed by their story that she tried briefly, during the first summer of Ollie's autism, to emulate the Son Rise approach. But at this stage it didn't work. Unlike Raun Kaufman, Ollie had not been born with autism. Rosie was still grieving for a non-autistic Ollie, and she could not bring herself to accept unconditionally the weird stranger he had become. I was *more* sceptical – too English, perhaps – to handle Barry Kaufman's evangelical prose, too aloof to listen to the guru, and I was wary of the apparent lack of a clearly defined curriculum. Nevertheless, we did consider seriously taking Ollie to America for an Option training course, even exploring the possibility of getting Edmond's cameraman god-father, Kees 't Hooft, to come and film the project for television as a way of raising the £8,000 or so which it would cost.

Then, right at the end of 1994 Rosie discovered *Let Me Hear Your Voice*, the account by another New Yorker, Catherine Maurice, of her success in rescuing her *two* children from the clutches of autism. She too, with the help of dedicated assistants, had worked long sessions, one-to-one, teacher to child, in a closed room, excluding every distraction of the outside world. The big difference was that her method was more overtly teacher-led and followed a form of behaviour modification developed at the University of California, Los Angeles, by a Norwegian psychologist called Ivar Lovaas. The 'Lovaas Method' as we came to call it, consists of a series of drills, where the child has to respond correctly to a given command to receive a reward. Starting from the simplest instructions, 'Sit down, stand up', the series builds into ever more complex drills, gradually teaching the child both to respond to language and eventually to use language himself.

Ivar Lovaas had plenty of critics. Some people dismissed his apparently authoritarian approach as being too mechanistic – more appropriate to training animals than educating children. Even Dr Rita Jordan, one of Britain's leading autism authorities, who had made a favourable study of Lovaas's work, warned me, 'It is very difficult for children with autism to develop a sense of self-autonomy and it seems to me that the training techniques which depend on cueing – while they can be very effective in building up skills – do nothing to address that fundamental difficulty.' Other commentators were dubious about his use, now abandoned, of 'aversives' – punishing children for non-compliance. In fact, when I spoke to Professor Lovaas on the telephone and when we observed him on a video, it was his gentle compassion which impressed me; most touching of all was the warm praise he lavished every time a child succeeded at a task. Whatever the criticisms, he had a track record of helping autistic children to acquire the rudiments of language and some understanding of human relationships, to the point where 43 per cent of one set of autistic children, according to Lovaas, lost virtually all their autistic features and went on to integrate happily into normal mainstream schools.

Those statistics begged all sorts of questions about just how autistic the children had been in the first place, what particular kind of autism on that huge ill-defined continuum they had exhibited, and how far their journey had subsequently continued along the normal educational road. But we didn't have time for cynical nit-picking. We had to try and unravel the tangled circuitry of Ollie's mind, *now*, immediately, before we lost him for ever. A few hours a week at nursery school might help a bit, but that still left several hours a day, and weekends and twelve weeks of school holidays. Now here was the kind of intensive intervention Rosie had been looking for − a rigorous system to help us re-engage our son and, quite apart from anything else, to provide a secure, predictable, manageable routine for his chaotically disrupted existence.

I finished Catherine Maurice's book on New Year's Day 1995. By the evening of 3rd January I had tracked down a phone number for UCLA and got through to Ivar Lovaas's department, where the secretary had just arrived for the first morning of the new term. She told me that there was a psychologist based near Oslo who had trained with Lovaas and was now helping parents set up home education programmes in Europe. She gave me his number and I faxed him a letter before going to bed that night.

Svein Eikeseth responded a couple of days later with an information pack and the news that he could give us two days' training in February, when he would be over in England helping a family in London, who could share with us the cost of his travel expenses. In the meantime we should appoint some assistants to work with Ollie and prepare his workroom. That morning we sent off an advertisement to the local paper:

PART–TIME ASSISTANTS WANTED
TWO HOURS PER DAY
This is a unique opportunity to train in the Lovaas early intervention method for autistic children. We need enthusiastic people, preferably reading psychology or education, to help us carry out this exciting new programme with our mildly autistic three-and-a-half-year-old son. In return for a commitment to September 1995, training will be provided by a member of Professor Lovaas's team from the Psychology Department of the University of California.

Pay: £4 per hour weekdays
£6 per hour weekends
plus travel
Please write with your CV and references

Somehow we were going to have to pay for all this. During that first fortnight of 1995, before the nursery debacle, Rosie was still hoping to run the home education programme parallel to the nursery school, with the special assistant – who had been recruited specifically to work with Ollie – helping us at home, as well as at school. But we were still going to have to pay additional helpers. We decided on eighteen paid hours per week and drew up a budget, to run for two years:

LOVAAS ASSISTANTS

10 hrs @ £4	=	40			
8 hrs @ £6	=	48			
		90 x 50 weeks	=	4,500	
		x 2 years	=	9,000	9,000

EIKESETH TRAINING & TRAVEL	1,700
AUDITORY INTEGRATION TRAINING	800
PAINTBRUSH THERAPY	1,000
DEBT	2,500
TOTAL	£15,000

The wages were as low as we dared offer and we knew that we would have to rely heavily on altruistic enthusiasm. Svein's very reasonable expenses covered one training weekend and one refresher course. The auditory integration training, to desensitise Ollie's distorted hearing, was scheduled for May. The 'paintbrush therapy' was yet another therapeutic desensitising nugget unearthed by Rosie's exhaustive explorations. The debt was the shortfall from the sale of Rosie's flat – a mortgaged liability which had barely maintained its price from the boom of 1987. But now that was sold, we could remortgage the Larkhall house to raise the £15,000. We were in business.

The advertisement did not produce a rush of eager psychology students, and some of those people who did apply seemed in need of therapy themselves – one woman wrote that working with an autistic child might help her 'to realise that my life can't be so bad after all'–

while others seemed just to be hoping vaguely that this might be a way of finding themselves. But there were also some promising potential teachers. Rowena, a young mother who was already working part-time at a local centre for autistic children, was keen to learn new ideas and said she could cover two of the weekend slots, so we enrolled her. Then we met Andy and Jo. They had both grown up in Merseyside, moved south to Glastonbury, home of all things alternative, and were now living in Larkhall with their seven-year-old daughter Bryony and one-year-old Pasha, who was to become a close friend of Edmond. Vegetarian, idealistic, peace-loving and gentle almost to a fault, their family seemed to demonstrate that rarest human quality – a total absence of malice. Andy worked as a part-time chef at a local home for disabled people and did odd bits of computer consulting. Disenchanted with institutional education, he and Jo were educating their children at home, with a dedication few parents can contemplate. On top of that huge commitment they were keen also to come and work with Ollie, and after a couple of meetings Rosie was convinced that they would be excellent teachers.

And so we began to establish a growing local network of generous spirits, without whom our life over the next few years would have been extremely bleak. Rosie was the leader and initiator; I was a kind of company secretary, doing what I could to help keep the machine running smoothly. Occasionally I did the precise opposite, upsetting the whole precious arrangement with a moment of crass tactlessness, leaving Rosie to repair goodwill. Occasional damage notwithstanding, she was adamant – and correctly so – that my role could not be purely secretarial and that I should do at least three actual teaching sessions a week with Ollie. So we started with

Rosie, myself, Rowena, Andy, Jo and, until diplomatic relations were severed completely with the local nursery school, their special assistant, Julie. By February, when Ollie's return to the school looked unlikely, we were putting all our effort into home education, with a typical weekday timetable looking like this:

8.00	**– 9.00**	**Lovaas work**
9.00	– 9.30	Play
9.30	**– 11.30**	**Lovaas work**
11.30	– 1.00	Play
1.00	– 1.30	Lunch
1.30	– 2.15	Play
2.15	**– 4.15**	**Lovaas work**
4.15	– 5.30	Play

In addition there was a weekly team meeting; Ollie also did two Lovaas sessions on Saturday and three on Sunday, giving him a total of thirty-four hours one-to-one teaching per week. 'Play' had to be supervised, either by Rosie, me, Edmond's carer, Tanya, or Ollie's Family Link worker, Siri. Supervision was particularly crucial during the mid-morning play session, so that either I or Rosie could cook lunch without Ollie clamouring around us and reaching dangerously for hot pans. Along with so many other perceptions, his sense of time had become scrambled, so that he had little concept of present and future, and found it almost impossible to wait for meals; one of my jobs that winter was to build an Ollie-proof gate (which had to be heightened frequently to thwart his ever more sophisticated climbing skills) between the open plan sitting-dining room and the kitchen. With Siri he always had a wonderful time, running and playing outside and, once a week, going swimming. He also went regularly with

Edmond to Combe Hay, on the other side of Bath, to ride Shetland ponies with my mother. Both boys had good balance, but Ollie in particular rode with a natural ease; he also jumped frequently off the pony without warning, as if it were just another tricycle or toy car.

For teaching we used the little bedroom at the back of the house which Ollie shared with Edmond. I had created it three years earlier by building a partition wall, leaving a box bedroom for Rosie and me, between it and the study. In the partition I had built a window for borrowed light; this aperture was now perfect for Rosie to observe and train the rest of us. We started tentatively in early February, trying to follow the Lovaas training manual, but we were really biding time until the Saturday morning when our Viking, Svein Eikeseth, arrived from Oslo.

He was like a big, blond, cuddly teddy bear and Ollie loved him immediately. We all sat round watching while he directed operations, sitting on the floor beside Ollie's little red table. Everything was geared to compliance – to understanding and responding correctly to precise instructions – and Svein was very specific about how space should be organised to achieve this. He placed Ollie's chair with its back against a wall, with the table immediately in front of it, and himself on the other side of the table, directly opposite Ollie, demanding attention.

Ollie smiled cherubically as Svein led him over to the chair and sat him down. Then giggled as this strange new man ordered, 'Do this,' and stood up. Giggled more as Svein repeated the instruction. Then rose to his feet himself with a little physical prompting. As he stood and smiled round the room, Svein roared, 'Goorrgh – good boy!' and handed him a raisin from the prepared box of rewards. Then repeated the process. Then started on sitting down. More prompts. More success rewarded. Soon Ollie was standing and sitting to order, without any physical prompts. We had a quick break, then Svein brought Ollie back to the table and got all of us to try the same procedure.

Then he asked Rosie for a bucket and a toy brick, the latter placed on the table. 'Do this,' he commanded, sweeping the brick into the bucket, then putting it quickly back onto the table for Ollie to repeat the manoeuvre. '*Good* boy!' Then, 'Do this,' as he shot his arms in the air, roaring 'Goorrggh boy' as Ollie imitated him straight off.

Ever since the autism diagnosis in the spring we had been trying hard to keep language simple, excluding extraneous sounds, and it was clear that Ollie still understood a lot. But there were moments of what appeared to be blank incomprehension – or, more likely, an inability to *act* on language. Now the idea was to start again from scratch, with a series of discrete trials designed to elicit specific responses to language. Svein started with a simple command, 'Stand up', prompting Ollie physically until it was quite clear that he understood what the words meant. Then he taught him 'Sit down'. Ollie performed brilliantly for a while, but then decided to remain standing, swaying and shaking with laughter, ignoring repeated commands to 'Sit down' and leaning towards Svein, giggling in his face, until Svein had physically to manoeuvre him back down. He repeated the commands and this time Ollie complied angelically. Svein handed him the Slinky for a quick reward play. Then took it back and repeated the drill. Again Ollie performed brilliantly and this time Svein swept him up into a big hug, repeating 'Good boy' as Ollie giggled with delight.

We stopped for coffee while Siri took Ollie to play

in the garden. Then back to work, with all of us taking turns at the table, Svein stressing the importance of swift, clear, precise instructions and responses, never allowing ourselves to get bogged down by truculent non-compliance, but giving a curt, unemotional 'No' to wrong responses, while enthusing ecstatically over successes, reinforcing those verbal rewards with little food treats or a special toy. He stressed the importance of positioning ourselves to be in control, with props ready, and as he moved on after lunch to demonstrate more complex drills he was like a conjuror, all hands, manipulating several toys at the same time as keeping Ollie's hands off the table. He was now attempting a more complicated verbal prompt, placing a brick and cup on the table, putting a second brick closer to Ollie and commanding, 'Put brick with brick.' Ollie repeatedly put the brick on the cup, so Svein modelled the correct response for him, covering up the cup with one hand and with his other hand directing Ollie to place one brick on top of the other.

We worked for the whole of that Saturday and continued through Sunday morning. Then on Sunday afternoon Svein drew up a detailed list of objectives, before setting off for London and leaving us to continue on our own. Inspired by his energy and precision, we made fast progress at first, advancing rapidly through a series of drills. Within a week or two Ollie was responding enthusiastically, particularly to rapid-fire instructions: 'Stand up. Sit down. Touch nose. Arms up. Stand up. Sit down and touch toes. Stand up. Jump. Turn round. Sit down.' Sessions were broken up into mini segments, with lots of breaks for playing. Because Ollie loved music we played cassette tapes, joining in the 'Hippopotamus Song' and getting him to do the actions to 'Row, row, row the boat', then progressing to 'Heads, shoulders, knees and toes'. I photographed a selection of toys so that he could start matching 2D to 3D objects. Rosie bought a whole series of jigsaws and other puzzles and made up colour cards. And, tentatively, patiently, she made the first attempts to coax individual vowels from the mouth of the son who had for the time being abandoned all speech.

The sounds took a long time coming, but Ollie's comprehension and matching skills seemed to blossom rapidly, and with them his confidence and happiness. Life seemed hopeful again, even if Rosie had had to make huge sacrifices to run the programme. There were times when she wished that autism would just go away and leave her to play with her younger son. And she was missing her cats. Molested ever more mercilessly by their tail-yanking tormentor, Ollie, they had been reduced to nervous wrecks, constantly fleeing through the cat flap or cowering anxiously on top of the piano. In the end Rosie had decided to find them a more secure home with a family on Sion Hill, one of Bath's most salubrious neighbourhoods. Coco and Chai settled instantly into their gracious new quarters without a backward glance, but for Rosie their departure was just another reminder of lost freedoms. I was less sad to see them go. I *had*, I suppose, liked Coco's sleek, genial insouciance; but Chai I had always found scrawny and neurotic. And jealous. She never forgave me for usurping her place in Rosie's affections. One morning during our first contented summer in Larkhall, waking serenely to birdsong and silver sunlight, delighting in my new-found domesticity, I turned my head and opened my eyes to find, not the beautiful face of my sleeping wife, but, interposed on the pillow between me and that golden vision, thrust right in my face, a puckered little pink feline anus.

Now Chai had gone and I almost wished I had tried harder to make friends. As for romantic wifely awakenings, during February and March I was mainly sleeping on the landing floor, so as not to disturb Rosie when I finally got to bed, usually at about four in the morning, after working through the night on the latest writing project. It was a large, ambitious coffee-table celebration of Himalayan climbing which I had taken over when the original author, Andy Fanshawe, died in a fall off Lochnagar in 1992. For two years the book had simmered in the background, but now the foreign editions were all tied up, publication date fixed and I had until the end of March to complete forty chapters, all illustrated lavishly with maps, diagrams and sumptuous photos. Since Christmas I had been steadily increasing the pace, revising Andy's original manuscript, writing several new chapters, checking facts, corresponding with photographers all over the world, and producing rough layouts for the designers. I enjoyed the hectic urgency of it, relieved to discover that I could still manage on three hours sleep a night if necessary. But the obsessive race to finish the book before departing on the Tierra del Fuego expedition left little energy for my early morning teaching sessions with Ollie.

One glorious red-letter Friday afternoon, 24th March, I typed in the final words of the introduction, copied the text onto a disc along with a final batch of photo captions, put the disc in an envelope addressed to my editor and walked over to the post office just as Anna and David Black arrived with their children for the weekend. I was free! As always with Anna and David, we ate and drank hedonistically. Spring was in the air and the children played in the sandpit, Edmond stuffing sand into his mouth for the sheer perverse fun of it,

Ollie playing alongside but not *with* the other children, comfortable with their presence, observing them with a quiet smile hovering at the corners of his mouth.

The following weekend we got a babysitter on the Saturday night so that Rosie and I could go to the Assembly Rooms and hear the brilliant young cellist Natalie Clein join the Allegri Quartet for a performance of the Schubert string quintet, on the night before I left for Tierra del Fuego. Imminent separation intensified Schubert's poignancy, and in the interval Rosie explained to an acquaintance that we were making the most of my last evening. The other woman blurted, 'You mean, in case he doesn't—' then went bright red and apologised as Rosie laughed, 'No, no, I've told him I'll say very nasty things about him at his funeral if he doesn't come back.'

Tierra del Fuego was the name Ferdinand Magellan gave to the intricate maze of islands and channels at the southernmost tip of South America as he sailed through his eponymous strait, forging a new sea route from the Atlantic to the Pacific. The fires he saw were the cooking hearths of indigenous Indian tribes – hunter-gatherers who lived off fish, mussels and crabs, and the leaves and berries of the dense forest which cloaks the land right to the water's edge. Now the Indians have all gone, most of them wiped out by European viruses to which they had no immunity, and the western extremity of Tierra del Fuego is totally deserted.

Sailing along the Beagle Channel into that desolate wilderness eight thousand miles from home felt almost unbearably melancholic. The names on the chart didn't help much: godforsaken little islets commemorating lost companions of Fitzroy and Darwin or, bleakest of all, Captain Cook's 'Bahía Desolada', where forest, sea and sky merged into relentless, sodden greyness. Perhaps it was restless guilt at leaving Rosie on her own to run Ollie's education. Or perhaps the disenchantment of an expeditionary veteran failing to revive the fresh anticipatory joy of earlier adventures, now that other more important events had taken over my life. Or perhaps it was just the weather, which was abysmal. Whatever the causes, it took me a while to drag myself out of this particular Patagonian slough of despond, pull myself together and enjoy my blessings.

The team was fantastic: Jim Wickwire was calm, dependable, optimistic; his old friend from K2, John Roskelley, once reputed for abrasive ambition, was now a gentler, mellower veteran with nothing to prove; Tim Macartney-Snape, who had been twice to the summit of Everest without oxygen equipment – the second time walking all the way from sea level in the Bay of Bengal – was a picture of competent strength. Then there was the ebullient skipper of our yacht, Charlie Porter, enthusing constantly about this remote primeval landscape of sea, forest and mountains which he had made his home. And there was his Cretan crewman and cook, Renos, who cheered us with huge steaks and spaghetti carbonara and, when we returned from squelching walks ashore, steaming cauldrons of mulled wine.

The obscure object of our perverse desires was Monte Sarmiento, a glittering confection of snow and ice towering south of the Straits of Magellan. We reached it after five days' sailing and Renos guarded the boat while the rest of us made base ashore and began to prospect a route through the forest. Freed from the soporific motion of the boat, perceptions shifted and I began to delight in the forest landscape – the gnarled silhouettes of the southern beeches, the crimson fuchsia-like pendant flowers of *Felicia buxifolia*, the peppery taste of the canella leaves from which the Indians used to get their vitamins, along with the bitter-sweet pink and white berries of the calafate – a kind of berberis which flourishes throughout Patagonia.

The team gelled, progress was made, summit attempts were planned. Then, descending steep ice one blustery afternoon, Jim was caught off balance by a blast from the Pacific, skidded out of control and smashed into a rock, wrenching his ankle. The following day the same thing happened to Charlie, dislocating his shoulder. After a long, farcical, agonising evening in a crowded tent, trying unsuccessfully, without morphine, to wrench Charlie's shoulder back into place, we returned – the fit and the walking wounded – to the boat. Charlie, Jim and Renos headed for Punta Arenas and hospital, leaving John, Tim and me to have one final, eleventh-hour, crack at one of Monte Sarmiento's twin summits.

It seemed selfish to be going back up without Jim, who had organised the whole adventure in the first place. On the other hand, I felt that we should try to finish the job we had come to do. So the three of us ploughed back up through the forest and on up the glacier to the top camp. Then, for the first time in three weeks, we were granted a whole day of fine weather to find a way up the previously untouched South-West Face to Sarmiento's west summit. At a purely utilitarian level, I felt pleased that the job was done, the objective reached, justifying, partly at least, my absence from home. At a deeper, almost cathartic, level I was relieved to have cast off the demons of Panch Chuli and faced up to my doubts and fears. The summit, for once, was the high-light of the climb – a moment of transcendent beauty with our mountain a shimmering jewel suspended above an endless expanse of land and water. That emptiness now felt comforting, not threatening – wilderness a source of solace not despair – our summit, for all its pointlessness, a moment of preciousness to be added to all those other treasured moments which give life at least the illusion of creative purpose.

Our glittering hour of glory was paid for with a hideous descent through battering wind-blasted snow, as Patagonia reverted to type. But the fight only intensified the satisfaction of returning to Jim's commandeered fishing boat, which was waiting down at the shore two days later to take us back to Punta Arenas. And then we parted for our different flights home, three of us leaving the southern autumn and returning to the northern spring. After four weeks away I was impatient to see Rosie and the boys, but I had to wait twelve hours for a connection in New York, so I got the bus into Manhattan and whiled away an afternoon at the Metropolitan Museum, post-Impressionists complementing the blossom in Central Park. I caught the night flight to Heathrow and joined the morning commuters on their journey into London, where I was booked to give an 11.00 a.m. lecture at the Civil Service College. Somehow I managed to submerge sweet domestic yearnings and project the required dynamic persona.

Then I was free, heading back west by train to Bath, impatiently ticking off Slough, Reading, Didcot, Swindon, Chippenham, then craning eagerly through the window to witness that brief glimpse over the river meadows of distant gables dwarfed by Lombardy poplars, before the train was swallowed up in the cuttings and tunnels of Brunel's masterful final approach into Bath. Fifteen minutes later my taxi left me in Larkhall. As I wrestled two large kitbags down the path I saw that our front door was open and the temporary flexible gate pulled across the path. A little boy was standing behind the mesh smiling. At first I thought he was Ollie, then realised it was Edmond, just two days short of his second birthday, grown bigger during the month I had gone. He looked me up and down for a moment before saying, 'Hello Dadda'; then another boy came out of the front door. He didn't utter any recognisable words but the 'aiyah . . . gaiyee' sounds he made were happy sounds, and when I said, 'Hello, Ollie,' he gave me a quick smile of recognition.

'It was so moving I burst into tears. I can't tell you how wonderful it felt. After all those weeks, he suddenly did it – "aaahh".' The children were in bed and Rosie was telling me about the big breakthrough while I had been away – Ollie's first successful copying of a specified sound. Like the wolf child of Aveyron in François Truffaut's *L'Enfant Sauvage* uttering his first faint human word, '*lait*', Ollie had strained every muscle in his face, struggling to achieve the exact co-ordination of diaphragm, larynx, mouth and lips, to emulate his mother. It was only one vowel, but it was followed soon by 'ee', 'oo' and 'mm'. Ollie was taking the first steps back to speech and he was enjoying the work, enjoying his own success.

My first weekend back home we took both the boys to the Botanic Gardens, turning a blind eye while Ollie climbed illegally up an irresistible Japanese maple, absorbed meditatively in bark textures and patterns of leaf, branch and sky. Then he ran over to a gorgeously blowsy flowering cherry, gathering armfuls of pink confetti from the ground and scattering it gleefully, then reaching on tiptoes to pluck fresh blossom from the branches. We headed towards the fish pool and a mischievous gleam came into his eye, so Rosie insisted, 'Edmond, take Ollie's hand . . . that's right . . . well done – you look after him.' And the two boys walked ahead, hand in hand, the younger protecting the older.

Later that week we had a phone call from Ollie's godmother Lizzie. Since January she had been desperately ill, at first semi-paralysed by Guillain-Barré syndrome, then stricken by leukaemia. Now she had started a round of intensive chemotherapy and was phoning from the oncology ward. She sounded terribly weak, but there was a kind of angry defiance when she complained, 'It's horrible: my body feels like a toxic waste dump.' The following week one of the friends who was looking after her, trying to cheer her with tempting alternatives to the dire hospital food, phoned, saying that Lizzie wanted to speak to Rosie. I could only catch muffled sounds escaping from Rosie's headphone, but I could hear the tears and the words 'I love you all.' She was very weak, all her disease-fighting white blood cells destroyed by chemotherapy. A few days later she caught a chest infection and died.

The funeral was on a radiant day at the end of May. The friend through whom we had first met Lizzie, Maggie Saunders, and her husband Victor – the same Victor who had saved my life on Panch Chuli – drove down from Scotland through the night with their son Hugo and arrived in time for a quick breakfast before we left for the Abbey. There was a terrible finality in the coffin resting so stolidly on its trestles at the head of the nave, but relief of a kind in the eloquent words of Father Philip Jebb, the Benedictine monk Lizzie had met and befriended, so unBritishly, in a train whilst immobilised by a points failure near Reading. And a kind of celebratory joy in the sheer number of people filling the Abbey. After the reception Maggie, Victor and I drove over to Bristol to do a couple of easy rock climbs in the Avon Gorge, savouring our aliveness, delighting in the fluid movement up the rock before returning to Larkhall for wine and supper.

Lizzie's death left a big gap in our lives, but made new connections. While helping tidy her house, we got to know Gail, a talented remedial masseur who had just mastered the art of 'zero balancing'. Self-indulgent quackery, I thought, until Rosie returned serenely from her first 'zee-bee' session. 'She's brilliant. I lie down on that couch, in Larkhall, and I go straight back to Africa.' So, every few days, Rosie escaped the nagging stress of nursing an autistic child and returned to the light and colour and carefree joy of her childhood in East Africa. Through Gail we got to know Shena Power and her fellow-cellist husband Bruno Schrecker, whom I had first heard fifteen years earlier in Oxford, playing Beethoven with the Allegri Quartet. Now in his late sixties, he was still with the quartet, performing frequently here in Bath and living almost next door to us in Larkhall. Often, walking past the tall gabled terrace where he lived – a scaled-up version of our own – we had commented on how much we would like to live there ourselves. Now, one summer night, we found ourselves in Bruno and Shena's garden, dining out under a velvet starry sky framed by an immense oak tree, with the burbling of the Lambrook at the bottom of the garden complementing Bruno's genial laughter.

That evening Rosie announced, 'We're going to live here.'

'What – turn Bruno and Shena out of their house?'

'No – we're going to live in one of these *other* houses in Grosvenor Terrace.'

I knew by now that when Rosie decided something it usually happened. Despairing of my stubborn resistance to change, she had already put our house on the market while I was in Tierra del Fuego, and sold it soon after I got back. We were due to move out in July, and I had agreed reluctantly that we had to find somewhere larger. We also needed a secure garden, because the present communal path, opening onto a road, was becoming ever more dangerous as Ollie got bigger and faster. A remote house in the country was a tempting idea, but with all the support systems we now had centred around Ollie, we really needed to stay close to the city centre. In any case, rural properties around Bath were prohibitively expensive. But perhaps Grosvenor Terrace would be possible?

In August two of the Grosvenor houses came on the market, by September we had managed to raise our mortgage to the absolute maximum (with the generous promise of additional cash from my parents to pay for some vital repairs) and in October we exchanged contracts on one of them, on the understanding that the current tenants would leave by the end of November. In the meantime we had moved out of our first house and were renting temporarily another house in the same Larkhall Terrace. Shifting just six doors down a gently sloping tarmac path should have been the easiest house move in the world, but unfortunately I had to do the entire job pushing our belongings on the boys' double buggy, hopping on my right leg.

The left leg was broken at Wintour's Leap, a cliff above the River Wye where I spent occasional evenings climbing. That particular afternoon of 28th June 1995, was one of the hottest in a very hot summer. The air was humid, the limestone clammy, and one stupid slip ruined my summer. I did not fall far, but just before the rope checked my plummet I clipped my left foot on a ledge, cracking the heel bone. At the hospital they told me I would have to be on crutches for three months.

Just as we were preparing for a sponsored bike ride to raise extra funds for Ollie's home education programme! And moving house. And trying to maintain the Lovaas sessions with Ollie. And having to manage without Edmond's work-experience carer, Tanya, who had suddenly left us without warning.

Rosie was justifiably angry about the accident, but this latest inconvenience seemed only to intensify her determination to explore every possible treatment for Ollie. In the spring he had spent a week doing Auditory Integration Training. Like so many treatments for autism, AIT lurked on the fringe of mainstream medicine – another of those slightly embarrassing poor relations excluded from the big happy family. Its methods were developed by Dr Guy Berard and Dr Alfred Tomatis and used successfully to treat the hypersensitive hearing of an autistic girl called Georgina Stehli. As she wrote in *The Sound of a Miracle*, 'People would bug me, I could hear them breathing and their stomachs growling across the room. Their voices were so high pitched they got on my nerves.' After treatment, her mother wrote, '[Georgina] told me that she was much more comfortable, that she no longer heard street noises three blocks away, or people flushing their toilets at the other end of the building, or the blood rushing through her veins.'

The proper sceptic might be rightly suspicious of a book about a 'miracle' written by the patient's parent. Our experience was that in this baffling, inconclusive world of autism, it was generally parents who got things done and that, just occasionally, remarkable cures – or at least profound ameliorations – were achieved. It is unlikely that Ollie shared Georgina Stehli's extreme hypersensitivity (both auditory and visual), but he was undoubtedly sensitive – painfully so – to some sounds, so it made sense to treat him. Rosie persuaded some other mothers from the local autism group to enrol their children and share the cost of getting a trained practitioner, Stella Carlton, to come and set up a temporary clinic in Bath. Stella was engagingly honest about the treatment, making it clear that none of the other children given AIT had made the same dramatic progress as Georgina Stehli. She also admitted that no-one was quite sure how the treatment actually worked: all they did know was that by listening through earphones to several sessions of modulated sounds and music, with certain frequencies removed, some autistic children lost some of their more acutely disturbing auditory sensitivity. So twice a day for ten days, we took Ollie to sit in a motel room on the edge of Bath and listen to what sounded like New Age music played backwards. Although at first it seemed to make him rather wild – perhaps because the world now sounded different again – after a few weeks he calmed down and never again had problems with loud sounds. AIT didn't cure his autism, but at least it made one aspect of his distorted world easier to manage.

Less effective was our experiment at the end of August, when a chance radio programme had the four of us decamping to an industrial estate in Kent to spend two weeks treating Ollie with hyperbaric oxygen. I knew of climbers whose frostbite injuries had been helped by hyperbaric oxygen, and the theory was that children with developmental disorders could experience the same kind of beneficial cell repair; some children with cerebral palsy, for instance, seemed to be benefiting. For Ollie it was probably, in retrospect, a complete waste of money, but at the time anything which offered even a faint hope of repairing his neural pathways seemed worth trying. So, twice a day, for two weeks, Ollie and I (Rosie was too claustrophobic) lay down on a tray and were slid into a pressurised chamber, to be infused for thirty minutes with pure oxygen.

With the fortnight's treatment costing £2,000 there was no spare money for a hotel, so we stayed at a campsite, oppressed by the smell of drains and by the shrill woman in the next plot who spent every spare moment, in her white stilettos, vacuum-cleaning her palatial tented atrium. We survived a week of this then telephoned Rosie's sister-in-law Shan, who lived reasonably close to the oxygen merchants and said, 'For goodness sake come and stay with us.' Right foot hopping heroically, left foot swollen and throbbing despite all the pure oxygen, I packed up the tents and we drove thankfully over to Jake and Shan's house, from where we commuted for the second week of hyperoxygenation. Then it was time to return to Larkhall for our follow-up training session with Svein Eikeseth.

All through the summer Ollie had continued his home education programme. At the end of May we had been able to report good progress to the senior educational psychologist. For example, the three initial 'receptive commands' – 'come here', 'sit down' and 'stand up' – had increased to include 'arms up, clap hands, hit legs, put in bricks, stamp feet, turn around, give cuddle, open door, close door, turn on light, turn off light, wave byebye, touch table, shake head, touch toes, open mouth, touch nose.' Sorting had increased to matching three-dimensional objects to their two-dimensional representations; his ability to copy simple two-brick structures had grown to magnificent sixteen-brick architectural fantasies – a thrilling advance from his obsessive lining-up phase, rewarded with lavish praise; and he had demonstrated the first embryonic hints of returning speech by repeating 'ooh', 'ahh', 'eee' and 'mmm' to order. Now, at the end of August, the list was longer, but the momentum had slowed and we all needed re-invigorating. On Saturday morning we all assembled with Svein in the boys' bedroom, with the video camera recording everything for future training.

Andy, our star teacher and the only volunteer remaining from our original recruitment, starts off with verbal prompts: 'Stamp your feet . . . look at me . . . touch table . . . clap hands . . . look at me . . . stand up and turn around . . . jump – now . . . look . . . go and knock on the door – no – knock on door – good boy . . . sit down . . . clap your hands . . .' Between correct responses, Ollie shoots sidelong glances at the newer teachers sitting around the room – Emma Finch, Emma Bird, Joanne . . . Then he starts giggling riotously, writhing and shaking himself off his chair. Andy manoeuvres him upright. 'Sit properly – good boy', and he sits calmly, angelic in maroon shorts and polo shirt, hands on lap, wide dark eyes alert. 'Say "ooh" . . . say "mmm" . . . say "ah" . . . say "oh".' He repeats each vowel perfectly, every facial muscle tensed in concentration, ending with a beautifully elongated 'ohhh'.

After a two-minute play break, Andy gets him back and arranges toys on the table. 'Push train . . . drink from cup . . . build with bricks.' Sometimes Ollie has to be asked two or three times before he gets it right. Svein interrupts: 'Just say "train" because the rest is just noise. The action is not important: what he is learning is the names of the objects. I notice that sometimes you use a lot of normal conversation. That is good, because that is how we talk. But with something new, just give the label.'

After lunch Svein gets the two new teachers to work with Ollie. One woman is hugely enthusiastic and Ollie matches her enthusiasm, standing promptly to order and rushing off in fits of giggles. Another novice has a turn, but when Ollie responds correctly her praise is rather lacklustre and he soon switches off. Time after time, Svein stresses the importance of praise and reinforcement. Late in the afternoon, tired after a long day's work, failing repeatedly to match objects, Ollie starts whimpering, then screaming with frustration. Again Svein tells us to give him good rewards for boring work. Rosie puts on the tape recorder and Ollie dances to the music, swaying contentedly.

On the Sunday I have a turn at the table. My task is a 'fine motor skills' exercise, with the aim of getting Ollie to draw a line across a piece of paper. At first I get it all wrong. The table is not close enough to Ollie. My prompting is too vague, and when Ollie does get close to success I fumble too slowly in the reward box. 'Get out the car!' hisses Rosie. Eventually I get it right, modelling the task for Ollie, helping him draw the pencil across the paper, then whipping out his favourite toy car and exclaiming 'Gooood!'

Then Rosie has a turn at brick building. With her there is immediate authority and firmness, as she gets Ollie sitting down to copy a building sequence. But there is also disappointment that he only manages a sequence of three bricks instead of the sixteen he was doing a few weeks earlier. And it is the same with imitated sounds: Rosie tells Svein that when she started to attempt repetition of whole words, Ollie lost individual vowels he had previously mastered. Svein reassures us by pointing out that the very fact that Ollie has managed to imitate sounds at all means that he has the potential to learn whole words and regain expressive language.

In a final pep talk before returning to Norway, Svein explains how we should organise the drills into a

Current Programme and Maintenance Programme, with mastered tasks going into the latter programme for occasional revision. He lectures the new teachers on punctuality and commitment. Again he stresses the importance of consistency, to avoid confusing Ollie, and the need to lavish him with praise when he succeeds. Then he leaves us, to continue on our own.

We waited five months before we could move into our house. The temporary accommodation was dark and damp. The carpets exuded stale smells of old cat pee, the gas cooker leaked and the kitchen tap dripped. At least the boys' bedroom was reasonably dry and airy and doubled as classroom for Ollie as we tried to keep up the momentum of his Lovaas programme, but it was hard to keep staff and ourselves motivated. And there were times when we just wanted to relax and play and pretend to be a normal family – the four of us pottering domestically – just being.

Looking back at video recordings, I see snapshot moments of quiet autumnal contentment. On a Saturday afternoon in late September we are all in our temporary sitting-dining room, sharing space with the tumble-dryer and freezer draped decoratively with Indian fabrics. Edmond sits on the pink-striped sofa, screwdriver in hand, helping his mother repair a video cassette. Ollie sits silently at the dining-room table, doing an alphabet jigsaw. There are long pauses between letters, as if it is too much effort to concentrate. Or to acknowledge us. But we pester him constantly, demanding attention.

'Say "Ollie".'

He gives a little smile and a faint 'O –'

'Say "hello."' Rosie repeats her request three times and eventually Ollie says 'Ugh'. Then he suddenly applies himself to the jigsaw, fitting seven letters in a concentrated burst of energy, rewarded by lots of 'Well done Ollie!'

Now the *Snowman* tape is repaired and playing on the television screen. Ollie continues his jigsaw to the sound of the elegiac piano chords accompanying David Bowie's opening narration; when Bowie's introduction finishes, Edmond takes over, chatting fluently, providing his own commentary to the film. Rosie gets out the octons and shows Ollie how the plastic pieces fit together. 'What a clever boy . . . look what Ollie's doing.'

As the Snowman sets off on his crazy midnight motorbike ride, Ollie is starting again on the alphabet. Then we reach the final dream sequence. Rosie laughs at the dancing Father Christmas and Ollie's face breaks into a wide engaged smile. He chuckles, 'Heeya . . . aiyeee . . . grgrhrh', opening and closing his right hand, pincering second finger against thumb.

A couple of weeks later, on a Sunday morning, Rosie is outside the back door, making rose cuttings for the new garden. As she dips scarred nodes in rooting hormone, the boys run backwards and forwards along the path, Edmond thrilled at chasing his elder brother. During brief moments of connection Ollie acknow-ledges his chaser. He looks slightly frail and wobbly in his check shirt, baggy pull-on trousers and black leather boots.

Later, at lunch, Rosie prompts him: 'Ollie, say "Mummy". Go on – say "Mummy".'

'Mmumm.'

'Well done!'

Then the boys are back outside, this time on the front path of the terrace. Edmond and Jay, the boy from Number Five, ride their trikes up and down. Ollie rides in parallel, alongside them but separate, giving them occasional sidelong glances. Then, while Edmond is cleaned up to go to Pasha's third birthday party, Ollie stands silently, contemplating the pigeons which belong to Brian at Number Seven. He smiles delightedly as they flap across the sky and exclaims, 'Aiyeeaiyeeaiyee'. Then, squinting slightly at the bright light, holds his gaze on the yellowing poplars, listening intently, no longer threatened by their rustle.

Another afternoon, at the kitchen sink. A huge grin escapes from the side of Ollie's dummy, as he stands next to Edmond and presses his face against Edmond's fore-head, disrupting his attempts at washing some toys. Edmond turns round and hugs Ollie, who runs fingers and thumb through Edmond's hair, stroking, feeling, exploring, then briefly clutching a whole handful of hair with a shriek of delight.

'Ollie's pulling my hair!'

'No he isn't – he's just stroking you.'

An evening in late October. It is bathtime and Edmond is busy playing with the baby doll – the one Ollie spurned when his younger brother was born. Edmond chants, 'Wash her face . . . wash her fingers . . . wash her bottom . . .' Ollie sits at the other end of the bath, long slender feet pressed together, hands stretched out to play with his toes. Rosie takes the doll from Edmond and tries to engage Ollie, putting soap in his hand, modelling washing movements along the doll's back and giving a Lovaas-style order: 'Do this.' But Ollie just pulls his hand away and returns to silent examin-ation of his toes. Edmond reclaims the doll and reiter-ates enthusiastically, 'Wash her bottom . . . wash her bottom . . .'

Bedtime, and Edmond stands in his cot, face pressed to the bars, rapt as Rosie reads the story about the naughty boy at the swimming pool. Then screams furi-ously when the story ends, while Ollie lies quietly in his bed, head on pillow, dummy in mouth, concentrating meditatively on his own settling down for sleep.

I always admired that meditative quality – his ability to draw in on himself and escape from all that was noisy, threatening or bewildering. At times it seemed crass to be attempting to disrupt his silent contemplation, pestering him with our relentless syllabus of behaviour modification. But when it worked – when he responded successfully and smiled delightedly at that success – it all seemed worthwhile. And in any case, he so often joined us voluntarily – watching, observing, chuckling at our laughter, trying to play with Edmond – that he clearly had a sense of belonging with us and wanting to communicate with us, perhaps even wanting to learn again how to make that interaction conform to normal 'appropriate' human behaviour. We owed it to him to do everything we could to try and help him make that return journey, even if that meant being very tough with him.

The toughness fell mainly on Rosie, who bore the brunt of the teaching and the organisation and whose world became increasingly confined. For me there were occasional escapes. In November I spent two weeks in North America, first promoting the new Himalayan book at the Banff Mountain Festival in Alberta, then flying south to give two lectures in Colorado, then over to Boston for another lecture, followed by a meeting in New Hampshire. In Colorado I stayed with Robert Anderson, leader of our 1988 Everest expedition. We climbed in Eldorado Canyon and on the Flatirons above Boulder, where the Rocky Mountains rear up at the western edge of the Great Plains. My broken heel was mended, the air was bright and crisp, the dark red sandstone dappled with brilliant yellow lichen, the distant higher mountains dusted with the first winter snow. All

that colour, space and movement felt gloriously liberating, but it was only a temporary uneasy release from
more important responsibilities. When I told Robert
about Ollie's autism he was astounded; the last time he
had seen him he had been a bright, talkative, completely
'normal' toddler.

Soon after I returned from America Rosie had to leave
me in charge while she drove over to Hampshire to join
her father, brother and sister at her mother's nursing
home. Ever since the accident two years earlier, Kay had
been withering under the onslaught of Parkinson's
disease and now the end was close. All weekend she clung
tenaciously to life and on the Monday Rosie had still
not returned. Siri, our Family Link respite worker, offered
to look after Ollie and Edmond while I drove north to
lecture at a business training course. That evening she
phoned me at the conference centre to pass on the
message that Kay had died.

The funeral was a week later, on the day we took
official possession of our new house. Siri took over again
while Rosie and I were away. It was a cold grey afternoon in Alresford and afterwards we all sought refuge
in a warm, bustling pub, eating and drinking until after
closing time. We finally headed back to the hotel, Rosie's
father, brother and nephew – three generations with
arms linked – weaving tipsily through the falling snow,
singing in celebration of a dear lost life.

And then, with little time for grief, Rosie was plunged
into the banality of another house move. While she
looked after the boys and packed up the temporary
home, I worked with the builders on the new house,
rushing to make it vaguely habitable in time for
Christmas. Frantic to complete the work in time, I hardly
noticed Rosie's concern about Ollie, who had become
rather thin, pale and listless. For him, moving house

could be deeply upsetting, so Rosie took the two boys to stay with our friends Keith and Pru Cartwright, while I supervised the actual move on 22nd December. Our builders' budget was now used up, so the next day I was working myself on fitting kitchen lights when Rosie arrived back and asked me to help Ollie in from the car. At the Cartwrights he had opened a wrong door and fallen down steps into the cellar and hurt his leg; he also seemed to have flu, and both Rosie and Edmond were feeling ill too.

I ate Christmas dinner alone in the half-finished kitchen while the others stayed in bed upstairs. Although no-one had spotted anything amiss on the X-ray of Ollie's leg, it still seemed sore. In fact both his legs seemed to be aching and he was loath to get out of bed. Later that week, when she had recovered from the flu, Rosie tried to take him for a walk, hoping that air and exercise might cheer him up. He kept stopping, and years later Rosie reproached herself for trying to make him continue. 'He kept asking me to carry him. Then he burst into tears, crying and crying, and I realised that he must be in terrible pain.'

Back at home he collapsed in bed, refusing virtually all food. We took him back to the hospital where a young doctor at A&E tried forlornly to make a diagnosis on a child who could not speak. All we could tell her was that his legs seemed very painful, although nothing had been noticed in the recent X-ray. He also seemed to have pain in his abdomen. The doctor had no answers, nor did our local GP, yet Ollie was clearly very ill. My brother Philip took one look at him, lying listlessly in bed, and agreed with us. 'He looks terrible – all pale and waxy . . . and so *thin*. Surely there must be something seriously wrong?'

While Ollie languished I spent much of the first
month of 1996 continuing to make our new house more
habitable, putting off the intellectual challenge of
unwritten articles and lectures while I immersed myself
in carpentry, relishing again the sweet scent of fresh
wood shavings. Less sweet were the toxic fumes of anti-
woodworm treatment, forcing us all to leave for a day
and stay with William and Fiona, Ollie's surviving
godmother. Searching for the bathroom in the unfamiliar
house that night, Ollie fell into a cupboard, re-intensi-
fying the pain in his legs. Back at our own now wood-
wormless house he returned to bed, where his Lovaas
teachers just sat with him, not attempting any work, but
providing what comfort they could. Increasingly he
preferred the security of our double bed to his own
bunk.

On 24th January one of the GPs from the local practice came to see Ollie, but was unable to explain his
condition. One of his colleagues came on the 31st but
was equally baffled. Two days later, having made elaborate babysitting arrangements, Rosie accompanied me to
Derbyshire for the farewell dinner for Maggie Body –
editor to numerous mountain-travel authors going all
the way back to the great explorer Eric Shipton – who
was retiring from Hodder & Stoughton. That was on
Friday evening. On the Saturday Rosie returned to Bath
while I drove on to give a lecture in North Wales,
intending to stay for some climbing on the Sunday. But
that night Rosie phoned to ask me to come home. 'I
can't bear it any more. He's just crying and screaming
all the time. *You'll* have to have a turn – it's driving me
demented.'

So I returned and took over for a while, stroking Ollie
when he would let me, otherwise just sitting quietly
beside him and getting him to drink some liquid. He

cried less on the Monday and I started work on some wood panelling. I had nearly finished the job when one of the GPs came on the Tuesday afternoon to examine Ollie. He could not tell the doctor what was wrong, but his eyes seemed infinitely sad, his face was palely cadaverous and his legs pitifully thin with sporadic little bruises. Rosie, who had so recently watched her mother sinking away, said categorically that Ollie was dying. The doctor listened politely but thought that there was no particular reason to admit him to hospital.

On Wednesday I prepared for a lecture trip to Scotland while Rosie sat with Ollie. By the afternoon she could bear it no longer and told me, 'Stephen, you must phone the doctor and *insist* that Ollie is admitted to hospital.' The hospital agreed to have him and at dusk I wrapped him in blankets and carried his skeletal body down to the car. Rosie set off with overnight things, leaving me in charge of Edmond.

Early on the Thursday I left Edmond with Andy and Jo, so that I could fly up to Aberdeen to give my lecture at the university to an enthusiastic group of students, who endeared themselves particularly to me by buying lots of my books. For an hour and a half I lost myself in projecting memories of the Himalaya, concluding with our epic retreat from Everest. Simon Richardson, an old Oxford friend living in Aberdeen, was putting me up for the night and the plan was to climb with him the next day, on the way to a second lecture in Glencoe. He was waiting at the back of the lecture theatre. 'That was good,' he said as we left the building. Then as we got into his car he announced, 'Rosie phoned. You've got to go back to Bath. There's a flight first thing in the morning and I've cancelled your Glencoe lecture. She said could you phone her when you get back to our house.'

We arrived twenty minutes later. I said a quick hello to Christine, then Simon took me upstairs to a telephone where I could talk in private, and gave me the hospital number. A nurse answered and went to fetch Rosie. She came to the phone almost immediately and said very calmly, very gently, 'Hello darling. I'm afraid that Ollie has leukaemia.'

Chapter Five

So Ollie was going to die. Like Lizzie. Like Ali MacGraw in *Love Story* – luminously healthy playing her violin in the Christmas concert, by spring whispering her wan adieu from a hospital bed. That was the plot with leukaemia: you died.

I tried to cry that night but no tears came – just a surprised sense of unreality. The same surreal disbelief transformed perception on the pre-dawn flight from Aberdeen. Didn't all these purposeful dark-suited businessmen realise what a momentous event had taken over my life? And now, an hour later, how can I be standing so mundanely at the Heathrow luggage carousel, waiting for that sack full of climbing trivia, while my son lies dying? I wanted desperately to see him and Rosie, but I still had three counties to cross. From Reading station I phoned the children's ward at Bath and a friendly voice answered. 'Hello. I am the consultant oncologist here. Ollie and your wife have just left for Bristol, so you need to go the Children's Hospital there. Ask for Oncology Daybeds.'

Children's Hospital. Those two words seemed so redolent, so self-consciously heavy with melodrama, as I announced them to the taxi driver at Temple Meads station. Ten minutes later he put me down on St Michael's Hill and there it was – three storeys of imposing, gabled Victorian Gothic, fashioned stolidly from Bristol's austere red-grey limestone.

Oncology Daybeds was a reassuringly modern annexe

at the side, all crisp lines, matt paint and pale beech furnishings. Rosie hugged me and took me into a darkened room where Ollie lay attached to drips. He whimpered and Rosie reassured him, 'It's all right, darling, we're not going to do anything.' I stroked his frail, vulnerable body, then we left him in peace and returned to the bright waiting room.

'They can *treat* him, you know,' Rosie said.

'So he might not die?'

'Yes – they can make him better. Apparently most of the children survive.'

So this *wasn't Love Story*! No harrowing deathbed scene – or *probably* not: at the very worst that was deferred to some distant date. Rosie went on to tell me what a relief it had been to get Ollie into the children's ward at Bath two days earlier. 'There was a very nice woman on duty who took one look at Ollie and said, "This child is desperately ill – we must find out what's wrong with him." At *last* someone was taking me seriously and *doing* something.' Ollie had been too weak to register fear at the bright lights and strange faces, or to resist the battery of tests to which he was subjected. The CT scan showed no visible brain abnormality, but microscopic analysis of his blood samples revealed a catastrophic invasion of rogue cells corrupting the whole vascular system to a point where the oxygen carrier haemoglobin was reduced from a normal healthy count of between 11 and 14 to just 3.2. Ollie really had been on the brink of death.

Now, here at the regional oncology centre in Bristol, he had to have further tests before starting treatment, as the registrar, Helen Kershaw, explained. She was calm, polite and articulate and had that rare ability to reduce complex science to its essence, explaining the essentials to the patient (or parent) without ever patronising; she knew how to sound optimistic without resorting to hearty bonhomie; most important of all, she exuded an air of total competence. Ollie, she explained, almost certainly had the commonest form of childhood leukaemia – acute lymphoblastic leukaemia, for which the prognosis was good: about 70 per cent of children pulled through. She now had to collect bone-marrow samples to confirm the diagnosis and determine which subgroup of the disease Ollie had, which would determine the exact protocol for his treatment. She also had to do a lumbar puncture to extract cerebro-spinal fluid and check that no leukaemic cells had infiltrated the central nervous system. Treatment would start almost immediately and for the next week or two Ollie would stay here, in Bristol. Afterwards treatment would continue at the Royal United Hospital in Bath.

Later that afternoon I returned to Larkhall to collect Edmond from Andy and Jo and take him home. I still felt dazed, not quite believing, as I told people the news, that Ollie really did have leukaemia. Only gradually, lagging several steps behind Rosie, did I begin to learn how the disease worked.

Central to understanding leukaemia was grasping the nature of blood itself. The normal healthy blood cells which sluice through the body – cleaning, oxygenating, fighting infection, repairing wounds, servicing the whole unimaginably complex machine – are replenished constantly, generated by the million in the bone marrow. These cells develop through several immature stages before becoming fully functional. In the various forms of leukaemia it is the precursors – in particular immature pale leukocytes (from the Greek *leuco*, white) – which wreak havoc by dividing clonally, proliferating in the bone marrow and crowding out normal mature cells to a point where the blood ceases to function properly.

In the case of Ollie's specific disease, acute lymphoblastic leukaemia, Mosby's medical dictionary states that it is 'a progressive, malignant disease of the blood-forming tissues that is characterised by the uncontrolled proliferation of immature leukocytes and their precursors, particularly in the bone marrow, spleen and lymph nodes.' *The Oxford Medical Dictionary* defines it as 'The clonal proliferation of immature lymphoid precursors. The characteristic cell is the lymphoblast.' A 'blast' is a type of primitive, immature blood cell.

Returning to Mosby, the following initial symptoms are listed: fever, pallor, fatigue, anorexia, secondary infections (usually of the throat, mouth or lungs), bone, joint and abdominal pain, subdermal or submucosal haemorrhage, and enlargement of the spleen, liver and lymph nodes. Ollie had shown many of these symptoms and it seemed incredible that they had rung no alarm bells, until we realised that in an average year only about four hundred and fifty children in Britain get leukaemia. Many GPs never see a single case in a whole career; few see more than one or two. With Ollie, autism may have compounded the problem, influencing the doctors subliminally to ascribe his lethargy and anorexia to some vague behavioural complication.

The precise cause of leukaemia remains a mystery. Rosie wondered for a while whether electromagnetic fields from a perpetually humming supermarket freezer unit, parked outside our temporary house the previous autumn, might have induced the cancer. But the latest global epidemiological study, of which Ollie was a part, has ruled out electromagnetic causes and concluded that one in twenty children are born with a genetic defect which makes them vulnerable. However, only one in two thousand actually develop leukaemia and, in an attempt to find the trigger mechanism, Sir Walter

Bodmer, chairman of the Leukaemia Research Fund's Medical and Scientific Advisory Panel, suggests, 'The most plausible explanation now seems to be a challenge to the child's immune system, quite possibly involving common infections, which cause cancerous cells to emerge. How such a challenge triggers leukaemia remains a puzzle to be solved.' All of which fits Ollie's history of a deteriorating immune system.

When Ollie's diagnosis did finally arrive, at the eleventh hour, it was almost a relief to be dealing with something so much more specific than the ambiguities of autism. Here was an immediately identifiable micro-biological phenomenon, as Mosby's dictionary describes: 'Peripheral blood smear reveals many immature leuko-cytes. The diagnosis is confirmed by bone marrow aspir-ation or biopsy and examination, which show a highly elevated number of lymphoblasts, with almost complete absence of erythrocytes, granulocytes and megakary-ocytes.'

Erythrocytes (Greek *erythros*, red + *kytos*, cell) contain the oxygen-transporter haemoglobin, megakaryocytes are cells that form platelets, essential for blood clotting. Granulocytes include the vital neutrophils, the white blood cells (not to be confused with immature leuko-cytes) which remove cellular debris and destroy bacteria; they are the disease fighters in whose absence even common infections become deadly. The mysterious bruises on Ollie's legs were a sign of low platelets; his deathly pallor was caused by catastrophic depletion of red cells; luckily no chest infection had exploited the dearth of white cells. As for the pain in his legs, the tibia and femur – the biggest bones in the body – house the body's main concentration of blood-producing marrow, and it was here that the corrupt cells had proliferated, swelling in the marrow cavity, pressing against the bone walls.

Until the early Sixties, diagnosis of acute lymphoblastic leukaemia was a virtual death sentence. Then developments in multi-agent chemotherapy began to cure children with the disease. However, 95 per cent of them subsequently relapsed and died when the leukaemia infiltrated their central nervous systems. Then in 1965 it was discovered that cranial radiotherapy dramatically improved the survival rate to about 50 per cent, but at the cost of damaging the brains of these very young children. By 1996, through a still evolving process of trial and error, chemotherapy drugs had improved to the point where about 70 per cent of children made a complete recovery, most of them without recourse to damaging radiation.

The prognosis is less good for acute myeloid leukaemia; nevertheless, treatment of childhood leukaemia is one of the great post-war medical success stories (the survival rate for ALL has now increased to over 80 per cent). As with most cancers, the mainstay of treatment is a cocktail of different cytotoxic drugs – chemotherapy – designed to destroy the rogue cells. Because with leukaemia it is corrupt *blood* cells which are targeted, most of the good blood cells are also destroyed and they have often to be replaced with transfusions.

All this was explained at a meeting with our consultant, Professor Tony Oakhill. He was very tall, with dark hair swept across a high brow, an engaging smile and an air of ease – ease with himself and ease with his patients. He clearly loved his work. He enjoyed being at the cutting edge, hypothesising, testing, refining, steadily improving the children's survival chances and the quality of that survival, here at one of the top research centres in the country. He explained about the three main treatment phases: first Remission Induction

– a ruthless eradication of all leukaemic cells in the blood system, which takes about four weeks; then a second campaign, fought in the spinal fluid, just in case any undetected traces of leukaemia should have penetrated – or be trying to penetrate – the central nervous system and get into the brain; finally Maintenance Therapy – a sustained campaign of aggressive defence, repeatedly zapping the vascular system to mop up any lingering traces of disease.

Tony – after asking permission he used our first names from the start – showed us the provisional charts he had drawn up for Ollie, with the different phases blocked out. He was relaxed and friendly, but without attempting to trivialise the seriousness of the situation. And, right from the start, having managed to track down only one other autistic child with leukaemia – in Utah – he made special allowance for Ollie's unique problems. He had read carefully the case notes made by Helen Kershaw, had noted the late onset of autism which he attributed to 'an insult' to the system. He then said that, in view of Ollie's particular neurological problems, he was recommending a less aggressive form of the second phase – the assault on the central nervous system. Cranial and spinal irradiation were nowadays only used if leukaemic cells were actually detected in the cerebral fluid. However, most children *were* routinely given intrathecal injections – injections into the spinal fluid – of one of the mainstay drugs, methotrexate; in Ollie's case, he thought it best, apart from two initial doses, to avoid this.

Ollie would, however, receive all the standard oral and intravenous drugs. For intravenous treatment, to avoid repeated pricking of arm and hand veins, most children have a 'wiggly line' attached permanently to a vein in their chest. A tap at the end of this line gives instant access for administering drugs and transfusions, and for taking frequent blood samples to check cell counts. Ollie would never tolerate a wiggly line: he would just rip it out. But there was a brilliant invention which could get us round this problem. The portacath is a kind of blood reservoir – a tiny hollow disc, the port, about one centimetre in diameter, connected to a plastic tube, the catheter, which is grafted into a vein beneath the collarbone. The disc is embedded in the chest with its top surface – a soft membrane – sitting immediately beneath the skin. Every time you need to access the disc reservoir – and the subclavian vein to which it is connected – you press a short needle directly through the skin and the membrane beneath. Although the skin has to be pierced, this direct access to the reservoir is much less painful than repeated pricking of vein walls. Once a particular treatment is finished, the needle is removed, the pinprick seals shut and the portacath remains safe, sewn in place beneath the skin.

In Ollie's case, a special numbing cream, lidocaine, was applied to the site before each treatment, to minimise the pain of needle pricking skin. But for the first few days, until he had gone into the operating theatre to have his portacath inserted, Ollie had to face the repeated trauma of needles piercing hands and arms. And a whole baffling new world of strange faces, bright lights, noisy machinery, crying children, chemical smells. And the endless procession of people in blue uniforms and white coats crowding around his bed.

On the Sunday night, the day after I returned from Scotland, he was moved up to the main oncology ward in the old Victorian building. There was, thank goodness, a spare cubicle available, where curtained windows created a bit of a haven. Rosie thought that this haven should be sacrosanct and that, amongst all the strange,

prodding, pricking, manipulating people, Ollie should at
least be able to trust his parents. So the sister agreed to
take him out to the treatment room for any unpleasant
procedure like inserting a cannula.

That night Rosie returned to Larkhall to be with our
neglected second son. I stayed in the cubicle to watch
over Ollie. I longed to sleep, but he remained resolutely
awake, lying in the semi-darkness, plugged into his trans-
fusion line. He was still terribly weak and would soon
become even weaker as the corrosive drugs coursed
through his veins. Apart from sitting up occasionally to
use his pee bottle, he lay quite still, dummy in his mouth,
thumb and second finger stroking endlessly a folded
corner of his snuggly. Incipient tears pricked my eyes. I
longed to fold his frail body protectively in my arms,
but knew that he would hate that. So I sat slightly apart
and eventually switched on the television.

They were showing a documentary about the family
of Alison Hargreaves, the mountaineer who had died on
K2 the previous August. I remembered the shock of the
early morning radio announcement – five people dead
near the summit, one of them British. Later that day
they had confirmed that it was Alison. I had visualised
the exhausted, gasping euphoria of the summit; the cruel
fury of the storm as they tried to descend too late, in
the dark; the harsh cold, rasping on parched throats and
gluing eyelids shut; the grey, iron-hard ice; the malevolent battering of the wind; and then the terrible violence
of sliding, bouncing, crashing through the darkness. Now
her widowed husband was taking the two children to
Pakistan, to those harsh, bright, austerely beautiful
Karakoram mountains where their mother had died.

I remembered the last time I had climbed with Alison.
I knew the exact date, 22nd November 1990, because it
was the day Margaret Thatcher resigned. I met Alison at

her home in Derbyshire. She was pregnant with her second child; the first, Tom, aged two, was playing with her in the kitchen. She seemed utterly content and it was clear that climbing took second place to her children. And yet she had a passion – a compulsion – which could not be ignored. And now the two children were motherless, Tom filled with sullen, silent loss, the younger Kate pointing cheerfully at a cloud above K2 and asking, 'Is that Mummy?' I grieved for the children, and for Alison's parents, and thanked fate for sparing me on Panch Chuli, and, for the time being at least, sparing Ollie, now at last sleeping peacefully beside me in the darkened ward.

For two weeks Ollie stayed in Bristol. He was taken down to the operating theatre to have his portacath fitted. A couple of days later, for the first time, we smeared a blob of the magic lidocaine cream onto the bump on his chest. Then told him how brave he was, as a nurse held the bump between finger and thumb of her left hand, and with her right hand pressed the short needle through the skin, then taped down its plastic butterfly wings to hold it in flat against his chest, then stuck a syringe into its attached tube junction and pulled back the plunger to draw out a testing column of crimson blood; then pushed in another loaded syringe to squeeze colourless Heparin flush into the portacath, ensuring that no tiny clots clogged this vital access to his vascular network.

Through this access port corrosive chemicals were pumped into his blood: cytosine arabinase, cyclophosphamide, etoposide and vincristine. This last drug, vincristine, is particularly corrosive and fatal if administered in any other way than intravenously. It derives from an alkaloid found in the Madagascar periwinkle, *Vinca rosea* (now reclassified as *Carantheus roseus* by those infu-riating botanical taxonomists), and inhibits cell division by binding to tubulin, preventing a cell from making the spindles it needs to move its chromosomes around as it divides. But as well as intravenous drugs, there were oral medicines – pills we had to crush and mix with fruit juice, then syringe into Ollie's mouth – thiogua-nine, oral methotrexate, mercaptapurine . . . Possible side effects from this cocktail included bone ache, loss of deep tendon reflexes, abdominal bloating, head-ache, fatigue, constipation, thirst, irritation of mucous linings and alopecia – loss of hair. And there was the corticosteroid, prednisolone, taken between cycles of chemotherapy to boost recovery, but in the process causing drastic facial bloating, swollen eyelids, headaches, ravenous appetite, hyperactivity and sleeplessness. And then there were the regular monitoring lumbar punc-tures, when the sudden change of pressure in the spinal fluid could cause painful headaches.

For these lumbar punctures Ollie had to be perfectly still while the hollow needle was inserted into the small of his back. At first he was sedated with a drug called ketamine, which merely put him into a brief trance. But on the third occasion it induced a fit; the doctor decided that ketamine was too risky and for all subsequent lumbar punctures Ollie had to have a full anaesthetic. So once a month he had to be deprived of food and drink, sedated with a pre-med drug and then wheeled into theatre, where I would play one of his soothing music tapes, stroke his head, then cradle its sudden sinking weight as the thick white anaesthetising juice was squeezed into his porta-cath. Then quickly I left him to the experts, returning later to the recovery room when he emerged groggily from unconsciousness.

For the first two weeks of treatment Ollie stayed in Bristol. Some nights, after tucking him up in his hospital bed, Rosie, Edmond and I would walk through the dark streets to the family house provided by the wonderful charity CLIC – Cancer and Leukaemia in Children. Later Ollie moved to the John Apley ward, the children's unit at the Royal United Hospital in Bath, where special CLIC units – Portakabins bolted onto the side of the building – provided basic family accommodation and a degree of isolation for the child so vulnerable to infection. Time after time, as good cells are zapped along with the cancerous ones, the chemotherapy patient becomes 'neutropenic': the neutrophils are so depleted that the body has no defence against common infections. So we had to syringe nystatin into Ollie's mouth to check ulcers, and Difflam (benzadamine hydrocholoride) to numb soreness. And when a 'neutropenic fever' took hold and his temperature rose above 38 degrees, he had to be put on the first line of antibiotic defence, with two further lines in reserve, should the first fail to check the fever.

All this Ollie had to endure without – as far as we could tell – a clear intellectual understanding of why it was being done to him, and without the speech to tell us how he was feeling. Photos from those early days of treatment show him sitting in the CLIC unit family room, with huge, dark eyes staring sadly from deep sockets, surrounding skin translucently pale – fragile porcelain beside Edmond's robust, ruddy, stoneware vitality. Every evening the two boys would watch *Rupert and the Frog Song* on the CLIC video player, so that the surreal kitsch of Paul McCartney's croaking operatic chorus remains indelibly associated with the rituals of chemotherapy.

Sometimes we would all eat in the CLIC unit. Then Rosie would settle Ollie into his hospital bed, say his prayers, kiss him goodnight and take Edmond home, leaving me on standby. Some nights I sat for ages beside Ollie, longing to escape to bed, or at least go and read a book. On one occasion I tried surreptitiously reading while I sat with him, but when I moved my hand to turn the page, Ollie whimpered bossily, his thin, weak arm held out to gesticulate – 'Don't move. Stay exactly as you are.' Stress and biochemical turmoil were intensifying his autism, so that the slightest change could be deeply upsetting. Resigned to a long wait, I sat utterly still, willing him to sleep, longing to end this enforced game of statues.

Not all our days were spent in hospital. Once the initial induction phase was over, Ollie spent most of his time at home, on daily oral medication. Blood samples could also be taken at home: one of the two specialist CLIC nurses, Eileen or Ali, would come every few days and wait patiently while we coaxed Ollie onto a kitchen chair, persuaded him to remove his shirt, wiped off the pre-placed lidocaine cream, and held his hand while the nurse felt his chest for the exact centre of the porta-cath. His face would pucker anxiously, then soften into a surprised, proud smile as the needle sank home, the blood flowed up into the syringe and we all chorused, 'Well done, you brave boy!'

Life returned to some kind of normality. I achieved sporadic bursts of work in the office space I rented in town. Or stayed at home Ollie-proofing the house. Now that he was more energetic again, we had to thwart his exploratory urges and compulsion to test every object to destruction. Bolts had to be fitted high on every door, staircases made safe, lockable gates hung between each of our four storeys, so that Ollie could be contained in one area at any given time.

Chemotherapy was working its magic and the cancer was in remission. But 'remission' was a relative term. In

1996 blood samples were still being assessed with traditional light microscopes, which could only detect an infestation of more than 5 per cent of cancerous cells. In other words, a child's blood could still be harbouring up to five billion cancerous cells, yet be pronounced in remission. Hence the need to maintain the relentless chemo bombardment for two or three years.

Since Ollie's treatment that blunt attack has been refined. Now, using molecular DNA techniques, it is possible to detect one rogue cell per 10,000, making the monitoring of 'minimal residual disease' infinitely more precise, allowing oncologists to vary the aggressiveness of each child's treatment according to individual risk. In Ollie's day it was still a case of blanket bombardment, with frequent visits to the John Apley ward for regular intravenous infusions, or for emergency care every time a neutropenic fever flared up. In hospital, as at home, he needed constant one-to-one care. We still had Siri and one or two of the Lovaas teachers to help out. But for much of the time Rosie or I had to be there. And things occasionally went wrong. On one occasion corrosive chemotherapy fluid spilt and burned Ollie's skin. Sometimes an inexperienced nurse would lose patience and rush to insert his portacath needle, holding him down and terrifying him.

Anxious and traumatised, he started again to smear faeces, on one occasion filthying his bed four times in one night. Timetables were not adhered to. Cover did not always materialise when promised, so that Rosie or I had to rush in at short notice to look after Ollie. His gluten- and dairy-free meals did not always turn up, or they were so late that Edmond was kept at the hospital, waiting up long past his bedtime. Things came to a head one morning when a doctor was trying to access Ollie's portacath for a blood sample. Ollie was terrified and

Rosie insisted that the doctor would just have to wait, all day if necessary, until Ollie consented. At which point the exasperated physician snapped, 'We can't have the whole National Health Service revolving around your son.'

We asked for a meeting with all the senior doctors and nurses on the ward. As usual on these occasions Rosie insisted that, in the male-dominated hierarchy of the NHS, I should do the talking, briefed thoroughly by her. So I arrived at the meeting with several pages of notes and put our case – or rather Ollie's case – as forcefully as possible. Right at the start, in Bristol, we had discussed with Tony Oakhill the philosophical question of whether it was actually right – whether it was ethical – to treat Ollie. We felt that, despite all the difficulties autism had created for him, Ollie had an enormous capacity for joy and that, given the good odds on success, we should try to save his life, even if that meant subjecting him to frightening treatment. But we should try to avoid any unnecessary stress. And people had to realise that Ollie was not just another leukaemia case: he had unique special needs, and Rosie knew better than anyone else in the world how to meet those needs.

I stressed that the hospital also had to consider the needs of the whole family. Rosie had to have time with Edmond; I had somehow to earn some money; the hospital would have to provide more cover to make those things possible. Then, returning to the most impor-tant issue, how to minimise the trauma of treatment for Ollie, I handed out our set of guidelines for approaching him:

1.   No grabbing and forcing.
2.   Maximum of two people in the room.

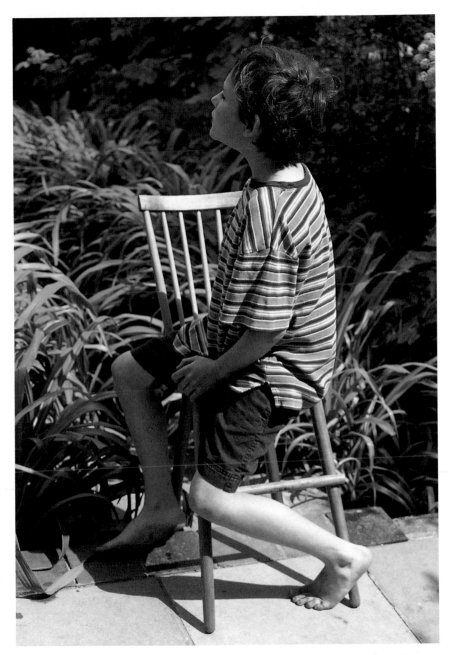

A special Ollie moment – balanced with exquisite precision on a tilted chair, lost happily in a private world of wonder. Summer 2001.
(*This and all uncredited photos © Stephen Venables*)

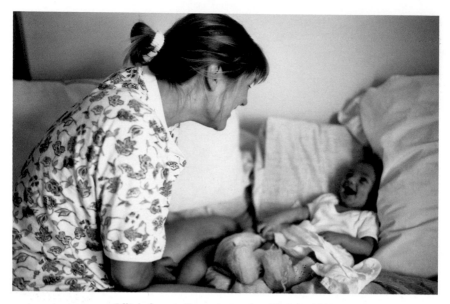

Ollie's first smile at six weeks old, July 1991.

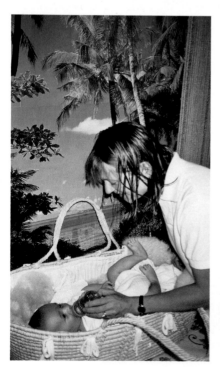

A few weeks later, enjoying breakfast in an exotically decorated Chartres café. Rosie has just washed out the grime from our night in a fleapit hotel.

The hardest wrench of the Panch Chuli expedition was missing Ollie's first birthday.

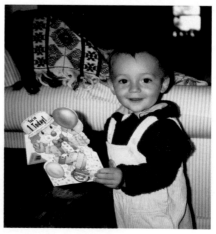

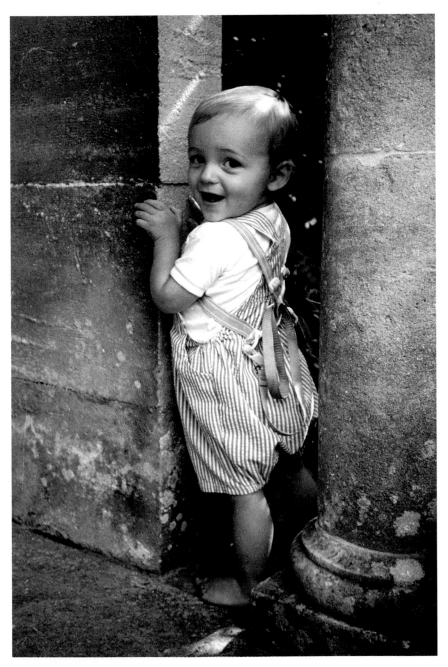

August 1992. I am still on crutches, recovering from the Panch Chuli accident. Ollie has just learned to run and is about to escape.

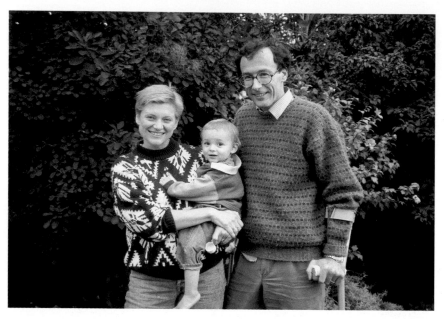

August 1992.
Fresh out of hospital, in my parents' garden with Rosie and Ollie. (© *Ed Webster*)

Christmas 1992.
The Elephant and the Bad Baby.

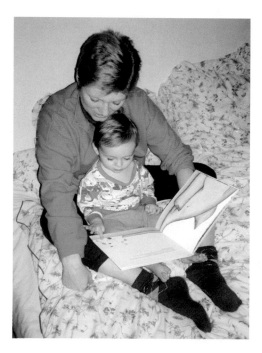

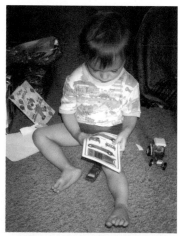

June 1993. Ollie's second birthday, one month after the birth of his brother Edmond.

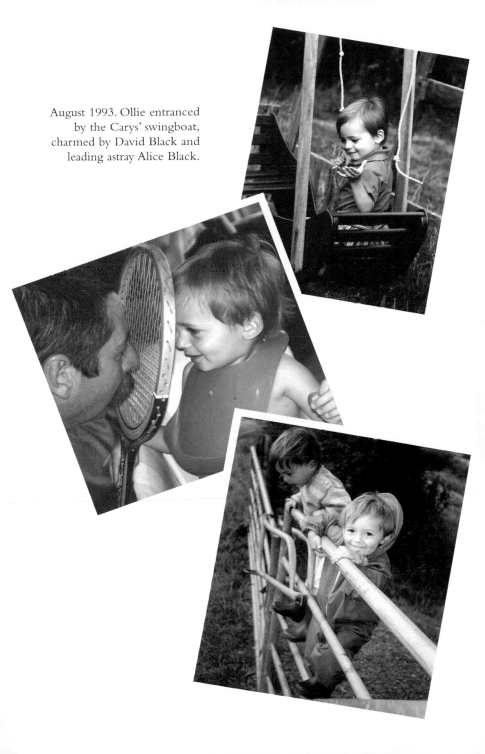

August 1993. Ollie entranced by the Carys' swingboat, charmed by David Black and leading astray Alice Black.

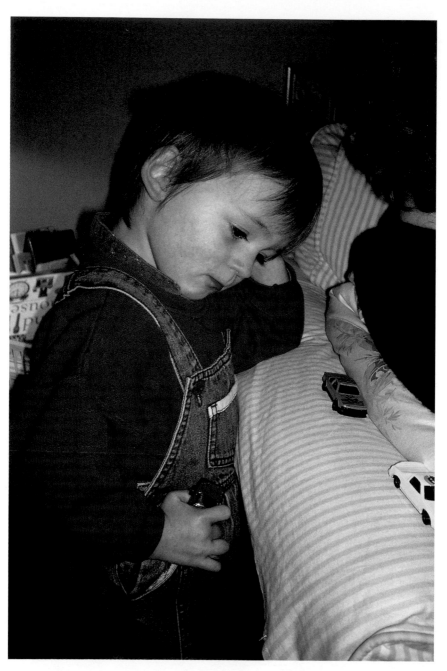

January 1994.
A new, withdrawn, anguished, autistic Ollie endlessly lining up his toy cars.

Already in 1993
Ollie had begun to
take refuge behind his
dummy and 'snuggly'.

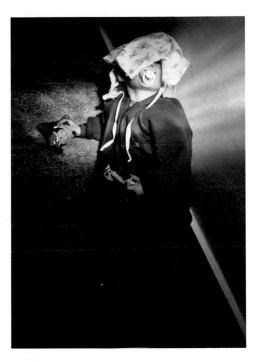

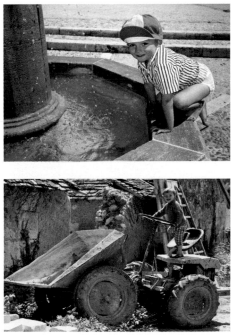

Dordogne. June 1994. Our last
proper family holiday for five years.
Despite the autism, the authentic
mischievous Ollie shines through,
escaping into a Bergerac fountain,
picnicking with Alice Black and
commandeering a dumper truck
on his third birthday.

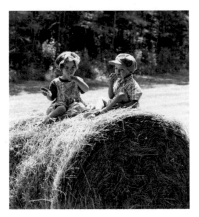

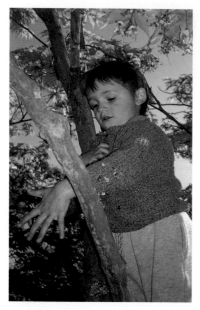

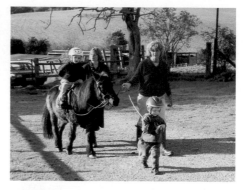

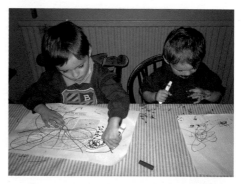

Summer 1995.
Ollie climbing in the Botanic
Gardens, riding with Granny
and drawing with Edmond.

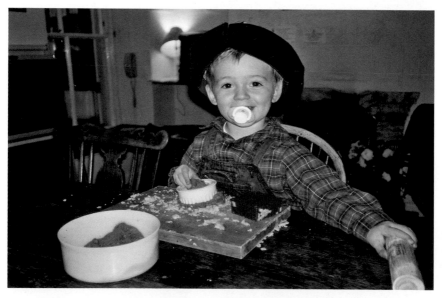

Ollie loved hats. I bought this Turkestani one in Gilgit. October 1993.

3. Make sure you have everything you need before you start.
4. Be calm and confident.
5. Be patient.
6. Be persistent. Be prepared to stop and try again. And again. And again.
7. No jabbering.
8. Don't try to fool Ollie or divert him: explain clearly and with signs what you want to do.
9. Ask his permission. Say 'please'.
10. Have lots of time available – and you will find you take a lot less.

Yes – we were the original Parents From Hell. Arrogant, perhaps, to demand so much from the beleaguered, attenuated National Health Service. Selfish to expect such special treatment for our son. But there was a history behind our bolshiness – the mismanagement of Ollie's birth, my unnoticed post-operative wound infection, the tardiness in acknowledging Ollie's autism, the almost fatal delay in diagnosing leukaemia – which made us determined that this time we should assert ourselves and champion Ollie's cause. We also felt that this lumbering, bureaucratic leviathan of a health service, with its impossibly ambitious promise of universal free healthcare, had to adapt, however inconvenient that might be, to the unique requirements of a very unusual child. And as his parents knew best what that child needed, it had to listen to those parents.

Perhaps it was unrealistic to expect from an over-stretched general paediatric ward the same expert care as in the specialist oncology centre in Bristol. Nevertheless, things did improve in Bath after our meeting. Ollie settled into the six-weekly cycle of maintenance therapy, and by April it was possible for me to

fly to South Africa for twelve days to earn some much-
needed lecture fees and replenish my dwindling reservoir of saleable mountain experience. Once again Paul
Fatti gave his time generously, taking me up one of his
remotest rock climbs, high on the basalt escarpment of
the Drakensberg – the Zulus' 'Barrier of Spears'. Then
I flew over to Cape Town to marvel again at its immense
sandstone cliffs, stay with old family friends, the Mills,
dash round the incomparable Kirstenbosch Gardens,
then hurry 8,000 miles home to Larkhall with a huge
bunch of proteas for Rosie, arriving on Saturday, 4th
May. The next morning I got out the video camera to
record Edmond's third birthday.

Morning sunlight pours in from the east-facing
garden as he sits happily on the little trampoline in the
kitchen, bent over a book, talking himself through *The
Tailor of Gloucester* . . . then gets up to paint at his easel,
periodically tasting the paint. Sibelius's violin concerto
plays on the radio. Ollie sits at the table, eating a gluten-
free pancake and making contented noises – 'Nyeh . . .
nyah'. Chemotherapy has reduced his hair to a thin skim
of grey fuzz. Rosie comes down and reads Edmond his
birthday book from godmother Joanna Cary. Later she
and Lucius come for lunch with their four children,
who help Edmond assemble the plastic sections of a toy
canal, from which Ollie will later meticulously remove
all the rubber seals.

Another May morning and Edmond and I are in the
train, setting off for the Bristol Sea Fair. Edmond provides
a piping commentary as we pull out of Bath station: 'Train
going now . . . all the leafs coming out of the trees now
. . . tunnel! . . . Out of the tunnel now . . . crane!' Suddenly
Ollie's wordless existence seems painfully diminished.

But a week later it is *his* birthday and regrets are
banished. My mother and I, Rosie, Edmond and Emma

Bird – one of Ollie's Lovaas teachers who lives in a barge on the canal and remains one of our most generous helpers – sit round the kitchen table. Lemon icing oozes down the side of the cake. Four candles stand on top; the fifth is being chewed by Ollie, now completely bald, sitting serenely at the head of the table. Rosie takes the chewed wax stump, adds it to the cake and quickly lights all five candles. As we start to sing 'Happy Birthday' Ollie laughs, gets up and runs out to the garden. So Edmond deputises, leaning forward from his plastic booster chair and blowing out the candles.

Another weekend. Another morning of sunny domesticity. Edmond crouches on the floor chattering bossily to his plastic minibeasts. Ollie sits at the table in stripy pyjama top, head golden smooth, eyes lost in concentration as he dips crisps in tomato ketchup. Then the ketchup is finished and he gesticulates with an open hand, 'Njah, njah, aiee!'

'Ollie – Ollie, look at me – say "please". Say "*please*".'

He gestures again with bent wrist. Then reluctantly looks up and makes eye contact, face muscles working overtime to produce a 'bheez' sound, surreptitious smile stealing from the corner of his mouth as he stretches out a hand to receive the rewarding ketchup bottle. Later, hunger satisfied, he gets down and stands at the easel, takes the brush in his left hand and adds big broad strokes of yellow and green to Edmond's painting. Then he runs laughing into the garden and Edmond takes his turn at the easel, adding a big red circle and explaining, 'It's a O for Ollie.'

Evening, and Edmond has gone to bed. Ollie, the older brother, stays up. Our old neighbours from Larkhall Terrace, Richard and Sue, have come round to see the new house. Dark gaps show between the floorboards. Woodchip wallpaper has been steamed off to reveal a crumbly hundred-year-old plaster patina. Ollie is in pyjamas, sitting on the sofa between Richard and Sue, quietly dipping crisps in some kind of dairy-free mixture. Then Richard hands him a crisp. Ollie holds it in the fingertips of both hands, studying shape and texture, sensing its sharp crinkly edge. Then he picks another crisp out of the bowl and hands it silently to Richard.

Richard almost died five years ago, when his GP dismissed complaints of chronic headaches and failing circulation, telling him cheerily just to 'let this lovely lady look after you at home.' Six hours later he was rushed unconscious to hospital with meningitis. Sue had to wait a fortnight before Richard emerged from his coma, profoundly deaf and disabled. Now, after five years nursing an invalid, she knows all the potential support systems and tells us about the St John's Hospital – a local charitable foundation which helped pay for alterations to her house. Perhaps they would help us too? We just need to present them with a one-off, practical, vital project which requires funding.

We *did* have a project. The garden. Our long narrow strip ran straight down to the Lambrook and it had still not been Ollie-proofed. It needed to be enclosed completely by seven-foot-high fencing. Solid weather-boarding would be too claustrophobic; wire chain-link too oppressive. We needed a light, airy framework for climbing plants (including lots of very prickly roses) which would eventually form an impenetrable jungle wall. So we presented the St John's almoner with a budget for willow-hurdle fencing and her committee agreed generously to cover ninety per cent of the cost, along with fitting wooden security bars to all the sash windows in our dangerously tall house.

The hurdles looked elegant – slender willow poles threaded vertically through bands of woven hazel, with the horizontal bands too far apart for Ollie to climb – and the long space they enclosed was now safe. But dull. Rosie's imagination and my hard graft transformed it into a series of terraces, separated by trellis fences (Ollie-proofed with chicken wire) and in one section roofed by pergola slats. Julian Freeman-Attwood, my ever-generous climbing companion from the South Georgia expedition, provided oak planking to edge paths and contain beds; friends of my parents donated immense slabs of Pennant sandstone that had lain in a Bath basement since the eighteenth century. Under Rosie's instruction I heaped excess excavated earth from the terraces into a huge mound. Then, when she said it looked boring, I rebuilt it with a spiral bicycle path leading to its summit – a kind of oval ziggurat. By the autumn the layout was almost complete, paths of rubble hardcore awaiting their top layer of compacted limestone hoggin, and the first shrubs and wispy saplings settling in for the winter.

The garden was now a safe sanctuary for Ollie. And for us. With travel ever more difficult, we could find fulfilment and fantasy in this little green space, with its enclosing backdrop of mature neighbouring trees – the glossy hollies which seeded themselves so happily in the limestone soil, the huge willow whose fur buds appeared like glistening raindrops in March, then softened in April to downy pale yellow; the horse chestnut's sudden rush to leaf in early May, followed quickly by exotic creamy candle flowers looking outrageously oriental beside the hesitant bronze unfurlings of Bruno's huge venerable oak.

We were lucky to be here but life with Ollie was still tricky. Illness and chemotherapy seemed to have unravelled all the progress of the Lovaas home education

programme. We had given up formal lessons and
although one or two of the teachers, such as Emma Bird,
were still helping with respite, we were running out of
funds to pay them. Rosie was exhausted and desperate
for more help. 'Don't worry,' telephoned the head of
CHADS – Child Health and Disability Services – 'the
cavalry's on its way.' This particular relief came in the
form of a local respite centre, where Ollie spent his first
two-hour session on 5th July. Over the summer he
returned several times, occasionally staying overnight,
leaving us free even to go away from Bath. But the separation was always painful and when he returned Ollie
often seemed withdrawn, even traumatised by the
strange, erratic, sometimes violent behaviour of some
very disturbed children and adolescents.

In September, while Rosie tried to coax Edmond out
of nappies in readiness for starting at a nursery class,
Ollie, now at compulsory school age, had his introductory visit to the local primary school unit for autistic
children. A new layer of soft, gorgeously smooth, velvet
hair now covered his head; but he still looked very
fragile, riding a tricycle round the enclosed playground.
For Rosie it was again a terrible wrench, handing this
vulnerable child over to strangers. After all the meticulous one-to-one Lovaas teaching of the previous year,
Ollie was now going to have to adapt to the one-size-
fits-all compromises of institutional education. While we
should have been grateful to the State for his expensive
place at a specialist unit (complete with taxi transport
to and from home), it was hard to relinquish control.

It also felt ironic. Earlier that year I had attended the
inaugural meeting of Peach – Parents for Early intervention with Autistic Children. This is a charity to
support the growing number of parents doing Lovaas
work – Applied Behavioural Analysis – with their autistic

children. Now, in September, I was doing a one-day hundred-mile bike ride, sponsored mainly by generous friends, to raise £4,000 towards setting up a staffed advice centre. Some of the autistic children had done incredibly well with ABA. Despite its apparently mechanistic approach, their speech was blossoming and they were making more sense of other people's baffling behaviour. Some were now moving on to mainstream schools, as we had hoped Ollie might do. But he wasn't. For the moment we had run out of steam, handed over to the nanny state, admitted temporary defeat. For the time being we all had just to survive, to get through the next phase.

So, when he was not feeling too ill, Ollie went to school on the south side of Bath, while Edmond started at nursery class on the north side. Quite often during the autumn term I was away lecturing, on one occasion fitting in a day's winter-climbing on Lochnagar in the Cairngorms, finally enjoying my date with Simon Richardson, postponed from the day Ollie was diagnosed with leukaemia nearly two years earlier. Then I had a few days in New York, as guest of the American Alpine Club. Then I was back home, working again on the house, installing more security bars around the stairs to thwart Ollie's latest leap in climbing standards, and preparing some of the house for long-awaited decoration.

Edmond took part in his first Christmas play, looking as shy and bewildered as all the other three-year-olds lined up on the stage. Ollie's term ended, and he came home with special presents for Mummy and Daddy, managed a hurried 'buh-bye' to the taxi driver and rushed upstairs to lick the paint off the Christmas tree decorations. Late after supper on Christmas Eve Rosie and I collapsed on the kitchen sofa. The BBC was showing a film on Antarctica produced by our friend Martha Holmes. Images of South Georgia brought back memories of our separated Christmas, seven years earlier, when life had seemed so simple and hopeful. Then we watched and listened to the midnight service from Salisbury Cathedral.

It was too much – the sublime early Gothic too painfully beautiful, the carols too suffused with melancholy, the joyful birth too overshadowed by future pain – and tears started to roll down Rosie's cheeks. We looked back a year to the day we had moved into this house, when Ollie had collapsed listlessly in bed, and Rosie sobbed, 'What a terrible year it's been; I wonder what the next one will be like.'

The following day the house burned down.

Chapter Six

No. Exaggeration. The house didn't actually burn *down*. But it was comprehensively torched. After lunch we switched on the Christmas tree lights next to the grand piano in the room at the back of the house. Then lit all four candles of the Advent wreath in the corner of the sitting room, near the bay window at the front of the house, where Rosie's gorgeous interlined crimson damask curtains from Larkhall Terrace were hung sketchily, still waiting to be refitted to the new house. Beneath them sagged an old synthetic sofa – a cast-off from friends – draped in more thick curtain fabric.

We unwrapped some presents until Ollie became agitated by the fragmentation of neatly wrapped parcels into a random jumble of torn paper, ribbons, toy cars, pencils, books, CDs. 'Poor Ollie, it's too much, *isn't* it?' sympathised Rosie, stroking his silky, now wavy, new hair. Then she turned to me. 'Would you take the boys downstairs for a bit, darling, while I go and have an LLD?'

Like Napoleon, Churchill and Thatcher, she had mastered the restorative power nap, and a Little Lie-Down would fortify her against the Christmas flu which had struck traditionally. So she went up to our bedroom directly above the sitting room and I took the boys down to the basement kitchen. I put on the CD Rosie's father, Robin, had given me for Christmas, then started washing up the lunch things. I turned up the CD player to compete with running taps, determined to enjoy the music. Mozart's A major piano concerto. K488. Memories of playing it myself in the summer of 1970. Or trying to. So familiar it was almost hackneyed. Except that that serene, sunny opening could never, ever, pall. To misquote Samuel Johnson, a man who was tired of K488 was tired of life.

There was a bump upstairs and I wondered whether Rosie had come down to fetch something. I carried on scrubbing the roasting pan. Piano and orchestra wove their contrapuntal filigree, boosted electronically to a lush travesty of eighteenth-century intentions. There was another thump from upstairs. Had I upset Rosie? Was the music too loud? A thud reverberated on bare floor-boards. Then another. Then a crash of breaking glass. What the hell was going on? Had some lunatic broken in?

I rushed upstairs and as I swung round into the piano room I saw the dark Christmas tree silhouetted against yellow flames which filled the sitting room completely, crackling and sputtering as they licked greedily up hundred-year-old walls of lath and horsehair plaster. A malevolent carpet of oily black smoke – reconstituted nylon sofa – rolled across the floor towards me. And as I stared despairingly at this hellish chiaroscuro scene, impotently furious at our neglect of the Advent candles, Rosie ran down the stairs towards me, shouting, 'Where are the children?'

'Er –' There was a ghastly heartstab of doubt – where's Ollie? – then I remembered that he was in the garden. As we ran down towards our children, the flames leapt across the gap from the sitting room and the Christmas tree erupted in a resinous crackle. Downstairs, while Rosie dialled 999, I grabbed the garden hose, pulled it through the kitchen and headed back upstairs – an angry

futile gesture defeated immediately by a now impenetrable wall of heat.

'There's nothing you can do,' Rosie shouted, 'we've
got to get out.' Another radiator came adrift upstairs
with a loud crash. Higher up, at the back of the house,
the boiler hissed and fizzed. Rosie took Edmond out
into the garden, where Ollie was on the mound, dancing
obliviously, staring up at the darkening midwinter sky. I
grabbed coats, jackets, shoes – anything I could salvage
before the whole house came tumbling down – and as
I rummaged in the cupboard I heard a shout and saw
Andy, owner of the Larkhall delicatessen, framed in the
doorway at the street end of the kitchen. 'Is anyone
trapped upstairs?'

'No – we're fine. Thank you – we're all in the garden.'
He ran back up the steps to the safety of the street and
a moment later the front bay window burst outward in
a fountain of glass shards and dancing orange flames,
almost singeing the eyebrows of Colin the publican,
standing outside the Rose & Crown on the far side of
the road. At the back of the house, committed now to
our willow-caged garden, we shuffled down to the
brook, Rosie slithering in the only shoes she had been
able to find – a pair of ballet pumps. At the bottom of
the garden we manoeuvred the children through the
gate, along the brook's clay bank and past the bottom
of Jill's garden, then handed them, one at a time, over
the fence into Roger and Rose's garden.

Ollie found himself in a strange house, surrounded by
strange people. But they were sensitive people who
found a quiet room where he could feel secure. Only
now that we were all safe from the blaze did Rosie allow
the shock to take hold, shuddering her body with painful
coughs. 'I think I swallowed some of that smoke,' she
wheezed. 'Thank God the smoke alarm in the boys'

room went off – I was fast asleep. Just a shame that all the other alarms we bought were still sitting in a carrier bag, otherwise I might have woken sooner.' She wheezed painfully, gasping for air, terrified by the first asthma attack of her life. Ollie hardly seemed to notice, but three-and-a-half-year-old Edmond hugged her protectively, then cried when a fireman clamped a yellow mask over his mother's face.

Oxygen calmed Rosie, as the fireman told us that the blaze was now out.

'What – already! That's incredible.'

'Well, the London Road was empty. Best day of the year to have a fire – we got to you in two minutes.'

We were lucky to live so close to the fire station. Another fifteen minutes and the whole house could have been destroyed. As it was, gas, electricity and plumbing were out of action. The ground floor was gutted completely and at the front of the house the flames had begun to pierce the floorboards above, melting nylon straps on the luggage we kept under the bed where Rosie had been sleeping. At the back, the open staircase had acted as a chimney, sucking the heat up two storeys, blowtorching ten decades of layered paint into a blistered carbuncular carapace. But worst was the smoke – the oily grey residue of metamorphosed petrochemicals insinuated comprehensively into every surface.

Number 6, Grosvenor Terrace was now uninhabitable. On Christmas Day. But within an hour of the fire, the people from Number 1, whom we hardly knew, came round to tell us that we could shelter in Bruno's and Shena's house. 'We phoned them in Norway – you know they're spending Christmas with Marius – and they said of course you can use their house.' Ian – I now discovered his name – and his two daughters helped me prepare the house, packing priceless cellos, bows and the whole of Bruno's antique glass collection into a locked room. Then, once the house was reasonably Ollie-proof, we went to fetch him, Edmond and Rosie. We had just settled in and were cooking some supper when the doorbell rang. I opened the door and a woman handed me a bucket full of notes and coins. 'We did a whip-round at the pubs,' she explained, 'so that you can buy some new Christmas presents for the boys.'

On Boxing Day we tried to take Ollie back to our own garden to play. But as soon as we entered the cold, dark, hose-doused basement he faltered, shaking his head. Even without seeing the charred carnage, he could smell the destruction upstairs and refused to go through the kitchen to the garden. Rosie, too, traumatised by swallowing toxic smoke the previous afternoon – so that she never, ever again smoked another cigarette – found the smell intolerable. Even after repeated washings, she declared much of our bedding unusable, could not bear to keep the boys' blackened bunk beds and had to jettison smoke-infused books from upstairs along with the irretrievably charred volumes downstairs.

I was less sensitive about the whole affair. In fact I rather enjoyed this new adventure, as we moved from Bruno's and Shena's house to spend New Year with Jake and Shan in Sussex, then returned to a temporary holiday let in a flat, then settled in a more permanent rented house on the other side of town, which became our home for the nine months it took to sort out the mess in Larkhall. When the insurance money finally began to come through and relieve our various emergency overdrafts, I was thrilled. We had cash to spend! On new books, new duvet covers, new sofas to replace the much-lamented 'frequent use' pink stripes. I had never bought a sofa before! Nor commissioned a new cherrywood fire surround, with carved hellebores to mirror the Victorian fireplace tiles which had miraculously survived the holocaust. Nor found that local joinery firm which could match the remnants of a unique architrave moulding.

Of course there were sad losses, especially the charred books which my mother spent hours inventorying, shivering heroically in the cold, boarded-up piano room. And the irreplaceable photo of Rosie's mother as a young Wren officer. And the poor old piano itself, first heated to God-knows-how-many degrees, then doused by a fireman's hose. But it was in need of a good overhaul, and the tropical birds and flowers Rosie eventually painted on its restored veneerless casing were an exuberant alternative to staid rosewood. Overall, despite the gigantic hassle, we benefited from the purge, and, yet again, we were touched by the generosity of friends and neighbours. We could have put it down to pity – people knew about Ollie's autism and his leukaemia – but it was something more than that: regardless of illness, Ollie always seemed to touch people's innate goodness. Even the loss adjuster, Jenny, felt inspired to stretch the terms of our insurance policy to the full, helping us to build something positive from the ashes of a stupid, careless mistake.

From our temporary mews house on the grand heights of Bathwick Hill, Edmond continued to go each day to his nursery class. Ollie, when well enough, was fetched by taxi and driven to his special unit. But often he stayed at home, watched by me, or Rosie or one of several new helpers. Social Services planned to recruit more helpers and in March made a video to show potential recruits what to expect.

★

Pale blossom jewels the black almond boughs and the Bath stone glows bright and warm. Two women walk along the canal towpath with a little red pushchair. The child in the pushchair is incongruously large – nearly six years old – with knees pushed high, and he has a dummy in his mouth. He wears a blue check lumberjack shirt, baggy trousers, and little leather boots. After the baldness of the previous summer, his hair is now long and luxuriant, with slightly curly pointed sideburns so that he almost looks like a little Orthodox Jewish boy. He has perfect baby teeth, but his face is clouded by a worried half-frown. His mother stops and asks, 'Ollie want to get out?' He shakes his head. 'No?' He rocks forward in go-faster motion. So they continue walking and he leans back in his chair, head lolling slightly with tiredness. But then he looks up at the sky with a glimmer of a smile. Then he rocks from side to side, shooting a sideways smirk at the tall, slender red-headed woman, Loulou, who says, 'That's a nice smile.'

Cut to a small dining room. The table is protected with an oilcloth and another cloth protects the carpeted floor. Rosie and Loulou sit at the table with mugs of tea. Rosie explains to camera, 'We have to remember that chemotherapy can make Ollie feel very ill. It can give him headaches or make him feel sick, or cause diarrhoea. But anyway, regardless of the chemotherapy, the world is a very frightening place for him, because he cannot see or hear properly and he cannot understand the things people are saying and the sequence of events – a bit like us arriving in China with everyone speaking an incomprehensible language and behaving in what seems an odd way. You have to remember that he is doing the best he can, and make the world as safe as possible for him. If you do that he can be very happy.'

There is a joyful shout – 'Oyeeoyee' – from the little

courtyard outside and we cut to Ollie running backwards and forwards, stopping at the end of each lap to
smile and shake his head. Then he gets on his tricycle.
Then off, briefly positioning it and squinting to sight
along the handlebars, before abandoning it for another
running lap of the courtyard, hands out to the side,
fingers splayed. Then he runs up to Loulou, arms
outstretched, and she sweeps him up, spinning him
clockwise, then anticlockwise, gives him a brief hug and
kiss, then puts him down for another run.

Back in the house Loulou qualifies this exchange. 'You
don't usually get the same kind of feedback you get from
an ordinary child, and that can feel rather demoralising
at first, but after a while you get to know what to expect
and to realise that in his way he can be very animated
and communicative.' Rosie chips in to warn that helpers
cannot make their satisfaction contingent on immediate
success with Ollie. 'They have to be able to accept bad
days. I think what I am saying is that we don't want
people with big egos. The people who are most
successful with Ollie are the ones who can stand back
a bit, be confident in themselves and not need to prove
anything.'

Loulou, who has nothing to prove, goes back out to
the garden, where Ollie climbs up, wraps his legs round
her waist and hugs her, then shrieks with delight as she
holds his arms and lowers him backwards, upside down.
He gets down and walks a few circles, holding her hand.
Then he runs over to the far corner of the courtyard
and climbs into the magnolia tree, balancing skilfully,
spreading his weight on thin branches. With one leg he
bridges elegantly across to a stone wall and reaches out
to the chicken-wire fence I have fixed on top of the
wall. He presses and shakes the wire, checking for weak-
nesses. Then he climbs down and continues his circular

tour of the courtyard, stopping briefly to tap his chin with the open palm of his left hand.

Back in the dining room, Rosie adds her instructional gloss: 'It's really important to remember that Ollie can move at the speed of lightning and all he really wants to do is to escape. He has absolutely no sense of danger whatsoever and has had lots of near misses, like falling out of an upstairs window, or dashing in front of cars or eating something he shouldn't. We try to anticipate the dangers so that we can move them before Ollie finds them himself.'

That recruiting video was initiated by Ollie's new social worker, Niki Smith, one of the most astute of the many disability experts brought into our lives by autism. We had discovered that there is a tendency in the world of 'Special Needs' for the professionals, probably unconsciously, to try to take charge, to patronise, to talk down, antagonising someone like Rosie who had grown up in Kenya, in an ethos of pioneering self-sufficiency. Medics, too, would occasionally infuriate with their demotic bonhomie. I winced every time some complete stranger of a nurse or doctor greeted me with a cheery 'Hello – are you Dad?' Rosie – again influenced by the comparative formality of her Kenyan Sixties upbringing – would simply hold out her hand and say, 'Hello – my name's Rosie Venables. And who are you?'

With Niki there was a refreshing lack of chumminess. Which doesn't mean that she was cold or aloof. Simply that she wasn't here to be our friend: she was here to do a job. Her attitude was, 'What can I do to help this boy? Please will you, his parents, tell me what would be most useful and I'll try to make it happen.' Top of the list of useful things was recruiting another carer to work long-term with Ollie.

For three years now, Rosie had been working non-stop, caring, protecting, teaching, inspiring, organising. Unlike me, she had had no restorative escapes. Now, at last, her chance came for a complete break. Her brother Jake, after several years' relentless grind, had turned his travel company into a seriously profitable success and was at last having a holiday himself, taking his wife and daughter to Kenya for a fortnight. He was also taking his father, Robin, who was finding the life of a widower a lonely business. And Rosie. For her it was an opportunity to spend some time with her father, and to escape the low grey skies of the little island she had never really come to terms with, returning briefly to the colour, space and rich scents of her African childhood.

Ever efficient, she drew up a timetable for her absence. Niki had not yet found her new recruit, and Loulou was tied down for the Easter holidays with her own children; but two young assistants from Ollie's special school unit agreed to do some holiday shifts, helping out Andy, Jo and Emma Bird, giving me some time to research and write an overdue *Telegraph* article. For Edmond's benefit (and perhaps Ollie's – it was hard to tell) I made a big wall chart, with a numbered square for each day of their mother's absence, and in each square a picture of a giraffe, or a lion, or a palm-fringed beach, or a photo of Rosie, or Uncle Jake, or Grandpop, reclining serenely in a big sun hat with gin and tonic in hand.

We saw her off at Bath station on a Saturday afternoon. On the Sunday, the day she and her family were flying to Africa, Ollie developed a temperature. By nine in the evening it had risen to 37.8° centigrade. I phoned the John Apley ward and they reminded me of the usual procedure. 'It sounds like a neutropenic fever. Keep checking his temperature and if it gets to 38 you'd better bring him in.'

At ten o'clock the thermometer hit the danger mark and I phoned Di and Ken, a South African couple who had a son in Edmond's class and who were always prepared to help with the latest Venables crisis. I smudged a large blob of lidocaine cream on Ollie's portacath site, securing it with a self-adhesive wound dressing; then packed emergency things (cassette machine, tapes, spare dummies, snuggly, wet-wipes, clothes, drinks), school clothes for Emond and overnight things for myself; then strapped the two boys into their car seats and drove round to Di and Ken. Rosie had only been gone a day, and as I settled Edmond into the strange bunk bed, his face crumpled with tears. I promised to be back in the morning and hurried on to the hospital.

'Hello, Ollie,' breezed the duty nurse cheerfully. Poor man – it was completely well intentioned, but disastrous. In the treatment room, attempting to secure a needle in Ollie's portacath site, he kept up a hearty banter, antag-onising Ollie to the point where he refused to have anything done. We decided to leave it for half an hour and retreated to a cubicle. Then I had to reapply lido-caine to the no longer numb portacath site. We returned to the treatment room. More noisy chat. More flinching, crying and head-shaking from Ollie. In the end, hating myself for doing it, I had to restrain him while the nurse finally pushed the needle home, and syringed out the samples needed for a full blood count.

By the time he finally got to bed Ollie was very distraught. I just longed for sleep. Before pulling out the parent's folding bed, I checked the windows of the ground-floor cubicle. The bottom one was locked. There was also a small upper window which was unlocked, but which seemed too small and too high for even Ollie to bother with. Harrowed by excess emotion, I sank heavily towards sleep, hardly aware of Ollie's restlessness on the bed beside me. I only registered dimly the metallic noise as he tested the lower window and then thought, 'Ah, good – he's settling down.' In the last moments of consciousness I held a brief, warm image of Rosie, happy in her aeroplane seat, somewhere over the Mediterranean, then slipped into the seductive embrace of sleep. I was woken perhaps an hour later by fresh night air on my face. 'Yes, it *was* hot – he's opened the top window,' I reasoned blithely as I turned over to go back to sleep. Then some dormant instinct finally pricked my complacency and I decided I had better just look. So I propped myself up on one elbow and glanced blearily towards Ollie's bed. It was empty.

White crumpled sheets. Above them the flimsy NHS curtain flapping accusingly. Cold night air invading the hospital sanctuary. I ran out into the corridor, pulling on trousers as I shouted at a night nurse, 'Ollie's escaped!' and ran out through the main door. What to do? Where to turn? Oh shit, shit, shit. Fuck. Perhaps he's still nearby? Quick – round the block, past the CLIC units. Here we are – the open window, eight feet . . . nine feet . . . ten feet up? What a jump! What a boy! Thank God it was a ground-floor window. Trample marks on the dewy grass. But no other sign of Ollie. Nothing. How long has he been gone – half an hour . . . an hour?

My only hope was speed, so I got the car and started driving round the hospital, processing past an endless litany of bright, modern, sans serif signposts, cheerfully advertising orthopaedic outpatients, maternity wing, cardiology centre, postgraduate centre, family services, laundry, accident & emergency, psychology, pathology, radiology . . . an endless, labyrinthine search-and-rescue nightmare. I tried every lane and cul-de-sac, did one final patrol of the perimeter road, then stared forlornly out into Weston, one of Bath's more affluent suburbs – an enticing hinterland of terraces, semis and large detached houses, with gardens, groves, hedges, flower beds, shrubberies, ponds, swimming pools, toolsheds, conservatories, two churches and a large cemetery offering limitless possibilities for exploration.

It was three o'clock in the morning and the streets were deserted. By now Rosie would be somewhere over the Sudan. What the hell was I going to say – oh, sorry, I was asleep? No – I didn't wake up when he climbed out of a high window, jumped ten feet to the ground and wandered off into the night, wearing only thin pyjamas, just as he was getting a life-threatening neutropenic fever?

Oh no, no, no. I've really fucked up this time.

I returned to the children's ward, where the hospital night manager had now arrived. She told me that the police were on their way. I asked her what time in the morning the local radio started broadcasting – perhaps we could put out an announcement? – and she looked very unimpressed, envisioning a PR disaster for the hospital. Then the police arrived. The senior officer said he already had a car searching through Weston and was also going to send out the sniffer dogs. Did I have a piece of clothing? All I could find were clean clothes smelling of Persil, not Ollie. So the two Alsatians were led to the dewy grass beneath the open window, but my own superimposed footprints had muddled the scent there. The dogs looked confused. Again I was taunted by images of Rosie over Africa. Then there was a crackle of distorted speech on the police officer's radio – 'Young boy . . . yes . . . brown hair . . . yes . . . no trousers?' He turned to me: 'I think they've found him, right over towards the Botanic Gardens, about half a mile away. Apparently he didn't have any trousers on.'

Oh Ollie! You wonderful explorer! You knew exactly where you were going, didn't you! What a brilliant boy! And what a fine escape! Proud, relieved tears pricked my eyes and a moment later the car drew up with Ollie inside. We never saw the pyjama trousers again, but I imagine that some mystified burgher of Weston found them discarded enigmatically beside his disturbed gold-fish pond and is still wondering how they got there. Ollie, with his acute sensitivity, could not bear the feel of wet cotton on his legs.

The night wandering did no harm, the first line of antibiotics quickly zapped the infection and after a couple of days Ollie came back to our temporary home, with its little courtyard garden secured by chicken wire. Then, a week or two after Rosie returned from Kenya, he perfected a new climbing move, managed to bridge over from one of the magnolia branches and disappeared. While Rosie called the police, I grabbed my bike and pedalled out onto Bathwick Hill – a broad, steep road where the cars came fast from around a bend, with little warning. There was no battered child in the road, but what about the canal? Ollie loved water and couldn't swim. I raced down to the towpath and patrolled the banks, scanning the canal's opaque brown surface and staring anxiously into dank dripping locks. Nothing. Heart pounding, calves burning, I pedalled back up the hill, exploring side roads and an area of open ground leading into fields. Cars passed. I had a sudden vision of Ollie, the beautiful enchanting boy, already ten miles away, imprisoned speechless and uncomprehending in the back of a strange vehicle, perhaps not even frightened, but smiling seraph-ically, seduced by the comforting rhythm of the motor car, untroubled by the strange man at the wheel.

Again the hot tears pricked my eyes and I began to draw up tentative funeral plans. I raced back to the house. Ollie had now been gone for half an hour and Rosie was distraught. Then the telephone rang. Someone had contacted the police. A boy had turned up in their garden . . . no trousers . . . about the right age . . . couldn't speak . . . seemed to fit the description, but his name appeared to be Charles Hudson?

'Charles Hudson!' Rosie thrilled. 'Yes – he's my ex-husband's nephew: Ollie's wearing his vest. Thank you *so* much.' Before she arrived with the pushchair to collect him from the elderly couple whose pond he had been investigating, a neighbour of the couple happened to drop in, took one look at the silent boy helping himself to food from the kitchen table and confirmed: '*I know* who that is! That's not Charles Hudson: that's *Ollie Venables*. Hello, Ollie, I used to be a health visitor when you were a baby.'

I added a new layer of chicken wire to the fence and domestic normality resumed. Edmond, approaching his fourth birthday, was thrilled to have his mother back from Kenya, watching and listening while he stood at the easel, talking his way through elaborate narrative paintings. It was April and after weeks of negotiation, rebuilding work was about to start on our own house; some time this summer we would all be back home. Ollie seemed to be coping stoically with the six-week cycles of chemotherapy. It was now fourteen months since his leukaemia had been diagnosed and he was still in remission. In another ten months the treatment would be complete and, with any luck, he would be cured for good. Now that the worst was over, Loulou was attempting short sessions of Lovaas work, resurrecting our efforts to salvage remnants of speech, supplementing his official school curriculum at the special school.

First thing on the morning of Monday 28th April I took Ollie into the hospital for one of his routine lumbar punctures, marvelling again at the dedication of the nurses who worked in the recovery room, monitoring and comforting the theatre patients as they emerged, often traumatically, from artificial unconsciousness. Sometimes Ollie cried with pain and confusion when he woke; today the anaesthetist seemed to have found just the right cocktail of drugs to ease his transition back to wakefulness. By lunchtime he was back home, playing in the garden.

On the Tuesday morning I was back at work in my rented office in town. I was on the telephone when Rosie suddenly walked in. She looked distraught and rushed straight over to Jay, whose office I shared, to ask if she could use his phone. Losing the thread of my own conversation, I heard her saying urgently to Loulou, 'He probably has a terrible headache. Give him some Calpol immediately – yes ten millilitres – and don't try to make him do any work.' I made excuses to my caller as Rosie put down Jay's phone, came over to my desk, and said very calmly, 'We need to talk – can we go outside?'

We walked out into the light and headed along Walcot Street, past the shop where we had bought the gorgeously upholstered Knole sofa, past Anil's sandwich bar, and the second-hand computer store and the woman who knitted the beautiful woollen hats and the framing shop and the discount shoe shop; and, as we jostled obliviously with the busy cheerful spring crowd, Rosie said, 'Ollie's had a relapse.'

Chapter Seven

'I don't know how they manage to do that job. It must be so harrowing to have to keep telling people such terrible news. Chris looked really shocked.' Rosie had been called in to the children's ward first thing that morning, as soon as the oncology registrar had received the lab results from the previous day's lumbar puncture. Leukaemia cells had been found in Ollie's spinal fluid.

'She said it was very, very serious and that we would have to think very carefully about whether we want to continue treatment. Apparently when children relapse in the central nervous system the prognosis is really poor. They have to start the treatment all over again . . . right from scratch . . . I'm not sure I can bear to make Ollie go through all that suffering if he's just going to die at the end of it.'

So this was the snub to our blithe complacency. All the time we had imagined Ollie cured, malignant cells had been lurking invisibly, waiting to infiltrate the precious fluid bathing his spinal cord and brain and add fatal insult to the enigmatic injury of autism. As we drove together back to Bathwick Hill – any attempt at work now seemed pointless – Rosie reminded me of the day the previous summer when Chris had questioned our decision for me to have a vasectomy. Knowing our genetic susceptibility, we had decided not to chance having another child with a significant risk of becoming profoundly autistic. Chris had just said simply, as she accessed Ollie's portacath for a routine chemotherapy session, 'Are you sure that's a good idea?'

Ollie was playing quietly with Loulou, his possible headache subdued with paracetamol. There was no outward sign of the fatal cancer and a miasma of un-reality hung over the next few days as we agonised about what to do. On Thursday 1st May, while Ollie had another exploratory lumbar puncture in Bristol, Tony Oakhill talked us through the possibilities. Again I admired his ability to be dispassionately objective, but sympathetic. He reminded us how fifteen months earlier he had recommended a conservative dose of intrathecal methotrexate; then reminded us why that decision had been made – out of concern for his already damaged nervous system. He explained that now the situation was completely different – now that we knew there was leukaemia in the central nervous system – the only serious treatment option was radical and aggressive: two full years, including repeated intrathecal methotrexate and high doses of radiation to the spine and brain. Short-term effects of radiotherapy included nausea, tiredness, aching and itchy skin; possible long-term effects included shortening of the torso, loss of cognitive skills and sterility. I am not sure whether at that stage he also mentioned cataracts and an increased risk of brain tumours; but he made it clear that this would be a gruelling journey and he told us that after a CNS relapse the odds on full recovery from acute lymphoblastic leukaemia were reduced drastically to about twenty per cent. He could only tell us about probable outcomes, not advise on whether to continue treatment; only the parents could make that decision.

On Friday, my birthday, we went over to Grosvenor Terrace, where the builders had finally started work, ripping out charred partition walls and scorched ceilings. Dust sparkled in the sunshine; outside in the garden cherry blossom fell like confetti on the earth I was raking smooth for turfing. In London Tony Blair revelled in his Wordsworthian new dawn as he posed with his family for the first time on the steps of Number Ten Downing Street. That night Angie (a school-leaver who had just joined our team of helpers) babysat while we went to hear Bruno performing with the Allegri Quartet. On Saturday afternoon I stayed with Ollie while Rosie trawled the annual flower show with his godmother Fiona. On Sunday evening my father dropped in for a drink and as he was about to drive off he leant out of the car window, put his hand on my arm and said, 'What a terrible decision for you to make. I can't begin to tell you what to do: I just wish there were something I could do to help.'

Monday was Edmond's fourth birthday. At breakfast he sat at the dining-room table unwrapping new carriages, engines, rails, points, sheds and bridges for his wooden train set. His little birthday tent was already pitched in the sitting room. Tuning in to the celebratory mood, Ollie emerged from the tent. Then jumped back inside, pulling the flap shut with a laugh – 'Gyaiyah! Aiyaiyee!'

It seemed impossible that a death sentence hung over this ebullient child. During the weekend Rosie and I had grappled inconclusively with our predicament. I felt that we had to respect Ollie's joyfulness. He had an extraordinary ability to bounce back from pain and suffering, to seize enjoyment, to grasp life. He probably had no concept of death – of an absence of life – but I felt that if he were able to imagine the possibility of losing life, and the notion of enduring pain and discomfort for a twenty per cent chance of *not* losing that life, he would say 'Yes – let's give it a try.'

Rosie was less sure. 'I don't know that we have the *right* to make him suffer like that. I think he's suffered enough already. And just supposing he *does* recover, what about the future? His life has been so diminished by autism. What's it going to be like for him as an adult, living in some kind of institution?'

'I know, I know. But I still think he has an incredible capacity for joy. And . . . I sort of think it would almost be *easier* just to let him die . . . the misery and sadness would be easier than all this struggle and uncertainty.'

'It wouldn't. It would be horrendous,' she insisted, 'it would be ghastly. Have you any idea what it's like when someone dies from a cancer?'

Later that morning we went into Bristol to talk with Tony Oakhill's fellow oncology professor, Philip Mott. He reiterated the possible side effects of treatment, reminded us that the only way to keep Ollie motionless for precision radiotherapy would be a general anaesthetic, repeated nearly every day for two weeks. We asked him again about the chances of success – of full recovery from a CNS relapse – and he put into context the limitations of epidemiological statistics. 'Yes, only about twenty per cent get through, but that doesn't mean that Ollie, the individual child, has a twenty per cent chance. Each case is different and for all we know it could be that *he* actually has, say, a fifty per cent chance.'

In the afternoon we put statistics aside to preside with determined cheerfulness over Edmond's birthday party, riding the toy train, lighting candles and singing in the rain at the bird gardens near Bath. In the evening Pru and Keith, Edmond's godfather, came for a drink. As a senior pathologist running the entire laboratory service for South-West England, Keith knew far more than us about our own predicament, but he made no attempt to guide or push us in any direction – was just quietly sympathetic, acknowledging that sometimes life was a bitch.

Rosie was coming round reluctantly to my point of view and by Wednesday morning she had agreed, uneasily, that we should resume treatment. After leaving Edmond at school we drove down the hill to the Royal United Hospital, parked, rang the oh-so-familiar security bell, entered the John Apley ward with its grimly cheerful bright colours, sat down to wait in the corridor and, at nine o'clock were asked in to the consulting room, where Tony Oakhill was waiting with the Bath team. I cut straight to the chase and said that we would like them to treat Ollie's CNS relapse. Rosie stressed how very hard this was going to be for an autistic child, reminding everyone again that Ollie was a unique child who required a unique approach. Tony then explained the rough timetable for Ollie's new protocol, announcing that the treatment would start with the first of many lumbar punctures on Monday 12th May 1997. If everything went according to plan, it would finish in the spring of 1999. It was hard to read his professional inscrutability, and I could have been completely wrong, but I thought that I detected a slight lift – a lightness of demeanour, suggesting that he felt we had made the right decision.

Once again the pages of Rosie's diary were crammed with a renewed concentration of pharmacological reminders: intravenous vincristine, cytarabine, epirubicin, asparaginase, etopiside; oral thioguanine, mercaptapurine, methotrexate; and IT MTX – intrathecal methotrexate, injected into Ollie's spinal cavity, under general anaesthetic, on 12th, 19th and 26th May; then 5th, 12th and 23rd June; then yet again on 12th and 21st July and 11th

August. This time the initial remission induction was even more aggressive. By the end of May Ollie was clutching at his head, removing handfuls of hair. By 6th June he was almost completely bald, once again wearing his blue Christopher Robin sun hat, smiling quietly to himself, surrounded by Now You Are Six cards and presents, as his teachers at the special unit sang 'Happy Birthday'.

Again I marvelled at his ability to shrug off pain and fear. And at Rosie's ability calmly to co-ordinate hospital, school, home helpers and family. In addition to all this, she had to spend much of May travelling down to Winchester to visit her father. During the final days of their Kenyan holiday he had complained of a cough and sore throat. Back at home in Alresford the cough grew more insistent and his chest became painful. For three weeks the pain intensified, with his GP showing little concern. In the end Rosie's sister Nonie went to visit Robin, saw how ill he was and took him straight to hospital, where he was told that he had lung cancer and would be dead within four months.

Later that week – the same week Ollie's relapse was discovered – I spoke on the phone to Rosie's brother Jake. 'Dad seems very philosophical,' he said. 'He says he has had a wonderful life and he's ready to die.' For Rosie it was almost a relief that her father would be spared knowledge of Ollie's relapse. 'I think that would have been unbearable for him,' she said, 'and he's hated being alone – he misses Mummy desperately. But I wish he could have lived longer, to see Edmond growing up.'

Rather than wait four months, Robin simply decided he was going to die straight away, just five days after the cancer diagnosis. With all her experience of interpreting Ollie's non-verbal communication, Rosie was the perfect nurse to ease her father's departure as his familiar loquacious flow slowed to a trickle, then dried up completely. While she took turns with Jake and Nonie at his hospital bedside in Winchester, I stayed at home, going alone to the Festival concert we had booked weeks earlier. A French violinist and cellist whose names I have long since forgotten joined the pianist Imogen Cooper for a glorious programme including an electric performance of Beethoven's 'Ghost' trio, then concluded with Brahms – the rich, warm, luscious B major trio, brimming with joy and love and sadness and the kind of indefinable yearning which only music can properly articulate.

Robin died two days later. At his funeral, as at Kay's, I was asked to read from the famous letter St Paul wrote to the Romans – '. . . neither death, nor life, nor angels, nor principalities, nor powers, nor things present, nor things to come, nor height, nor depth, nor any other creature, shall be able to separate us from the love of God . . .' Again, afterwards, we celebrated defiantly, drinking a little too much wine, the middle-aged siblings reminiscing about the parties and the fun and the adventure of their African childhood. I remembered Robin's infrequent visits to Larkhall and wished that I had cherished more the life of the scholarship boy from Lancashire, who went so proudly to Oxford in 1937, only to have his youthful optimism shattered by the terror of war as he was forced to leave Oxford for five years, eventually to drop death on the heads of the young men and woman of Dresden with whom he had recently sung such happy beer-fuelled songs on a walking holiday in Germany . . . wished I had heard more stories of his time in the Fleet Air Arm at the Siege of Malta . . . what was it really like in the rear turret of that lumbering Swordfish, as the deadly Messerschmitts swooped in on you over the black waters of the Mediterranean, and every other plane in the squadron was inexorably shot down? And what about the times you went drinking ashore, hoping that your odiously heroic pilot wouldn't round you up for another extra mission? And what about those days after the war, as a young colonial officer going on safari, in the bush for weeks at a time, entertained by the paramount chiefs of Northern Rhodesia as you acted out the final days of the British Empire, sustained by an idealistic belief in the power of education and the values of European culture?

Rosie and I returned to Bath, to a summer dominated by Ollie's oscillating health. At times he was fit enough to go to school, to go swimming, to join his grand-mother at the local stables, riding ponies. Often when I took him in for his lumbar puncture he was manic, watching for opportunities to dash out of his cubicle and snatch food from startled neurotypical children in the main ward. Maintaining 'nil by mouth' was a wearying challenge, and I always took in a screwdriver to close off the valves on all the water taps. Sometimes television helped and Ollie would rock meditatively to music, until the wall-to-wall pop drove me demented and I switched over to the news, on one occasion finding myself curiously moved by Governor Chris Patten's red-eyed departure from Hong Kong, while Ollie lay peace-fully beside me, sedated at last by midazolam, now that a slot was ready in theatre.

Then the porters arrived and off we went. The two nurses checking Ollie's name tag. Trundling down the familiar corridor, Ollie happy to be on the move. Through the big swing doors to theatre reception. Then the final double check of name tag against the notes, which seemed so bureaucratic until one day Rosie and I visited a special school where there was a severely retarded child who had gone into hospital for a lung operation and come out with part of her brain missing. Whenever possible, *I* took Ollie into theatre, because Rosie found it very distressing. We had a good routine established, with the minimum possible number of green-overalled staff, all requested not to attempt any well-intended jollity, nor to bombard Ollie with super-fluous words. Everything was kept as calm as possible, with one of Ollie's soothing early music tapes playing as the thick white juice sluiced into his portacath. But even so, it always felt like a little death as he slipped away, so utterly vulnerable.

In July, at the low point of one of his chemotherapy cycles, drained of white blood cells, Ollie developed a serious neutropenic fever just as Edmond was exposed to chickenpox at school. Three spots appeared on Ollie's chest and although no-one could be certain they were chickenpox, he was put on the standard prophylactic drug, aciclovir – the best hope for checking what could, in his neutropenic condition, be a fatal illness. For a week his temperature raged as he lolled listlessly on a hospital bed, isolated in a cubicle. By the second week he was on the third and final line of antibiotics. By day, Rosie drew up a timetable of two-hour shifts for herself and our various helpers, including wonderfully compe-tent, serene Kate Hillard – the result of social worker Niki's careful search; by night I took over, sleeping beside Ollie on the hospital floor.

One morning, as his temperature began at last to drop, an ambulance came to take us both to Bristol – to the central oncology centre. In a huge waiting room, surrounded by elderly cancer patients, Ollie wandered backwards and forwards, searching restlessly for food, oblivious apparently of his lingering fever. After an hour or so I persuaded him to get onto a spare trolley and began wheeling him backwards and forwards, but, fever notwithstanding, he kept jumping off. Frazzled and weary, I wheeled him into the contained space of an empty treatment room, where he got off the trolley and started emptying cupboards. Then at last the radiologist we had been hoping to see appeared at the door.

'This boy looks very ill,' she said. 'I can't do anything with him today. And, in any case, I had him booked in for two weeks' time. There seems to have been a mix-up . . . I'm *terribly* sorry that you've been kept waiting all this time for nothing.' That sincere, direct apology – for a mistake which was no fault of hers – was very impressive. As was the trouble she then took to explain what she would be doing when Ollie was fit again. Under general anaesthetic, his head and torso would have to be measured very precisely, using a tattooed dot at the top of his spine as a reference point for various masks which had to be made specially. These masks would shield his internal organs from frying, as she directed a series of precalculated radiation doses along different sections of his spine and skull, zapping thoroughly any malignant cells the intrathecal methotrexate had failed to mop up.

After a long wait, Ollie and I were ambulanced back to Bath. Soon his temperature dropped to normal and we returned home, where domestic calm resumed until one hot Sunday morning, barefoot in the tiny cluttered kitchen of our temporary home, preparing some squid for lunch, Rosie knocked her elbow dyspraxically against the heavy Sabatier knife resting on the edge of the worktop. I heard a resoundingly unfeminine 'Fuck!' as the carbon steel tip, smeared liberally with oxidised metal fish juices, speared Rosie's big toe. 'Quick – get the first-aid kit,' she shouted, before subsiding green-faced on the staircase, staring at the crimson welling from the neat puncture in the top of her toe.

'Why isn't there any bloody iodine?' she moaned accusingly, then perked up as she remembered the endless scrapes of her resourceful, accident-prone African childhood. 'Hydrogen peroxide – that's what we need! I think there's some in the laundry cupboard.' I found the bottle and poured some liquid onto the wound. Edmond watched, entranced, as his mother fizzed and frothed, pink at the toe.

I made some tentative remarks about stitches, but Rosie was adamant that the last place she wanted to visit on a hot crowded Sunday afternoon was the RUH Accident & Emergency ward. So we just protected the toe with a plaster and tried to ignore its earthward droop. But two days later, taking Ollie into Bristol for his radio-therapy measurements, Rosie kept tripping up over her droopy digit. With all the authority of someone who had long since lost a big toe, freezing it stone dead, along with three of its neighbours, on Everest, I insisted, 'The knife fell *across* the toe – it must have severed the tendon. Why not get someone here to look at it?'

So while I took Ollie into Oncology, Rosie dropped in to Accident & Emergency, where they confirmed a severed tendon and referred her back to Bath for an operation. It was like old times, with roles reversed, as I took her into the RUH orthopaedic department and settled her into the familiar ward.

She came home the next day. It had taken the surgeon seven hours to retrieve the tendon, which he found halfway up her calf. He sent her home with a tempo-rary metal spike protruding from the repaired toe, and a warning not to bang into anything – fine advice, perhaps, for a genteel spinster living alone in a spacious apartment, but hardly realistic for the mother of an autistic child. Within half an hour of getting home Rosie had jabbed the spike three times, on each occasion almost fainting from the pain. 'What you need,' I announced, 'is one of those things they put on rabid dogs: you need a foot muzzle.' Which was quickly improvised with pliers, some wire coat hangers and an orthopaedic shoe. Thereafter Rosie strode boldly forth, her left foot caged securely against jostling children.

On 18th August Ollie started radiotherapy. I watched on a closed-circuit screen as the radiologists positioned the masks over the inert little body, lying prone in the theatre, looking so fragile and vulnerable. The session only lasted a few minutes, requiring a minimal dose of anaesthetic, so that recovery was much quicker than after a lumbar puncture, and with no residual pain. By the third morning Ollie had grown so accustomed to the routine that he walked straight into the theatre, jumped giggling onto the X-ray bench and pulled off his shirt to reveal the expectant portacath tube. Come on – time for my happy juice!

Rosie meanwhile had had her toe spike removed excruciatingly without anaesthetic and, accelerator foot newly unmuzzled, had driven Edmond over to Henley to stay with our Cary cousins – the same cousins from whose upstairs window Ollie had tumbled. When I phoned in the evening to tell her how brilliantly Ollie was coping, she sounded pleased but fraught. 'A terrible thing's just happened,' she quavered. There was a pause as she spoke away from the telephone, 'Yes please, Joanna, another glass.' After a restorative swig she spoke to me again. 'Edmond's just hanged himself.'

'What!'

'Hanged himself in that horse chestnut tree with the swing. Thank God I was there to rescue him.'

The two of them had been climbing, Rosie on a higher branch, when Edmond slipped and fell. There was a loop of rope tied beneath the branch, next to the swing, and he fell through this loop. Rosie heard a piercing shriek and looked down to see him dangling from his neck, legs kicking the air, lips screaming purple. Newly mended toe forgotten, she leapt out of the tree, scrabbled to her feet and lifted Edmond's thrashing weight out of the noose, hugging and kissing him as tears poured down her cheeks – tears of relief mingled with terror at what might have happened if she had been further away, or if the muscles of his neck had not been stiffened defensively by screaming. For the next two days in the Carys' adventure-training zone Rosie never let Edmond out of her sight.

Ollie's radiotherapy came to an end. Back in Larkhall, determined to complete the house rebuilding before the start of the autumn term, I blustered and fretted, antagonising builders and decorators with my demands for perfection. During the final week I worked non-stop on the house myself, and early on the morning of Sunday 31st August I was tiling the bathroom when the radio announced that Princess Diana had been killed in a car crash. A week later, on a bright Saturday morning with the first tingling of autumn in the air, as we settled back into our new phoenix home, all four storeys – even the stair treads (you don't have stair carpets with an autistic child) – painted in zingy optimistic yellows, reds, greens and blues, we watched the funeral on the television. I had grown tired of the public hysteria – the maudlin sentimentality, the interminable media chatter, the vindictive carping at the royal in-laws – but as the coffin processed out of Westminster Abbey to John Tavener's anguished harmonies it was impossible not to be moved.

Another week. Another funeral. This time Mother Teresa's, glimpsed on a television at New Delhi airport as I arrived with the six brave clients who had signed up for the first of my new 'Venables Ventures' adventurous holidays. The Ventures subsequently proved short-lived, unable to develop without serious amounts of cash, staff and advertising, but they made a bit of money and this first trek, to a region on India's northern frontier called Kinnaur, was a chance for me to return to the Himalaya, five years after the accident on Panch Chuli. Four of the party – Jill and Jane, and their respective husbands – were complete Himalayan novices. They delighted with their enthusiasm, rising to the challenge of a whole new set of experiences – like eating fried chapattis, curd and searing lime pickle for breakfast; clambering over an immense landslide which had just dammed the Sutlej river, destroyed the Hindustan–Tibet Highway and wiped out an entire village; wading streams; being woken up by avalanches; stomping with Himalayan villagers in their annual flower festival dance; being blessed at a Buddhist nunnery; climbing over a 5,000-metre-high pass; and surviving an impromptu, suicidal taxi drive along the Great Indian Trunk Road during the Friday evening rush hour, when we missed the train back to Delhi.

It was good to see the Himalaya afresh, through others' eyes. Good also to have with us my old Mumbai friend Harish Kapadia. He asked about Ollie. Said why didn't we all come and stay in Mumbai for a few weeks, doing yoga, eating healthy vegetarian food, soaking up the soft seaside warmth? I prevaricated and Harish asked if Ollie would be frightened by all the brown faces. No, of course he wouldn't, I laughed, but at the moment it would all just be too difficult. Leaving aside the immediate imperative to complete his leukaemia treatment, there were all the problems of travelling: with an autistic child like Ollie you had to plan every move, always checking for unexpected dangers and terrors. At home we had a system – a routine which made life manage-able – and for the time being we couldn't conceive of disrupting that.

After seventeen days away, I resumed my place in that system. Edmond was now back at school. Ollie, when the chemotherapy regime allowed it, went to his special unit, delivered and returned by taxi, sitting in the back of the car with a kind woman employed by the local education authority to help Special Needs children. Most of the children at the unit were more able than Ollie; some of them had quite extensive speech; some were beginning to spend time in the mainstream school alongside the unit. Ollie, by comparison, seemed to struggle with the demands even of a special school. Even tasks such as simple jigsaws seemed now to defeat him. Frustration made him tearful. Nausea, itching and stab-bing pains, induced by cytotoxic drugs, intensified the frustration. One day he came home with his white shirt stained red. A note from the head said, 'Don't worry, it's not *his* blood.' In a moment of tearful fury, he had bitten his teacher on the chin.

At home occasionally, banging his clenched hands against the side of his head, he would advance on Edmond, grinding his teeth, pressing his face angrily against his brother's. Several times, thwarted by Rosie or me over forbidden food or a locked cupboard, he tried to bite us. The best response was calm avoidance, holding his arms firmly, and manoeuvring him to a quiet place, where he could sit and recover, dummy in mouth, fingers stroking the folded edge of his snuggly, until he achieved a kind of Zen-like trance. When he had recovered completely, Rosie might sit with him and gently stroke his head. Edmond, too, would often sit with him, roles reversed, comforting his elder brother, showing him the pictures in one of his storybooks, or laughing at a Pingu video, delighted when Ollie let slip a surreptitious smile or a loud 'aiyee' at the animated penguins' made-up language.

Despite the frustrations, Ollie was often happy at school. One of the assistants later told us about his brave efforts to make words: 'We used to keep a supply of satsumas on a high shelf. Ollie never tried to climb up and steal one (and we knew he could), but would come with his little face screwed up with concentration and say "owinge pees", and was ecstatic to receive a treat. He would peel it delicately and separate all the segments before gobbling it up and running off.' That charming desire to please was his default mode: like every other human being, he loved to succeed and, unautistically, to please others. And he had a gentleness which could even influence the other children: 'We had a boy called George – a chunky burly boy who barged his way through the day taking no prisoners. One day Ollie was happily riding his tricycle when a gust of wind blew off his cheeky hat and sent it bowling across the garden. George spotted it and pounced on it; we waited, holding our breaths, as he marched over, the hat held in his two hands, arms outstretched towards Ollie. He stopped, smiled at him and planted the gentlest kiss on Ollie's poor bald head and then replaced the hat with the utmost care, before storming off to create mayhem elsewhere. We had never seen George's gentle side before – it took Ollie to winkle it out – and it really thrilled George's whole family when they heard.'

Gentle, radiant, calm, charming, flirtatious . . . he could be all these things; and he could be manic, hyperactive, testing, *exhausting*. By the evening Rosie and I were usually longing for Ollie's bedtime. Often we would both bath the two boys together, Edmond getting out first to ride bumpily on my towelled knee for 'This is the way the farmer rides' (just as I and all my brothers and sisters had done with *my* father) shouting 'Again Dadda!' while Ollie had a final splash, sliding backwards and forwards, sloshing gallons over the side of the bath. Then we would settle them down in bed, Ollie often wearing a chest harness and reins attached to the bedhead, to stop him wandering. However, his perennial bowel irritability, exacerbated probably by chemotherapy, was playing up that autumn of 1997 and we were having ever more frequently to change shit-smeared sheets, sometimes several times a night. So for a while we abandoned the reins.

One evening Ollie was quite unable to settle, so we just left him the run of the top two storeys (locking my study and our bedroom). The stair gate between the ground floor and first floor was shut, its top now extended by another six feet to thwart Ollie's improved climbing skills. Rosie and I slumped in the sitting room, determined to enjoy a break from child-minding. Ollie crashed and thumped upstairs. We read our books.

The crashing and watery sloshing got louder. 'It's your turn, darling,' Rosie pleaded. So I went upstairs and found Ollie skidding on a vertical skating rink, an entire bottle of detergent emptied over the varnished stairs. I mopped and skidded, cursing my elder son. After half an hour's swabbing the lethal slick was removed and Ollie held up a protesting arm as I locked the bathroom door. 'Sorry Ollie, it's too dangerous. No more water play.' His only reply was a manic laugh.

We settled down again, this time in the piano room, immediately at the foot of the stairs, where Rosie had some sewing to do. Ollie appeared at the stair gate. 'Unhh . . . unhh!'

'No, Ollie. Time for bed.'

'Unhhh!'

'Oh for goodness sake, Ollie, *go to bed.*'

He laughed and disappeared back upstairs. Rosie
resumed her sewing as the noise continued above. But
after ten minutes peace descended and we dared to hope
that Ollie had gone to bed. Then we heard him again
on the landing, immediately above us. There was a soft,
susurrating 'ssthhhwubb'. And another 'ssthhhwubb', this
time landing on the lower stairs, inches from Rosie's
head. 'Oh *delightful,*' she groaned, as another soft, moist
turd lobbed down from the landing. 'Faecal hand
grenades – my favourite! Come on then Stephen, let's
get mopping.'

Ollie's bladder was also used for inventive naughtiness. Once a week we took him to the new music
therapy centre in Bristol, where a man of impeccable
gentleness tried to engage him with a beautiful array of
percussion instruments. Ollie loved music – everyone
knew that – but in this particular circumstance, where
the therapist was trying to entice him into active partic-
ipation, he only wanted to be naughty, trying repeatedly
to pee in the hand drum. Naughtiness was infinitely
more fun than compliance. Or was this just Ollie's own
relentless logic, which interpreted every hollow object
as an obvious pee bottle?

So much of the time with Ollie we were guessing at
motivations, trying to understand enigmas. But, as 1997
came to a close, for all the laughing interludes, there was
a pervasive sense of struggle – of Ollie finding everything too difficult. He seemed increasingly distressed by
attempts to make him conform to 'normal' life. For all
his success with the satsumas and his enchanting effect
on burly George, school was too much for him. A
circular letter sent out to parents towards the end of the
autumn term warned that some children, struggling to
cope with the curriculum, might have to move. No

names were mentioned but it was blatantly obvious, looking at the checklist of expected skills, that Ollie was well short of the mark. When the kind taxi woman brought him home on the last day of term, laden with present and cards, we felt that he would probably not be going back in January.

The first new hair, again gorgeously velvet smooth, had just sprouted on his head but he looked desperately pale, with dark shadows under his eyes. For hours at a time he slumped on the sofa. When Angie, the immensely popular helper who was now leaving us to go and work in the Alps, came to say goodbye, Ollie was pleased to see her – was comforted by her presence – but sat very quietly beside her, a look of weary sadness in his dark, dark eyes. Toys, puzzles, jigsaws . . . none of them seemed to hold much interest, and it seemed that the cranial radiotherapy *had* damaged cognitive skills. It had also destroyed the left-handedness he inherited from my father; such manual skills as he now had – and they were dwindling fast – were transferred to his right hand.

Illness hadn't just destroyed skills. The relentless assault on mind and body seemed also to have beaten down even Ollie's boisterous confidence. When Edmond sat down on the floor beside him, eager to help, completing Ollie's laborious jigsaw or brick structure with casual ease, Ollie walked away, sad and hurt. At school, quite apart from problems with the curriculum, he felt cowed, to the point where on a non-school day he whimpered if we drove anywhere near the familiar buildings. He had become a timid, cowering, nervous wreck.

Most distressing of all was his soured relationship with Rosie. At times now he could hardly bear to look at her, perhaps blaming her – the mother who ought to protect him – for all the frightening treatments inflicted on him over the last two years. We seemed to have travelled back down a long dark road since glimpsing that promised land three years earlier, when we had embarked so hopefully – and at first successfully – on Ollie's home education Lovaas programme. When we received the quarterly newsletters from Peach, the charity we had helped to set up, it was hard not to feel bitter when we read about other children progressing, some of them to the point where they could now attend mainstream schools. With Ollie we were simply surviving from day to day, just trying to make life bearable for him, not knowing how long that life was likely to continue. We had reached rock bottom.

Or would have done, if Rosie had not, yet again, been searching for some new way forward. School, she reasoned, was not working; so Ollie needed to stay at home. But we couldn't just have him wandering round the house, pleading for food, rummaging in cupboards, emptying bottles, turning on taps and generally driving us demented: if Ollie was to be at home, we needed a method – some kind of educational structure which would occupy him and keep us sane. We had tried the Lovaas method and that had proved successful until leukaemia turned everything upside down. What we needed now was something much gentler, less demanding, more child-centred. What about the Kaufmans' Son Rise programme, which we had considered seriously when we started this autistic journey three years earlier? Perhaps now was the time to consider it again? But how to find the £8,000 or more for a training course at the Option Institute, even if a week's slot were available? We had extended our mortgage to the maximum to buy Grosvenor Terrace, there were no spare savings and I was unlikely suddenly to become a successful investment banker overnight. Of course there were ways of finding money, but they would take time and Rosie wanted to get started *now*. We needed an instant miracle.

The very next morning we got our miracle when the quarterly newsletter from the National Autistic Society arrived in the post. Inside was a Stop Press announcement: because of the huge number of enquiries prompted by a recent BBC documentary on the Son Rise programme, the Option Institute was coming to London, in January, to run a collective Start-Up course for parents, at a cost of $995 per parent or carer. At the current exchange rate that would cost just £1,243 for the two of us. With childcare and travel, the whole thing would come to under £1,600. We could find *that* much, surely. 'I can stick at least half of it on my Access card,' Rosie announced cheerfully. 'Let's do it!'

So after Christmas, we embarked on our new adventure, unsure how we were going to find the money and staff and energy to run a full-time home education programme in a specially adapted room for an indefinite period of time, but just knowing that somehow these things would happen.

We paid our fees and a highly efficient professional-looking information pack arrived from the Option Institute in Massachusetts. The course would take place over five days, starting on 12th January 1998, in Edmonton. 'Where on earth is Edmonton?' Rosie asked as I groped myopically through the London A–Z. 'Ah . . . here . . . just off the North Circular. It's probably only twenty minutes from Ealing . . . perhaps Anna and David would have us to stay.'

Our five days' absence had to be planned meticulously. A carer had to sleep at the house each night. Edmond had to be driven to and from school, fed, bathed and put to bed. Ollie needed constant one-to-one care from 6.30 a.m. when he woke up to 7.30

p.m. when he went to bed. Monday and Tuesday would
be spent in hospital, first in theatre having a lumbar
puncture, then in the children's ward on intravenous
drips; Elaine the CLIC nurse would visit Larkhall on
Wednesday and Thursday to give him further cytarabine injections, before removing his portacath line.
Rosie had to plan menus for the five days, leaving all
the food – including food for overnight carers – in
the fridge. During the week before departure, Rosie
and I stayed up for hours each night, juggling the
timetable until every two-to-three-hour shift was
filled. Then we typed individual, detailed, unambigu-
ously bossy instructions for each of our helpers – even
Siri, the wonderfully calm, dependable family link
worker who had been with us since Ollie's autism
diagnosis.

SIRI
Sunday 11 January
7.00 p.m. – overnight. With Ollie and Edmond at
Grosvenor Terrace.

Monday 12 January
OLLIE NIL BY MOUTH

6.45 a.m.	Ollie and Edmond up. LIDOCAINE on Ollie.
	Put on eczema ointment and dress.
	Edmond dress and prepare for school – see list in kitchen.
7.45 a.m.	Leave Edmond with Sue.
8.15 a.m.	Ollie at ABC ward for lumbar puncture.
	Lunch – Give 7.5 ml CO-TRIMOXA-ZOLE and check with nurses about THIOGUANINE.

12.30 a.m.   Nurse takes over at John Apley ward.

Tuesday 13 January

1.00 p.m.   Phone John Apley (824821)
                       to see whether Ollie has
                       left.

1.30 p.m. – 4.00 p.m. With Ollie. If at John Apley,
                       please make sure that nurses
                       have given his line a HEP
                       flush, in case he pulls it out.

4.00 p.m.   Andy takes over at
                       Grosvenor Terrace.

Wednesday 14 January

10.00 a.m. – 12.00 a.m. Take over from Emma.
                         With Ollie at GT.
                         Andy takes over at 12.00.

7.00 p.m. – overnight   Take over from Kate for
                         overnight. Ollie in bed.
                         Edmond home at 7.00 for
                         bath and bed.

NB EDMOND HAS BEEN IN A CHICKENPOX
HOUSE AND MUST NOT HAVE CONTACT
WITH OLLIE BEFORE WASHING AND
CHANGING CLOTHES.

Thursday 15 January

8.00 a.m.   Edmond and Ollie up for breakfast.
             Give Ollie mouthcare and
             THIOGUANINE (check RUH notes)
             after food.

9.15 a.m.	Andy takes over with Ollie. Drive Edmond to RUH for ear test. Then school.
3.00 p.m.	Take over from Andy. Edmond back at 3.30 (no chickenpox routine today).Supper, bath and bed. Give mouthcare and THIOGUANINE if necessary (see RUH notes). Please use OILATUM PLUS (2 capfuls) in bath. Keep water shallow because his line is in. Use eczema soap substitute. Pat dry: don't rub. Eczema ointment all over before putting on pyjamas.

Friday 16 January

7.15 a.m.	Edmond up for breakfast.
8.15 a.m.	Catherine collects Edmond. PLEASE PUT OUT RUBBISH FOR COLLECTION. Ollie – CO-TRIMOXAZOLE (7.5 ml), mouthcare and THIOGUANINE (if instructed) after food.
9.30 a.m.	Kate takes over.
3.30 p.m.	Take over from Emma. Edmond back from swimming by 5.00 p.m. Supper – 7.5 ml CO-TRIMOXA-ZOLE and THIOGUANINE if instructed. Mouthcare. Eczema procedure at bathtime. Stephen and Rosie home by 8.30.

Eczema was Ollie's latest challenge. A very helpful dermatologist from the hospital had taught us how to minimise its aggravation, but it was yet another complication in Ollie's daily care, written up in the notes, alongside details of mouthcare, nausea relief, itching relief, pain relief and regular antidotes to constipation. Oral chemotherapy drugs Rosie left in pre-prepared, labelled syringes in the fridge, with warnings not to spill any drugs on skin as they could be corrosive.

All this responsibility our brilliant carers had to take on for very modest pay. Some of that money was covered by Social Services and by Ollie's disability grants, but additional care for the five days cost us £300. By the Sunday afternoon, as we took turns to pack for London and made a final round of co-ordinating telephone calls, Rosie and I were completely exhausted. At tea time Rosie escaped for an hour to wallow luxuriously in a steaming bath laced with aromatherapy oil. Refreshed and fragrantly marinated she came back downstairs, forgetting to lock the bathroom door. Half an hour later, going up to collect my toothbrush, I was assailed by an overpowering olfactory cocktail. Choking despairingly on a pungent Mediterranean and oriental blend of rosemary, lavender, rose geranium, cedarwood, mandarin, vetiver, sandalwood, patchouli . . . I picked up all the little brown glass bottles from the bottom of the bath; every single one had its cap missing and had been tipped down the plughole.

'Ollie!' Rosie screamed.

'What's he done, Mumma?' piped Edmond eagerly.

'Oh *Ollie* – you wretched boy – my *one* little luxury . . . did he really get them *all*?'

'I'm afraid so.'

'That was about two hundred pounds' worth. How could I be so stupid to leave the door unlocked? Oh well, I suppose, in the great scheme –'

The front-door knocker announced Siri's arrival and

a few minutes later, fraught and frazzled, we escaped the madhouse and set off for London to learn again how to love our crazy, beautiful, exasperating, bottle-tipping elder son.

Chapter Eight

We arrived too early the next morning at the Edmonton conference centre, so Rosie and I went round the corner to wait in a greasy spoon café. As we sipped our weak Nescafé the room filled and the regulars glanced suspiciously over their *Suns* and *Daily Mirrors* at a swelling crowd of self-consciously middle-class intruders. They all looked fraught and I whispered to Rosie, 'Who do you think all these weirdoes are?'.

'Autistic parents.'

'Ah . . . yes, of course. Do you think *we* look that weird?' And, sure enough, at nine o'clock we all found ourselves in the same registration queue, directed upstairs by smartly groomed young Americans.

'They look like Mormons,' whispered Rosie.

'They can't be: they're Jewish.'

We all gathered in a purple, brown and lilac 'banqueting hall' smelling of unwashed feet. Husbands and wives were instructed not to sit together. Rosie and I both lurked sceptically, several rows back in a sea of faux Louis Seize chairs; separated from my wife, I ignored my neighbours and stared impassively at the dapper young man who appeared on stage to welcome us and then deliver a rousing eulogy, introducing Barry Neil Kaufman.

We all watched warily as 'Bears' Kaufman strode on in tailored black trousers, immaculate tie and broad-shouldered, double-breasted dogstooth jacket, to dominate stage centre, sweeping the audience with a confiding twinkly smile. He pivoted on his heels, tall and erect, turning frequently to profile his magnificent great beak of a nose, microphone caressing badger-striped beard, catching every modulation of his rich baritone. He spoke of miracles and unconditional love and of happiness being a choice. Three hundred parents bristled suspiciously and after a few minutes Bears stopped.

'Look at you all,' he laughed. 'So *this* is British reserve.' He scowled, hunched shoulders and folded his arms defensively. We all laughed with him and soon we thawed, allowing the master showman to tell his tale of turning preconceptions upside down – of his wife, Samahria, spending day after day, week after week, shut in a bathroom with their autistic son Raun, studying every tiny nuance of his bizarre rituals, following him, entering his world, learning from him, accepting him unconditionally. By creating that total trust, Samahria Kaufman was able gradually to entice her son out into the world of other people; by studying minutely his motivations, she managed eventually to encourage him into the first brave efforts at speech.

Raun Kaufman emerged completely from his autistic world. He became 'normal' and did extremely well at university. Now he himself teaches at the Option Institute his parents founded. Few – if any – Son Rise children have replicated that total transformation. But in a sense that didn't matter. In his opening session, before moving on to practical teaching methods, Bears was engaging us all in a profound 'attitoodinal' shift, inviting each of us to see our autistic child not as a tragedy but as a very special gift – as an opportunity for growth. Towards the end of the session he invited members of the audience to come up on the stage and speak about their children. There was a brief frisson of embarrassment while grown men burst into tears, but that embarrassment quickly melted as three hundred people allowed themselves to be drawn into a profound and necessary catharsis, letting flow the fears and tensions, the aching sense of loss and the 'why me?' disappointments.

After lunch I sat at the front and by tea time I was teacher's pet, arm shooting up regularly to ask questions and volunteer ideas. Back in Ealing that evening, as we glugged our wine and chattered manically, David Black said, 'What a transformation: last night you two looked completely finished.' On Tuesday we again arrived early in Edmonton, this time eager for work. Bears alternated sessions with fellow teachers from the institute, including his gorgeous daughter Bryn, who herself is adoptive mother to an autistic child. Time and time again they hammered home the importance of the 'Three Es' – Energy, Excitement, Enthusiasm – modelling those qualities infectiously themselves. 'My God these people work hard,' I thought humbly, as they enthused us through a series of lectures, demonstrations and workshops, backed up with extensive music, props and video clips.

The core of the programme was 'Bonding through Acceptance' – the fundamental principle that we had to join our autistic children in their worlds, not in a spirit of reluctant shoulder-shrugging cynicism, but joyously with – yes – energy, excitement and enthoosiasm. They stressed the importance of seeking eye contact at every possible opportunity; of reacting with shock, surprise, delight and laughter to our children, showing them theatrically that their actions can get a response. They taught us to look for clues, responding immediately to the slightest request from the child, encouraging him or her to utilise other people. On 'Joining' they reminded us how Samahria Kaufman had copied her son's obsessive plate-spinning: 'Whatever this child chooses to do is the most important thing in this moment. It may be curative and it is in some way of value to this child. We must respect and trust this child's choices.' Everyone has his own autistic self-stimulating 'stereotypic behaviours': did we know that JFK had a thing about rocking chairs and kept one in the Oval Office? Bryn exhorted us to be 'happy detectives', joining curiously, seeking clues. She told us about the autistic girl who banged her head repeatedly against a partition wall, always in exactly the same place. The therapists realised eventually that the girl was choosing the most sonorous section of the wall, equidistant between deadening studs; with that understanding they got her a drum kit and enticed her gradually to transfigure the headbanging into more varied, creative, manual drumming.

Bryn then talked about crying, encouraging us not to reward whining. This didn't mean we had to be callous; we just had to project a sense of calm strength whilst remaining impassive, showing that 'crying is not the magic that moves people'. By the same token, we had to respond immediately, exaggeratedly, to the tiniest hint of cheerfulness or, better still, an attempt at speech. Because, ultimately, this was all leading towards the second basic principle of 'Inspiring Growth'. Here the teachers showed video clips of their colleagues in Massachusetts building on children's activities, improvising with all the inventiveness of a theatre workshop student. They demonstrated the importance of gaining eye contact before making a verbal request. Then they moved on to 'initiating' – encouraging us to take the lead in some new play, when we had established the necessary rapport. And, most important of all, they stressed the importance of teaching language – not just words, but a love of communication – always aiming to create situations where the child is rewarded for speech.

What became increasingly apparent was that, for all its child-centredness and flexibility, the Son Rise programme was actually quite interventionist. It created situations where the autistic child was encouraged to expand his repertoire, to interact with other people, to join the neurotypical world. In its own way it was just as rigorous as Lovaas's Applied Behavioural Analysis programme. It just started from a profoundly different premise and right now, with Ollie at his most withdrawn and traumatised, the philosophy of total acceptance seemed the most appropriate.

All the parents and carers on the course had been asked to bring photos of their autistic children. Rosie and I had forgotten ours and had been miserable on the Monday morning to see all the photos pinned up on a board, minus Ollie. We had phoned Siri, asking her to fax a copy of a shot taken the previous summer of Ollie smiling luminously in his sun hat, and when it arrived on the Wednesday we were thrilled to see his face up on the board with all the other children. Time after time, during the week, amidst all the practical teaching tips, we were reminded that these children were why we were all here and that, ultimately, 'the "experts" do not and cannot know your child as well as you do.'

By the end of the week I felt a deep admiration for Bears Kaufman, the Billy Graham of the autism world. On the final Friday morning he began by describing the time his father had telephoned to tell him that he had terminal cancer. How he had responded by telling his father that that was wonderful news. How his father had said, 'I knew you'd say something like that: that's why I phoned *you*, not one of the others.' For the whacky son, the successful advertising man turned teacher, even his father's impending death was an *opportunity* – a chance to explore and grow closer.

In the final session after lunch we were all asked to write a letter to our child (or children – some parents had two or even three autistic siblings) telling them how we felt about them. As we sat composing our outpourings of love, Bach's Air on a G String began to play softly, then Albinoni's Adagio, then Pachelbel's heart-wrenching ground bass. And probably Barber's Adagio for good measure. One of the institute staff circulated amongst the gold chairs with a box of tissues.

Shameless emotional manipulation? Maybe; but this wasn't an intergovernmental trading standards conference – these people were here to reconnect us with the most precious things in our lives. Driving back west down the M4 that evening, five days on from our fraught departure, spilt aromatherapy oils were forgotten. We couldn't care less whether Ollie had tipped a thousand pounds' worth down the plughole; or *ten thousand*. We were just desperate to see him – and Edmond – again.

They were both in bed, Edmond asleep, Ollie staring quietly into the semi-darkness, stroking his snuggly, with a faint smile hovering at the edges of his dummy. 'Hello my darling boy,' Rosie whispered, stroking his velvet head, 'we're going to have a wonderful time together.' He looked straight at her, sat up and put his arms round her neck. Thrilled by that fleeting moment of love and acceptance, Rosie emailed Bryn to tell her the good news. Bryn just emailed back, 'A hug . . . a wonderful hug!!!'

Now came the hard part. It was all very well to spend five days in a conference centre being enthused by professional inspirers, but how were we actually going to survive the next two or three years running our own home education programme, seven days a week, fifty-two weeks a year? We needed money, staff, equipment and a specially adapted playroom. And, somehow, our 'normal' life with Edmond had to continue parallel to the Son Rise programme.

The Option people had recommended enlisting unpaid volunteers to help with the teaching, with each teacher doing a minimum of three two-hours sessions per week: through the sheer positive force of our enthoosiasm, we would find people willing to come for nothing and share Ollie's new adventure. Rosie and I were not so sure about that. Yes – we might get some voluntary help, but we were also going to have to pay some of our staff. And find them. Helpers came and went. They moved away, went to university, got jobs, got pregnant . . . At the moment we only had a small nucleus of potential teachers. Either Andy or Jo, who had worked on the Lovaas programme, could probably be enrolled; and we had Kate, employed since the previous summer by Social Services. But she was only with Ollie for six hours a week. Siri, the family link worker, would still take Ollie out for regular play sessions, but didn't want to get involved in the Son Rise programme. We needed more people. And more money. We needed more support from Social Services and, now that Ollie was not at school, we had to persuade the Local Education Authority not only to sanction a highly unconventional educational programme unknown in Britain, but to help pay for it as well. Ollie's place at the Margaret Coates Unit, including the cost of taxi transport, had cost over £11,000 per year; why shouldn't some of that money be redirected to his new home education?

Serious lobbying was called for. First we needed the backing of autism experts. I wrote to our old friend Dr John Richer, in Oxford, and to Dr Rita Jordan at Birmingham University. She had made a comparative study of the Lovaas and Option methods of teaching autistic children and, despite some reservations, had made favourable comments about both. She and John Richer both agreed to write letters of support. As did Dr Kenneth Aitken in Edinburgh and, in Bristol, Dr Alan Kellas, who happened to be a great-nephew of Alexander Kellas, the famous mountaineering medic who died in Tibet during the British Everest Reconnaissance Expedition of 1921.

Next we enlisted our MP, Don Foster. We feared that, as a former mainstream educationalist, he might be hostile to the whacky Son Rise philosophy, but as soon as we met him in his smoke-filled Bath office (now, he assures me, smoke-free) we knew we had a powerful ally. 'Please understand,' he started, 'if I don't spend time saying how desperately sad all this is. I'm not here to offer sympathy: my job is to try and get things done.' He thanked us for our letter, which laid out exactly what we wanted and why. Then he said, 'I'll certainly write to the LEA in support. I also need to speak to the head of Special Education: I'll ring her on Monday.'

'That's fantastic,' Rosie said as we walked back to the car, 'the *power* of an MP – he can really make things happen.'

In the end, though, it lay in the hands of the education chiefs. Julie Taylor, Ollie's former headteacher, offered generously to back the Son Rise idea and at her suggestion we outlined our case in writing, stressing the uniqueness of Ollie's case.

26 January 1998

Mrs Julie Taylor
Head of Margaret Coates Unit
Fosseway Infant School

Dear Mrs Taylor

<u>Oliver Venables – annual review</u>

As you suggested, we are sending these written comments in preparation for the meeting on 4th February.

Although Ollie seemed gradually to be making progress at the Margaret Coates Unit, since he suffered a relapse of his leukaemia in the central nervous system last May, he has been on a more aggressive chemotherapy protocol, which has made it impossible for him to attend school regularly. The breakdown in routine has been extremely stressful for him and it has become obvious that, in his current state of health, he cannot cope with the demands of the Margaret Coates Unit and we do not feel that any other institution is suitable. However, we cannot just leave him doing nothing, as some of the time he is well enough to learn. We therefore wish for the time being to educate him at home.

Earlier this month we paid to attend a start-up training course run by the Option Institute. The course was excellent and convinced us that the Option Son Rise Programme is the best approach for Ollie's unique situation (he is the only child in this country with autism and leukaemia). The programme, which has been assessed favourably by Rita Jordan, is the only one we know of which can be used seven days a week, both at home and in hospital, and can run whether he is ill or well.

When Ollie is ill he cannot cope with the demands of a typical school-type programme, even at home, and this causes a lack of continuity, which as you know causes him great distress. That is why the Option approach seems to be the answer. It is particularly appropriate for Ollie for the following reasons:

1. By adopting a consistent approach with a regular team of helpers, Ollie's education can be continuous both at home and in hospital.
2. Predictable continuity will rebuild his confidence.
3. The unthreatening, child-centred method will compensate for the enormous stress of continuing medical treatment.
4. Because of Ollie's illness, we have to be with him for long spells of time, so it makes sense to have an educational programme designed specifically to be run by parents.

Ollie's chemotherapy still has over a year to run. If he has no further relapse and makes a good recovery we hope that he will be able to return to school. In the meantime, however, we feel the best solution would be for him to be educated at home, because any kind of institutional education could only be intermittent, recreating all the stress he suffered last term. We feel that the Option Son Rise Programme gives Ollie the best chance of a predictable, unthreat-

ening education, applicable whatever his health,
at home or in hospital. This continuity is vital
and we are prepared to work very hard to achieve
it. However, we cannot run the programme alone
and we will need additional helpers each to work
at least eight hours a week.

We would like to stress that we do not regard
this programme as an alternative to the Margaret
Coates Unit; we want to do it because Ollie's
leukaemia does not allow him to attend the unit,
and we hope sincerely that one day he will be able
to return.

Yours sincerely

Stephen and Rosie Venables

February 4th arrived and we all assembled in the head's
room. The meeting got off to a sticky start, with a lot
of talk about limited resources and the danger of estab-
lishing precedents. Then David Niven, head of the Social
Services team, interjected, 'We seem to be hearing a lot
of talk about what we can't do. Why don't we discuss
what we *can* do?'

'Good on you, David,' I thought gleefully.

'Ollie is a unique case,' he went on, 'and we need to
find imaginative, flexible solutions to his problems. The
Social Services would welcome a partnership with the
LEA.' Then he brought in his reinforcement, Niki Smith,
Ollie's actual social worker. Then Simon Lenton, the
ponytailed community paediatrician, added all the institutional clout of his consultant status, stressing the
disruptive effects of chemotherapy and the need for a
different kind of education. Hilary Gould, the tireless
social worker for Malcolm Sargent Cancer Care, made
an impassioned plea for Ollie to be given 'quality time'.
Jill Lambert, the speech and language therapist, stressed

the need for a consistent education which could be delivered both at home and in hospital.

It was fantastic: all these incredibly busy people making time to come to this meeting. All for one boy. And we wanted all that money to be set aside just for him. Yet again I was reminded of the huge *cost* of disability.

In the end we got the promise of ten hours paid help per week from Education, matched by ten hours from Social Services. It wasn't as much as we had asked for, but it was a valuable compromise. The following November we asked for an increase to thirty hours. Education money, were offered fifteen and, again with support from our MP Don Foster, pushed the LEA up to twenty-five.

At home meanwhile, we had been adapting Ollie's room. The Option principle is to make the playroom a place where the child feels completely safe and in control. There are no carpets to dirty, no precious china to break, no fences to escape over; there is no reason here to say 'No': the child is in charge. And free from distractions, so that the teacher – that other person trying to join the child's special world – becomes the most important thing in the room. However, the room was not completely empty. My mother donated some money for buying special toys. I built the recommended high shelves, too high for Ollie to reach easily, encouraging him to *ask* for specific toys. We ordered a six-foot-high wall mirror to maximise eye contact and to reinforce Ollie's sense of self; and a phenomenally expensive sheet of one-way mirror glass to replace a door panel, for discreet observation and training. My father built a set of plywood rostrum blocks and ramps. I hung a rope ladder from the ceiling. Marcel Wagner, a distant descendant of the composer, who runs a flooring business, donated a precious day to come over to Bath and fit the recommended padded linoleum floor – waterproof, gentle on the knees and, as instructed, in a plain pale colour devoid of distracting flecks or patterns. Ditto the walls, which were already a fairly neutral pale yellow.

All this cost money and again we were shameless in seeking funds from every possible charity and trust. We had already booked places for Rosie and two other helpers on a refresher 'Maximum Impact' training course in the summer, and the first available slot – August 1999 – to take Ollie and ourselves over to Massachusetts for a week's further 'Intensive' training and observation. The budget over the next eighteen months, excluding any payment to teachers, was just under £12,000 and all that money came from generous donors, ranging from the stranger who sent £10 after reading a newspaper article about Ollie, to the charitable trust which donated £2,000.

'Ask and it shall be given unto you.' Our local printing shop agreed to run off for nothing two hundred copies of the recruitment poster laid out by Rosie's graphic-designer sister, Nonie. The wording was cheesily provocative – 'Come and join Ollie in his adventure'; the picture was the best of a hundred frames shot in his newly adapted playroom, when Rosie and I spent a morning in the room clowning with Ollie, taking turns to shrug off English reserve and turn the room into a crazy theatre workshop. Ollie rode on our backs, escaped up his new rope ladder, stuck the empty waste-paper bin on our heads . . . and he *laughed* with infectious delight. The selected shot pictured Ollie and Rosie, laughing at each other, engaged one hundred per cent, through the rungs of the rope ladder – quintessence of attractive, zingy fun – reinforced by the wording which stressed that working with this autistic child was an opportunity *for the volunteer.*

The poster *did* attract some volunteers. But we also had to recruit proactively, through official channels. Through Social Services we found Adrienne, who had a real talent for the work. Through Bruno and Shena we met Matthew, an ex-pupil of Bruno's, who played the cello divinely but wanted to try something completely new. It was now spring, the programme was up and running, and Ollie was spending most of every day in the room, being introduced to increasing numbers of new people. Each new teacher was handed a shiny plastic dummy and a piece of towelling, then taken by Rosie into the room. At first they were told simply to sit and observe, trying to copy exactly what Ollie was doing.

Ollie was understandably defensive. He sat silently, dummy in mouth, staring into the middle distance, second finger of his right hand stroking with articulated precision a fold of his snuggly. The new teacher sat at a discreet distance, watching and copying, thinking, 'how clever – how brilliant to have discovered all by yourself this serene meditation.' (This talent of autistic people to create their own protective comfort is well documented. The autistic agricultural research scientist Temple Grandin, famous for her empathetic design of stress-reducing slaughterhouse systems, has described how she observed the comforting effect of firm pressure on cattle; and how, realising that she too drew comfort from a firm enclosing pressure, designed her own special squeeze machine, into which she climbs whenever she needs its reassurance.)

So we taught our teachers to respect Ollie's comforting rituals, knowing that sooner or later he might stand up and circle the room. And the teacher would follow. And perhaps, after a few turns of the room, Ollie would stop and look at himself in the mirror. And, if he were feeling brave, he might allow himself a glimpse of the teacher's face – her direct gaze mediated protectively through the mirror – and, if he were feeling extra brave, he might let slip a tentative smile. Which was the cue for the teacher to return a bigger, more theatrical smile and say, perhaps, 'Lovely smiling, Ollie!'

Even with Rosie and me, Ollie often started sessions in defensive mode. Ten minutes might pass before the first tiny subcutaneous ripple at the corner of his mouth heralded a wish to communicate. With new teachers it could take several sessions. As Rosie told each new recruit, 'You must remember that for Ollie it requires great courage to look someone in the eyes – especially a complete stranger.' She made them stay low, walking on their knees when they followed him round the room. Matthew, a large man well over six feet tall, had to stay *lying* down and it took several sessions before Ollie would allow him even to sit up. But then the connection was made and Ollie's innate boisterousness burst through the protective shell. Soon he was riding high on Matthew's broad back, a gleeful knight spurring on his trusty steed, riding faster and faster round the room, master of his universe.

Matthew had a natural flair, helped by a healthy disregard for convention. A Larkhall friend told Rosie one day, 'I've just seen a very large man walking barefoot down to the bus stop with a dummy in his mouth. Ah, I thought, he must be something to do with the Venables.'

Our school sixth-formers were more conventional. I recruited them at the beginning of the summer term, visiting five different schools to give presentations. Public speaking was, after all, my job: if I couldn't persuade a few lively teenagers to come and join us I might as well give up.

I took a projector and opened with an arresting shot of my friend Ed Webster dangling over a man-eating crevasse at 22,000 feet on Everest, told them very briefly about my mountain adventures, then moved swiftly on to our infinitely bigger adventure with Ollie. Told them about his autism. And the leukaemia. How he nearly died. But also told them about his spirit, his courage, his laughter. Showed pictures of him playing in his room, laughing from his rope ladder, sticking a waste-paper bin on his father's head. Then explained the Son Rise principle and what we were trying to do with him. Stressed the rigorous observation and note-taking we had been taught by the Option people, the importance of our weekly team meeting, the chance to develop skills – we were offering an opportunity, not a duty.

The next stage was for potential volunteers to come to our house, observe Ollie through the one-way mirror, and have a pep talk from Rosie. She gave them more detail – enough detail to put most of them off. She also warned them unequivocally of the emotional risks: 'Although he can be incredibly difficult, people *like* Ollie. They become very fond of him. If you work with him, you will probably come to *love* him. But you need to know that there is a strong chance that his leukaemia will come back: it's quite likely that he will die. So you need to consider quite carefully how you would feel if that happened.'

We were asking a lot of these seventeen-year-olds. Most of them lost interest, but we did end up with five sixth-formers – Annabelle, Jo, Elise, Sarah and Michael – who proved brilliant. At a purely functional level, they were reliable and punctual. But they were also bright

and imaginative. And able to shrug off potential embarrassment with remarkable maturity. Rosie warned all
new women teachers not to wear low-cut shirts: Ollie
could not resist a finely articulated cleavage, and the
bigger the bosom the bigger his delight. Once a rapport
was established, gleeful energy allowed to blossom, he
might suddenly try an exploratory grope; and even
complete strangers were not immune: dashing out of the
room one day to find a potential volunteer off guard on
the landing, he thrust his hand straight down her low-
cut dress. We never saw her again.

The girls who decided to stick it out coped brilliantly,
rebuffing any inappropriate attention with firm indif-
ference. Michael was presented with a different potential embarrassment. During his very first session in the
room he was sitting at Ollie's little table. Beside him sat
Rosie, a woman probably the same age as his mother,
giving a bit of feedback. Ollie was not feeling at all
nervous or withdrawn today. In fact he was quite manic,
positively *seeking* attention, circling provocatively round
the table, eyeing the seventeen-year-old and his mentor.
Suddenly, with no warning, he thrust himself between
Michael and Rosie, pulled down his shorts and flopped
a provocative penis down on the table – 'What d'you
think of that, then?'

'Poor Michael,' Rosie laughed at supper that night. 'I
felt so sorry for him. Anyway, he was magnificent. He
didn't bat an eyelid. If he gets into his medical school
he's going to be a brilliant doctor.'

Michael *did* go to medical school the following year
and we were confident that he would be a very sensitive physician. We had become increasingly demanding
of the medical profession, encouraged by the Option
staff to be more forceful on Ollie's behalf: one of the
central tenets of the Option philosophy was to be

unashamed in going after what you want. This didn't mean you had to be rude and aggressive – you just needed to be assertive.

Things had not gone very well at the Royal United Hospital. It was partly personal chemistry; partly, we felt, an inability of the system to give Ollie the kind of care he needed. Things came to a head early in 1998 when Ollie's neck seemed to be hurting. Rosie was fairly certain that something was wrong with his portacath – with the invisible tube inserted into the subclavian vein. An X-ray was considered but then dismissed and the problem was attributed to a side effect of the drugs. So vincristine, one of the most powerful and effective chemotherapy drugs, known occasionally to cause a stiff neck, was withdrawn. But the problems with the porta-cath persisted; soon after that another chemotherapy drug, instead of flowing into the vein, oozed out of the portacath into the surrounding tissue. The toxic fluid eventually burnt away the skin and back at home we noticed that the little portacath drum – the short cut to a vein leading straight to the heart – was exposed to the open air.

Rosie had a scary drive to Bristol for an emergency operation to remove the emerging portacath. As the surgeon pulled the plastic tube out of the vein where it had lodged for two years, he was startled to find that it was badly rucked. No wonder Ollie had been so uncom-fortable. Rosie's instinct had been correct.

A few days later I took Ollie back to Bristol to have a new portacath fitted. He would need a cannula inserted into his hand for the anaesthetic. The operation was on a Saturday, late in the afternoon. None of the team had met Ollie before and I explained to the anaesthetist that it was vital to keep everything quiet in theatre. I also requested very specifically that she should come up to the ward and fit Ollie's cannula before he arrived in theatre.

In the event, the porters arrived suddenly, without warning, to whisk us down to theatre, where Ollie was greeted by a phalanx of loud, chatty, green-masked strangers. He whimpered, 'Noo, noo, noo,' and scrabbled up into the corner of the trolley, trying to escape. I calmed him, then persuaded him to hold out his hand as I wiped off the numbing lidocaine cream. But he was watching warily. The moment Chief Green Mask started to unwrap the sterile pack and reveal the cannula, he shrank back, clutching my shoulders.

'Yes, I know, Ollie. Just try to be brave.' I stroked him. Told him again how brave he was. But he just shook his head, 'Noo, noo.'

'You'll have to hold him,' said the anaesthetist.

'Well, I'll try,' I agreed, hating my weakness. But Ollie just screamed and pulled his arm away.

'Look, this isn't working. I'm afraid we'll just have to give him gas,' said the anaesthetist. 'It'll be very quick.' Ollie kicked and thrashed and cried, fighting hopelessly to try and fend off the cold rubber mask. But as it sealed around his face he was forced to gulp gas and his terrified eyes closed. As the anaesthetist pushed the cannula into his now inert hand I left the room, trembling with anger – anger at myself, at my weakness in allowing these people to terrify my son.

An hour or so later I was called down to the recovery room. Ollie was kicking and screaming. Later he calmed a little, but as we wheeled him up to the ward he started screaming again. Back in his cubicle, he refused to settle on the bed, but jumped down and rushed screaming into the corridor outside. I ran after him and carried him back. Again he jumped up, pushing as I blocked the door, beating his hands against me, his face blotchy

crimson-white with furious terror. Then he started grabbing at the bandage on his left hand. I pinioned both
his arms but he wrenched himself free, pulling frenziedly
at the bandage, ripping out the cannula, flinging it on
the floor. As I wrestled him onto the bed, crimson blood
spattered my shirt. I held him tight, whispering, 'I know,
I know, Ollie: it's horrible, I know.'

At last the screams subsided into exhausted blue-
lipped sobs. I handed him his dummy and snuggly, and
pressed the play button on his cassette player. Soft femi-
nine voices began to intone:

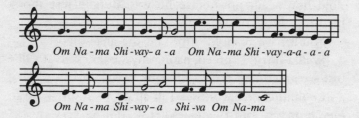

Om Na-ma Shi-vay-a-a   Om Na-ma Shi-vay-a-a-a-a

Om Na-ma Shi-vay-a   Shi-va Om Na-ma

Then again – 'Om Nama Shivaya-a-a . . .' and again and
again. Loulou had given him this tape and its repetitive
legato always had a soothing, hypnotic effect. Peaceful
at last, he lay on his side, eyes open, focused meditatively
on his pale thin fingers stroking the folded edge of towel.
He lay like that for perhaps an hour, absorbed totally in
his own autotherapy, until the terror demons were
banished and he could drift safely to sleep.

I was so angry about the fear suffered by Ollie that
I wrote a formal letter of complaint to Professor Mott.
I could understand perfectly well the reasons for the
gas mask – last operation on a Saturday evening,
theatre about to close for the weekend, necessity to

sedate the child quickly and safely, etc etc – but if we were going to continue treating Ollie's leukaemia we had to avoid subjecting him to that kind of anguish. If the anaesthetist had done as I asked, Ollie could have been enabled to drift fearlessly to sleep.

The timing of this Bristol fiasco was ironic because, assertiveness reinforced by our Option training, we had just arranged to switch all Ollie's oncology care from Bath to Bristol. Professor Mott sent back a very conciliatory letter, and with all Ollie's subsequent treatments we never again had to go through that kind of trauma. In fact people were so patiently indulgent towards the awkward Venables family that I sometimes felt guilty about the excessive demands we made of the National Health Service. But then I reminded myself that our job – our *only* job – was to do what was best for Ollie; nothing else mattered.

The long haul continued and Rosie often had to nurse Ollie on her own while I disappeared to earn money. In March an intensive chemotherapy week coincided unfortunately with one of my mini lecture tours. All day on Tuesday I chaired a meeting of the Mount Everest Foundation in London; then in the evening I compèred the London premiere of the new Everest IMAX movie, with a marathon party to follow. Over breakfast on Wednesday morning I interviewed Chris Bonington for a forthcoming book, then drove up to Newcastle for an evening lecture, followed by another lecture at St Andrews University on the Thursday evening. By that stage Rosie was desperate for help and she phoned to ask if I could return straight away. So, limiting myself reluctantly to a single post-lecture pint of beer, I set off at eleven p.m. to drive 450 miles back home.

★

At home we had to ensure that Ollie's special room was a secure haven. Apart from now rare visits to hospital, he spent most of every day here, from breakfast to bedtime. (Later, when it became increasingly difficult for Edmond to sleep in the same room, Ollie's bed was moved into the playroom, so that he lived here almost twenty-four hours a day.) We did however, diverge from the Option formula by building garden breaks into the timetable: even if this diluted the intensity of one-to-one interaction I was adamant that Ollie must have time in the fresh air. He also had time each week to go out for runs and walks with Siri. Each garden session was followed by a snack upstairs, to ease the transition back to his room. Breakfast, lunch and supper he also ate in his room, with whichever teacher was on duty sitting beside him on the floor.

So the room became his world and we tried to enter that world with eager, joyful, sensitive, creative enthusiasm. Often I failed – failed that leap of the imagination. But at other times, when I managed to be one hundred per cent present, living totally in the moment, I was able to delight in every nuance of Ollie's play. In my notes for the team meeting on 13th May I recorded three sessions with Ollie – half an hour on Friday, one and a half hours on Saturday and one hour on Tuesday. Although he took refuge behind his dummy for eighty per cent of the time and spent about forty per cent of the time stroking his snuggly, he also gave me spontaneous eye contact for over sixty per cent of the time. On the Tuesday he imitated me, playing the triangle, bamboo rattle and xylophone, exercising fine motor skills. Gross motor skills – and his greatest motivation – were demonstrated by climbing onto my back, stamping out rhythms on the floor, bouncing on the trampoline and climbing alone onto the top shelf. Genuine interaction was achieved through piggybacks, running round in circles and five minutes' shared play with his toy cars. New for me, that week, was Ollie bouncing on the trampoline, circling around me as I sang 'Round and Round the Garden', playing with the musical instruments and looking at both himself and me in the mirror.

Everyone had to keep detailed records of their sessions. From their notes, we recorded at the Wednesday evening meeting every activity which Ollie had enjoyed that week: being chased, having his feet eaten by a human crocodile, looking in the mirror, being looked at, playing with water, emptying containers. However bizarre, however unconstructive an activity might seem, we had to join in enthusiastically – even if we were just tipping Duplo bricks out of a box. At this particular meeting we then discussed possibilities for quiet activities – looking at books, playing with toy animals (getting them to pretend talk) singing, feet and hand games . . . Rosie then reminded everyone to reward Ollie for his brave efforts at engaging with us: gasping with surprise when he did something funny, telling him 'what a lovely smile!' or 'what gorgeous eyes you've got!', being genuinely excited by his games, singing songs about him looking at us. And she reminded everyone that a few months ago, Ollie had not been able even to *look* at strangers; now he was not only tolerating all these new people, he was actually *enjoying* them. This Son Rise experiment had changed his life profoundly.

The Wednesday team meetings were deliberately upbeat. But they were also a chance to try to resolve problems. Ollie loved to climb up onto the top toy shelf, then to jump down into the arms of whichever teacher happened to be with him. But with new volunteers he might spend an entire two-hour session sitting on the shelf, aware that most of the women could not actually reach him. (Nor were most of them strong enough to lift him down.) In the end we decided that I would have to build an additional shelf, closing the Ollie-sized gap, forcing him to stay at floor level, available for communication.

With chemotherapy drugs still irritating his bladder, he needed frequently to go out to the lavatory on the landing. This served a useful purpose − by waiting for him to attempt the word 'open' before sliding the high bolt on the playroom door, we could encourage him to speak − but it also became an increasingly distracting obsession, to the point where he was going constantly in and out of the door. In the end Rosie telephoned the Option Institute for advice. 'Get a Portapotty,' they told her, so off she went to the local camping shop and Ollie's new flushing chemical throne was installed in the playroom. Now, if he needed a pee or a pooh, there was no need to go outside. It just fell to Rosie or me, every few days, to relish the delightful task of emptying and cleaning the Portapotty.

There was just one memorable occasion when Ollie managed to unscrew the main valve and empty the contraption himself. We were having tea in the kitchen, ignoring the normal audio-buzz coming through the intercom from Ollie's room, until we heard the voice of Elise, one of the sixth-formers, cutting through Ollie's manic laughter with a slightly harassed request for help. We rushed upstairs to find her marooned in a sea of raw sewage, calm, smiling and determined that nothing would deflect her from 'choosing happiness'.

The summer weeks passed. Elise survived her trial by sewage. She and the other sixth-form volunteers became full members of the team. Then we were joined by Alison Jones, a young mother who was expecting her second child and worked with Ollie right up to the last few days of her pregnancy. Every timetable slot was filled so that all day, every day, Ollie 'worked' in his room, meditative silence alternating with boisterous noise. At the team meetings we noted his decreasing reliance on self-stim-ulating rituals and his growing confidence. But Rosie had also to remind people not to expect too much. On 15th July she wrote in the record book: 'Ollie has just finished his latest intensive chemo and is neutropenic, so he is not feeling very well. He is also on steroids, which can make him very manic and very hungry. If he seems unhappy, check on when he last had paracetamol – he may have a headache.' Two weeks later he felt much better. Everyone commented on how much more he was talking, how affectionate he was becoming, how he was starting again to say 'Mummy'. On 5th August we noted that he had reached the least traumatic part of the chemo cycle and was very communicative and cuddly. But there was also a reminder not to push him: 'If he wants to lie quietly, just be a calm comforting presence – don't feel you have to rush him into exciting activities.'

'Inspiring growth' could wait. For the moment it was quite enough just to know that Ollie was *happy*. 'It's incredible how different he is,' observed Rosie. 'At *last* he can do what he wants. Do you remember how thrilled he was when he first saw me copying him – sticking a jigsaw piece in my mouth – and his little eyes lit up with surprise as he thought, "She's doing it too – it's all right!" and he was thrilled. If he wants to bite his toys he can. If he wants to sit on the shelf for two hours he can. If he wants spend all day emptying cans he can. And it's working: now that he feels safe he *is* actually starting to do more constructive play. And he's letting us join in. He's allowing complete strangers to come and sit in his room . . . he's just completely transformed.'

That week Rosie took Matthew and Adrienne, two of

our star teachers, to the Option refresher course in London, keen to build on their enthusiasm. When they returned Matthew began to lead some of the team meetings. As well as thrashing out practical details, we had to do a lot of confidence-boosting and reinforcing of 'attitude'. There were theatre workshop sessions – how many different things can you do with this toy brick? How many different ways can we celebrate success? What new songs can we learn? – and visualisations where, for instance, Matthew (who had a charismatic flair for these things) might lead us along a path, through a dark mysterious forest to a cave where we discovered Ollie, sitting in a glow of warm candlelight, utterly calm, happy and serene.

Often Edmond would sneak downstairs to peep at us from behind the piano. 'What about me?' the five-year-old was saying. 'Why all this attention for Ollie?' Rosie had explained to Edmond what we were trying to do with Ollie. Often she took him into the playroom to share supper with his brother and to join his play. And she reminded him of all the things he could enjoy which were denied to Ollie. But however much Edmond understood that, he was bound at times to resent the way our lives revolved so unmistakably around the programme.

I too sometimes questioned the intense focus on Ollie, felt almost embarrassed – 'how presumptuous to expect all these people to pour all that loving energy into *my son*' – but then reminded myself that, whether they were being paid or were doing it voluntarily, they had all *chosen* to work with him. We just had to be grateful for that dedication and provide the leadership to sustain everyone's belief in the programme. In fact that leadership fell increasingly to Rosie, particularly in the autumn of 1998 as I prepared to leave again for the Himalaya.

Chapter Nine

We came round a corner and there it was – that immense curtain of ice, eight thousand feet high, pale blue, hanging in the sky, filling the head of the valley. Then clouds shifted to reveal a final pyramid, another three thousand feet higher. Ten years earlier I had stood there, on top of the world; and now I was returning, not to climb the mountain, but just to walk to the foot of its mighty Kangshung Face on this anniversary trek.

This was a job, I kept telling myself – half my trek-leader's fee had already been paid into our bank account and the other half was due on my return home – but it was also a nostalgic indulgence, a celebration, an escape. This eastern approach to Chomolungma, the mountain we call Everest, was a journey of pure enchantment, crossing high passes to enter one of Tibet's most sacred *beyuls* – special sacred landscapes. On the pastures high above the Kama river the ground was luminous with cerulean autumn gentians. Late that afternoon we reached another crest where stone cairns were silhouetted against a backlit vision of glittering braided torrents, pouring down from one of the greatest mountain amphitheatres on earth.

We descended to the valley bed and then climbed for two days, to arrive, panting in the sharp crystal air seventeen thousand feet above sea level, at the sparse meadow which ten years earlier had been my home. Here, in the spring of 1988, Sherpa Pasang Norbu and Kasang Tsering had tended our base camp. From this haven we had set off across a glacial rubble wasteland to advance base, and then on, in a series of tentative exploratory probes, up the immense wall above. To this meadow, with its welcoming smell of damp spring earth, we – Ed, Paul, Robert and I, accompanied by doctor Mimi and photographer Joe – had returned on an afternoon of soft redemptive rain from the greatest adventure of our lives.

Ten years on, tears of sweet remembrance pricked my eyes. Our Everest adventure, with its simple routines of rock and ice and ropes and karabiners, its harsh physical effort and its sense of wondrous discovery, now seemed so innocent and naïve. Life had become so much more complicated, the adventure infinitely more challenging.

The next day some of the anniversary trek team accompanied me three or four miles up the glacier for a closer look at the towering battlements and ice gargoyles of our 1988 'Neverest Buttress'. Then we all headed back down the Kama valley and up to the turquoise lakes of Shurima – the Lama's Throne – before leaving the *beyul* by another high pass decked with prayer flags. We drove round to the famous Rongbuk monastery on the north side of Everest, where Bill Norton donated to the monks a photograph of his father being blessed at the same monastery, with George Mallory, in 1924. Then drove east to the great monastic centres of Shigatse, Gyantse and Lhasa, before flying south, back over Everest, to Kathmandu, where thousands of beautifully dressed Hindu children thronged the streets for the festival of Diwali. Here I spent every spare scrap of cash on propitiatory gifts of lapis lazuli and silver and leopard's eye to take home to my beautiful beleaguered wife.

I arrived on Wednesday evening, envisaging a warm

welcome at the weekly team meeting, followed by a celebratory supper. But the sitting room was empty. Downstairs, Rosie was collapsed on the kitchen sofa, ill with flu. Matthew was with her. 'Sorry, darling, I'm afraid I haven't done any supper and if you want some wine you'll have to go and buy some. Kind Matthew has been helping out. I couldn't face a team meeting this evening.'

The boys were both asleep in bed. Edmond was fine. Ollie's programme was going well and there had been no dramas with his chemotherapy. But Rosie was exhausted – ground down by the relentless strain of running the whole show on her own for four weeks, without a moment's respite. Month-long foreign trips were a bad idea.

We had booked a break, thank goodness, planning to go away for Edmond's half-term holiday, just three days after my return. Overnight care was fixed, Rosie's daytime slots filled, timetables finalised. On Saturday morning, anxious not to upset Ollie, we slipped quietly away, driving through autumnal floods to Nantcol – a house in the Rhinog mountains, near Harlech, which I had not visited for years.

It was a chance at last for Rosie and me to give Edmond undivided attention. A chance to sit and read to him beside a glowing fire, listening to the rain lashing the ancient slate roof. A chance to take him scrambling up the flanks of Rhinog Fawr. A chance for him to smell the peat and heather. A chance, in his brand new size-three rubber rock slippers, to balance and edge up the blocky roughness of the Harlech gritstone. A chance to escape the gates and locks and timetables and special menus and meetings around which life in Larkhall revolved.

On the Wednesday afternoon, in pouring rain, we explored the old manganese mines just below Nantcol.

Edmond and I were descending a ramp of slick rock, ahead of Rosie, when we heard a scream. I climbed back up and found her whimpering with pain. She had slipped onto her outstretched right hand, cracking the wrist with an excruciating Colles fracture. Back at the house we telephoned a doctor who advised us to head for Dolgellau. So south we drove, down the coast, through Barmouth, up the estuary and over the bridge, reaching the hospital an hour later.

'Oh, no,' lilted the duty sister, 'no X-ray facility *here*. You'll have to go to Porthmadog.' So back into the car. Back north, this time up the east side of the Rhinogs. Headlights piercing the driving rain. Lorry spume lashing the windscreen. Eyes straining through the darkness to read the Celtic signposts. After an hour we roll into Portmadoc, to be told there is no accident and emergency department. 'Oh no – it's either Wrexham or Bangor you'll be needing.'

Back into the car. Edmond tired and fractious. Rosie weeping with the pain. Another hour of relentless black rain. At last we sweep into the new Bangor hospital, hopes raised by deceptive modernity. Yes – this is where we should have been directed four hours ago. There *is* an X-ray department. Edmond and I sit in a bleak waiting room, assailed by a televisual orgy of post-watershed violence, while Rosie disappears. She is seen by a young South African doctor. He has to reduce the fracture, which will be very painful. The plasterer has gone home, so he will put the plaster on himself.

She emerged an hour later, heavily drugged, arm encased in gleaming plaster of Paris. During the ninety-minute drive home through torrential rain, she kept asking, 'Where are we? Where are we going?' And repeatedly demanded sustenance: 'I must have soup.' So, at two o'clock in the morning, when we at last got back to Nantcol, I sat her in front of a bowl of soup, tried to hold her head up, and told her to get drinking.

'Why have you given me soup?'

'Because you kept asking for soup.'

'When did I ask for soup? How late is it?'

I gave up on the soup and put her to bed. Only in the morning, when the morphine wore off, did the pain return. By the time we got back to Bath, three days later, it had focused exquisitely on the very point of the fracture. Something seemed to be pressing hard on the broken bone. The local orthopaedic experts did an X-ray, assured her that the fracture had been correctly reduced and persuaded her not to risk damaging the mend by changing the plaster: she should keep it on for six weeks.

She endured stoically for four weeks, then announced she couldn't stand it any longer. So I rummaged in the garden shed for the Felco secateurs and applied finest Swiss precision engineering to the grimy graffitied plaster, snipping carefully up the side of Rosie's withered arm. The relief was immediate and as we peeled back the plaster we found a hard, angular ruck of gauze folded against the precise line of the fracture.

Unnecessary pain from shoddy plastering was depressing. Far more upsetting, when we returned from Wales, was to hear from Matthew that he didn't want to work with Ollie any more. He couldn't give any clear reason: he had just had enough, lost interest, run out of steam. All that charismatic enthusiasm – all that magic energy which had so delighted Ollie in the playroom – had burnt out. Rosie realised, now that she had been running the Son Rise programme for over six months, that that was going to be the biggest, most draining, challenge – sustaining the enthusiasm and belief of our helpers. And each time someone left, a replacement had to be trained from scratch.

Wendy Morris had already turned up while I was away in Tibet. Recruited by Ollie's social worker, Niki, Wendy proved to have real staying power. She herself had been a social worker in London. Now in Bath she was doing part-time trampoline instruction at the city sports centre, including the class Edmond attended every Saturday morning. She was robust and happy to operate on the weird fringe. But also she had the kind of quiet, patient, compassionate serenity we were looking for, and the confidence which allowed her to be trained by Rosie – a younger woman – without taking umbrage: there was no ego to flatter or seduce with the gratification of instant success.

That was good, because with Ollie the rewards were subtle and fleeting. Three years on from contracting leukaemia, bombarded with radiation and cytotoxic drugs, his abilities to 'develop' and 'progress' were still very shaky. There was no dramatic, forceful, ascending graph – just a wavering line with a faintly discernible upward trend. Our helpers had to eschew all the popular management clichés about growth and progress and definable goals; rather than make their satisfaction contingent on 'success', they had to savour every moment for its own sake, 'be present', follow every tiny, enigmatic behavioural nuance of this mercurial child and take delight in the minutest achievement, even if that achievement was just a fleeting smile of recognition.

That was asking a lot of our helpers. At the end of December another of our star teachers, Adrienne, disappeared without notice, leaving a gap in the timetable. The gap was plugged and the programme continued, providing a sustainable structure for life in Grosvenor Terrace. We rejoiced at Ollie's increasing ability to accept strangers into his life, his faith in fellow human beings restored. He became more confident and more playful. During his now rare visits to hospital, as the leukaemia treatment approached its end, doctors and nurses commented on his increasing eye contact.

He was also now much more energetic, thriving on a completely dairy-free and gluten-free diet. It was expensive – soya yogurt, for instance, costs much more than the milk equivalent and gluten-free flour is hideously expensive – and it required a lot of effort; almost everything had to be cooked from scratch. But, given our increasing knowledge about the toxic additives poured into most processed food and the inability of the autistic metabolism to handle those toxins, we were better off cooking with raw materials, including lots of vegetables and lots of meat and fish, enlivened with herbs and spices. Ollie loved strong flavours. He also loved fish. And he was heartily carnivorous. On Sundays he usually came down to the kitchen to join Rosie, Edmond and me for Sunday lunch, devouring hunks of roast lamb or chicken and, given half a chance, picking the carcass clean afterwards. For pudding he usually had fruit, yoghurt, jelly or plain chocolate.

The hard thing was to keep this relentless culinary production line on track. Ruthlessly efficient, Rosie drew up a two-week-menu plan, giving Ollie sufficient variety and us a clear idea of exactly what to cook, when. She asked Tony, our local greengrocer, if he would deliver fruit and vegetables. She organised another kind volunteer for a while to do the supermarket shopping, leaving her free for the constant round of recruiting, training and feedback, with just an occasional window of opportunity for time with Edmond.

My Everest trek had given me a break and my other work provided frequent escapes from autism. For Rosie the pressure was relentless. So at the end of 1998 I phoned up her brother, Jake, and asked if his company could offer a good deal on a week's sunshine. He was predictably generous and organised a very affordable week in Tobago for Rosie. Then, in February 1999, he took both Rosie and Edmond to Antigua for a week's Caribbean indulgence.

In March I took Ollie into Bristol for his final round of intensive chemotherapy. He loved riding in the back of the car, comforted by the engine's rhythm and the familiar, predictable view out of the window. Charlcombe Lane, Lansdown racecourse, the long line of beeches silhouetted on the hill above Wick, Junction 18, the M4, the M32, the now nearly finished new children's hospital and the final steep climb up St Michael's Hill . . . these were the familiar reassuring elements of our personal landscape.

At Oncology Daybeds they always gave Ollie a smiling welcome and they always had a private treatment room ready, obviating any need for him to cause mayhem amongst the 'normal' children in the main ward. Every time without fail he took an opportunistic swipe at the forbidden glutenous biscuits on the nurses' station, as I herded and jollied him into the treatment room. There, sticking as far as possible to Option principles, we allowed him to be in charge, turning on taps, indulging his passion for water play, making a terrible mess for three hours while cytotoxic drugs and restorative fluids were pumped through a long line into his portacath.

Then one day in March 1999 it all came to an end. Tony Oakhill told us that for the moment Ollie would continue to have occasional blood checks, with clinic visits at increasing intervals. We all knew that the odds on another relapse were high, and that with each relapse the odds on a complete cure lengthened drastically; but for the moment Ollie was free from the relentless cycle of oncology. He looked fit and strong and we had to base our life on the assumption that he would stay that way.

Spring. Again the glistening willow raindrops swelled and softened to downy yellow. Again we were startled by the sudden speed of the horse chestnut's sticky buds bursting into leaf. My Australian Sarmiento companion, Tim Macartney-Snape, came to stay on my birthday. We spent the morning climbing in the Wye valley, then returned to the garden, where Ollie was playing on the mound with a young Andalusian woman called Maite, yet another new helper in the long line of recruits.

We took Edmond for an early evening walk up Solsbury Hill, our closest escape from Bath's muggy pollution. The boys had both been coming up here since they were babies. Countless times I had run all the way down from its flat summit, a boy in each hand, leaping over grassy anthills; slithering, sliding, falling; during winter bogging down in the quagmire we called Passchendaele; reinserting tiny feet into tiny wellington boots; then in the next field waiting patiently while Ollie poked his finger meticulously, fascinatedly, in every single cowpat; then running on, down, down, down to Larkhall, where we would strip off drenched mud-caked clothes and go upstairs for a hot bath.

But today Passchendaele was dry and the first skylarks were singing invisibly above the buttercup summit of Little Solsbury. Tim gave Edmond a guiding hand as he solved a rock-climbing problem on the little limestone outcrop near the top. Then we returned to Larkhall, where Ollie was now back in his room, playing with Maite. A few days later the Social Services team came to make a video of Rosie working in the room with Ollie, to show to future potential recruits.

Ollie wears red tracksuit bottoms and the indestructible crocodile-patterned polo shirt which I bought three years earlier in Cape Town. His hair is thick and glossy with a slight wave and, approaching his eighth birthday, he has new oversized teeth and gaps in the front of his mouth, obscured for most of the time by his trademark dummy. Rosie follows him on her knees, circling the room, also with a dummy in her mouth. Suddenly Ollie takes her hand and she exclaims, 'Oh – taking my hand – that's nice!' He smiles. Then drags his little blue chair over to the window and climbs up, staring through the whitewashed glass at the opaque whiteness outside. Then leans across to Rosie to be lifted down. Then sits on the chair.

Rosie sits beside him on the floor and he holds out a foot to be stroked. He picks up a toy animal, holding it fastidiously between thumb and third finger. Rosie goes and gets her own animal, then returns to Ollie, holding the animal with one hand and stroking his foot with the other.

There is an atmosphere of calm contemplation. Then Ollie turns to Rosie. She gives him a beaming smile and he smiles back. Trying to initiate language, she asks, 'Shall I squeeze feet? Do you want me to squeeze? Shall I? Squeeze? Squeeeeeeze?' Ollie makes an approximate sound, so immediately she squeezes both feet, which he loves. Then she tries a different tack: 'You want more? More?' Ollie laughs, then pulls out his dummy to say 'Mmuh'. Immediately she takes his two long slender feet in her hands.

Ollie swings round off the chair to kneel opposite Rosie, taking her hands, all the while looking into her face, smiling and burbling. She responds, 'That's nice: you're squeezing my arm. Squeeze.'

Then she stops. Ollie gives her an importuning look: 'Unh . . . unh −'

'More?'

'Mmh −'

'More?'

And this time he says a clearer Mmuh, and she takes his feet in her hands again. They continue this game for a while, then suddenly he flings himself to the floor, grabs his snuggly, and settles into the foetal position. Rosie lies behind him, snuggled into the same position. They stay like this for a minute or two, then suddenly Ollie leaps to his feet and a new activity begins . . .

This was a child who six years earlier, before neural unravelling set in, had been talking in sentences and starting to read. On the face of it we had little progress to report. There had been no sudden, biblical bursting back into speech − barely even a repeat of the incremental learnings achieved during the behavioural Lovaas experiment. But we had to avoid those kinds of comparisons − forget about who Ollie wasn't and celebrate who he *was*. We had to admire his serenity and emulate his delight in tiny, apparently inconsequential, details. We had to cherish his laughter, thank him for every smile. And applaud his gigantic efforts to articulate words, as he tried so hard to make the necessary connections between brain and facial muscles. Above all, we had to be thankful that, after all the trials of the last three years, he seemed happy.

Rosie, in particular, was thrilled by what our Option training had done for Ollie. 'It really has made the most profound difference. If you think how miserable Ollie was that Christmas, before we went on the course . . .

I don't think he trusted anyone any more. Do you remember how he couldn't even bear to look at 'me? Hardly let me even touch him? And now, he's just so much more happy and confident and cuddly. He even *hugs* me again.'

Inspired by the Social Services team, I took more videos of Ollie that summer – not in his room, but roaming in the garden during his breaks from 'work'. The first clip is from mid-June, soon after Ollie's eighth birthday.

We find him in the kitchen, checking the dishwasher for any leftover scraps of food. Then he fills a cup with water and sidles out to the garden, drinking on the hoof, dummy temporarily hooked over his little finger. Then he returns to the kitchen and grabs a bottle of sun lotion, running off with a chuckle of naughty delight.

He runs barefoot, legs swishing the lush day-lily fronds. Round the corner, glancing backwards to check that he is being chased, past the metallic purple allium globes. Through the arch, past a luscious clump of blue irises, down under the pergola, which drips roses. Another provocative backward laugh, as he leaps down two steps, past the swaggering Régale lilies and *Rosa mundi*. He races round the mound then heads further down the garden to the climbing frame, where he balances four feet off the ground, feet stretched heel to toe along the narrow metal bar.

He looks up at the willow fencing, long since reinforced with chicken wire and extended twelve feet high to thwart repeated escape attempts. Beside the Lambrook our young tulip tree is palely luminescent against the darkening horse chestnut where a thrush calls, 'Pwhee pwhee . . . cchh cchh . . . terteeetee terteetee . . . nadeep nadeep nadeep . . .' A pigeon coos. Ollie rocks on the frame, sucking the lid of the sun-lotion bottle, holding its base delicately in outstretched fingers. He looks along the bottle at the dappled garden. Then suddenly exclaims in a joyous crescendo, 'Ooh blaiyah . . . num mum nyum mummm . . . eryah yaiee yaiee *yeh*!'

He jumps down and runs back up the path. Later the sequence is repeated, this time with an empty gin bottle. It is the same bottle I brought back recently from a business trip. Gordon's Export. 80 proof. A whole litre – an unopened treat. Until Ollie tipped the lot into the day lilies. Wendy noted that on this occasion Stephen, despite all his intensive training with the Option Institute, did not 'choose happiness'.

There were other tippings. There were tulip bulbs which failed mysteriously to sprout in the spring; only much later, when I dug them out and smelt the oily fumes of white spirit, did I realise what Ollie had done to them. There was the tub of tomato plants at Number Three, watered comprehensively with creosote when Ollie escaped one day to rampage amongst the neighbouring gardens. And the frequent postings – of carving knives into Jill's garden at Number Seven, of Duplo bricks into Tamara's garden at Number Five, and of my never-seen-again climbing boots, presumed washed down the Lambrook and out to the River Avon to drift inexorably westward to the Bristol Channel.

But today there are no gaps in the fence and Ollie is playing harmlessly with a now-water-filled gin bottle. He balances high on the climbing frame, both hands free to pour some of the liquid into his mouth. He tips the rest onto the ground, draining the bottle then holding it high in one outstretched hand, admiring its translucence as he half rotates on his perch, crying joyfully, 'Mmummrhaargh . . . mmummrhoorgh ghrghrghr . . .'

Later that summer . . . Ollie races down the path. Then runs back up, with his slightly ungainly sideways lurch. He settles on the paved terrace outside the kitchen and takes a watering can over to the water butt. He gestures at the tap and shouts, 'Unhh, unhh, oiee!'

'Ollie – would you like some water? Yes?'

He turns round and smiles, 'Unhh.'

I show him how to turn on the tap. Then ask him to turn it off. He sprinkles some water from the can, then turns it round to drink from the spout. Then grabs his bike with the stabilisers, and rides it back and forth, rocking sideways and exclaiming, 'Byeoouhh . . . ohloiee ahaieeyoiee . . .' Then wheels it down the steps to the next paved terrace, where he plucks shiny crinkly leaves from the pittosporum bush. Then runs down to the climbing frame, where he hangs out on both arms, rocking, bouncing and laughing through his gappy front teeth.

A woman's voice approaches: 'Ollie – time to go in now.'

'Hah!' He laughs and shakes his head.

I say, 'Ollie. Ollie – I think *Alison's* coming. She wants to *play* with you.'

'Guh. Ahugh. Gaiee! Oiee-huh-huh.' He laughs uproariously and feels his tooth gap with an outstretched finger. Alison appears, a smiling face framed by ringlets, carrying her plateful of bait. 'I've got a *snack* for you, Ollie.' He jumps down with another laugh, runs past her and shoots up the garden path. Alison follows more sedately with the plate of jam-spread gluten-free biscuits, and a moment later both of them are settled on the second floor in Ollie's room.

August comes. Last year Edmond, taking an autistic lesson from Ollie, snapped every single bud off the day lilies. This year he has allowed them to mature and blossom into exuberant orange trumpets, complemented by the outrageous purple of clematis Jackmanii. Saturated colour under a powder blue sky. Edmond, with breastplate and spear, bosses Pasha on the mound. Ollie, with his shirt off, twin portacath scars still shiny on his chest, plays his own contented tricycle game behind the mound.

A September morning and Edmond, Pasha and Ollie all sit on the kitchen sofa. Bob Marley is playing on the hi-fi. Edmond tries to help Ollie with a matching game of coloured pegs in a board, but ends up doing most of it himself, while Ollie rocks contentedly to the music.

That evening Edmond and Rosie sit at the kitchen table painting brilliant rectangular colour patterns (Rosie is going through her grid phase – 'my little autistic obsession'). Ollie, his day's work finished, sits on the sofa, lost happily in the *Snowman* video. Anne Hambrick, an education student from the university whom Ollie adores, comes down from writing up her Son Rise teaching notes. As she makes for the door, Rosie says, 'Ollie – say goodbye to Anne,' and he looks up from the screen to mouth, 'Mhh-bhh.'

We spent almost the whole of that summer of 1999 at home. I was writing a book on the Panch Chuli Himalayan debacle, so I tried to put in at least four hours every morning, working in the quiet house of some friends, often driving Edmond to school before clocking on. He was doing quite well at school and liked his new Welsh form teacher – 'when she talks it's like flowers dancing'. That left Rosie to keep Ollie's routine running smoothly. But for one week we both escaped. To paradise. The previous summer I had been best man at the marriage of my South Georgia Expedition friend, Julian Freeman-Attwood, to Emmy. This year they invited us to join them at Emmy's father's gorgeous house on Corfu, for a week of tranquillity and sybaritic spoiling. Julian had known Ollie since he was born and had followed all his trials with great sympathy. He also knew how hard up we were and quietly sent a cheque towards the cost of extra childcare during our week away.

But as the day of our June departure drew close we began to wonder whether this was a good idea. Once again we were up late every night, typing out detailed instructions and timetables. Rosie was on the phone all day long, juggling extra helpers for both Ollie and Edmond, who would have to be driven to and from school and supervised during the evenings. Our South African friends Di and Ken, Rosie's most generous allies at Edmond's school, had now left Bath and moved to London, where Ken was busy building the Millennium Dome. Edmond's best friend Frank had also left with his parents. Most of the other parents seemed unhelpful, their generosity usually in inverse proportion to the size of the gigantic, chrome-plated four-wheel-drive tanks which they seemed to find necessary to get around Bath's narrow congested streets.

I had grown up in a milieu where children regularly stayed in each other's houses and shared car lifts, or bicycled. It was assumed that parents would help each other out. These Nineties mothers seemed very different. Attempts to share the ferrying to and from Edmond's gym class had already drawn surly responses from one mother, making Rosie reluctant to ask again for help; but I persuaded her to try. Surely they would understand how desperately she needed this break for just one week?

Not a bit of it. There was tittering outrage at the mothers' genteel coffee morning. Before setting off in their gleaming machines for a hard day's shopping, they despatched an emissary down to Larkhall to tell Rosie, 'Some of the other mothers are getting rather fed up with being used as a free taxi service.'

'Oh, are they? I'm so sorry to hear that.' Rosie fixed the nervous messenger with a charming smile and continued, 'Well . . . you can tell your friends that they are a lot of selfish bitches and that as far as I'm concerned they can all fuck off.'

In the end, seventy-year-old Bruno, despite a busy schedule rehearsing for his swansong performance of the Elgar Cello Concerto, offered heroically to do some of the lifts. Then Ollie's godmother Fiona offered to have Edmond to stay, said she would drive specially to his school morning and afternoon, and added gleefully that she would make a point of scowling at the offending mothers. Bless them all. We dashed to Gatwick to join the midnight package scrum, and collapsed onto our plane. Sitting next to me was a woman with candyfloss hair who asked if I had been to Corfu before.

'No,' I answered, 'not Corfu. In fact I haven't been to Greece at all for twenty years.'

'Greece?' she exclaimed. 'I thought we were going to Spain – I've changed all my money into pesetas.'

After two hours we were offloaded into the smoky hellhole of the Corfu arrivals lounge. But once our luggage was secured we were whisked away, down to the silent dawn sea front of Corfu town, where a motor launch was waiting. A throaty roar, and we were off, a white arrow slicing the sea, silver-smooth between blue mountains. After fifteen minutes we reached Kanonas. A little bay, with a jetty and eucalyptus leaves crackling on the pebble beach. Chattery birdsong amongst ancient olive trees. Leggy pelargoniums tumbling rampant over sculpted limestone. A fig tree pendulous with purple fruit. And a silent mosaic courtyard leading to our bedroom where white linen lay smooth and crisp under a great tented mosquito net.

I loved it, every minute of it. Lazy honey and yogurt breakfasts beside a burbling fountain. The walk to the pool, bare legs brushing the pungent rosemary, bees humming in a thyme lawn. Tubs of agapanthus. White-hot stone against a cobalt, topaz, sapphire sea. My first sailing for decades, skimming the waves in single-handed Lasers. And the faster thrill, new for me, of riding the speedboat's turquoise wake on juddering skis. The evening Bloody Marys, sharp and icy beneath the wisteria, looking out past billowy blue-grey olives to pencil-sharp cypresses dark against the bare gold hills of Albania, Julian enthusing eccentrically about bigger, remoter mountains in the far wilds of Tibet and Antarctica.

There were other treats that summer, adding a glow to our work with Ollie. I spent several evenings on the piano, accompanying Bruno as he rehearsed his Elgar. What a thrill to be allowed to play with this hugely experienced professional and one-time pupil of Casals! There was *Manon Lescaut* at Glyndebourne with Jake and Shan – a chance to suffer vicariously the desolation of Puccini's exquisitely sad final scene, before escaping to drink and laugh and enjoy our huge blessings. There was a weekend trip to Washington to do a talk at the Smithsonian with my old Everest friends Robert Anderson and Norbu Tenzing. Then, back in England, there was the eclipse of the sun, when all the Son Rise teachers had a day off and we made an 'alpine start', rising at three a.m. to beat the traffic and drive down to Devon. We arrived in good time and took Ollie and Edmond for a walk down to the beach. Then we returned to the viewing field we had selected, had a huge picnic brunch, and waited excitedly. At first it was disappointing – no darker than an average rainstorm. 'Is this *it*?' I asked scornfully.

'Just wait patiently, darling,' Rosie answered. 'Look how all the birds are going home to roost – I'm sure that something more is about to happen.'

Ollie stood eager and alert on a hay bale, watching, listening, smelling the air, mystified but entranced. And then suddenly the darkness fell on us like a great weight – a whole two-hour nightfall contracted into a few seconds. After a brief pause, far out to the west over Dartmoor, a fiery red sunrise, flickering between dark clouds, swept across the land, racing towards us. Prosaic daylight resumed and the magic ended. Exhilarated by what he had just witnessed – and noticing our momentary lapse in concentration – Ollie jumped down from his bale and ran laughing down the field, glancing back over his shoulder to check that Edmond and I were obliging with a chase.

A week later we took Ollie to Heathrow airport to rehearse our departure for America: our turn for a week's intensive training at the Option Institute had finally come. The money was raised, the course paid for and the flights booked. I had written to several airlines outlining the potential difficulties of flying with an autistic child and explaining exactly what we needed to do to minimise the stress for Ollie (and his fellow passengers). Ammy Sandhu at United Airlines had sent by far the most helpful response, so the dubious privilege of welcoming Ollie aboard fell to United Airlines.

On this dummy run, we simply drove to Heathrow and wheeled Ollie's pushchair into the main departure hall of Terminal Three, just to get him used to the huge crush of people, lights and noise. Ammy came down to introduce herself and confirmed all the arrangements for the Saturday flight. The next day we drove down to Pembrokeshire to leave Edmond staying with the Blacks in the Preseli Hills. Then on Saturday morning Matthew the cellist (still a great support and friend to the family) drove Rosie, Ollie and me to Heathrow.

Ammy had done a wonderful job. We were whisked through fast-channel security and escorted straight to the business-class lounge. I felt a brief pang of pity for the regular clients whose companies had paid a small fortune for exclusive tranquillity; then reminded myself that we had just to concentrate on Ollie's needs. Rosie settled him calmly on a plush sofa while I went to the bar to fetch him a fruit juice. But he became restless, so someone found us a quiet room. There he could create private mayhem, eating mounds of crisps and other gluten-free snacks, tramping food into the carpet, laying waste to the room. We mumbled embarrassed apologies when the time came at last to wheel Ollie through to the plane, boarding last, minimising the wait for take-off. Ammy had secured three adjacent bulkhead seats, with no passengers in front of us; we just hoped that the row behind would be tolerant.

Ollie was brilliant. He sat back in his seat, between the two of us, and only a brief flicker of alarm crossed his face as the engines roared for take-off. Once we were airborne and cruising Rosie opened our voluminous hand luggage, stuffed with emergency drinks, food, towels, wet-wipes, spare clothes, books and the brand new toys she had bought as special surprise treats for the journey. The distraction technique worked well for the first half-hour, but by the time the main meal (special gluten/dairy-free for us) arrived, Ollie was getting restless. As Rosie and I unwrapped our cellophane packs, both his arms shot up, flinging trays in the air and spattering the bulkhead with food.

The stewardess just smiled and helped us calmly to clear up, and we ate what we could salvage. I then squeezed out of my seat to take Ollie to the lavatory. We settled back down. Rosie gave Ollie his headphones and switched on a music tape. He relaxed for a while, but when the stewardess brought coffee it was showered liberally around the cabin. I apologised profusely to the people behind us, who smiled sympathetically. Then the stewardess returned with two balloon glasses. 'I think you need these,' she smiled, handing us each a large brandy.

At Boston a special assistant smoothed our way through the thrashing crowds and within half an hour of landing we were being helped into the car which Frankie Whitehead, a Bostonian friend from Bath, was lending us for the week. Her Boston neighbour drove us out to the suburbs, showing us where to return the car the following Saturday, then left us to it.

There was a brief, bluffing hiatus, as I tried to work out how to drive an automatic car, and then we were off. That night we barricaded ourselves in a pre-booked hotel room, sleeping for three hours until Ollie, adhering religiously to Greenwich Mean Time, woke us at two a.m. Five hours later I went blearily downstairs and, after much experimenting, managed to extract some breakfast from a machine. Then we packed the car and headed west.

It was a gorgeous drive through a gentle, wooded landscape. Settled in the back car seat, Ollie was in heaven. At midday we stopped to go for a walk in the forest. It was good to have this special time – the three of us together, unrushed, free from all hassle. Of course it had been a wrench leaving Edmond behind, but he could have his own special times later.

That evening we reached Sheffield, beneath the

wooded hills marking the State border between
Massachusetts and New York. The Option Institute stood
in a grassy clearing, set back from the road. The Son
Rise houses were a few hundred yards below the main
house and refectory, one assigned to us, one to another
English family we met later in the week. We took Ollie
straight to the big playroom and he fell delightedly on
some giant building bricks. Later, while Rosie settled
him in bed, I searched the kitchen drawers for a
corkscrew. After a fruitless search I unpacked my
penknife and used that. It was only as Rosie and I sat
drinking that she spotted the notice: 'No alcoholic liquor
to be consumed on the premises please.'

'Oh well,' she beamed determinedly, 'it'll be good for
us to go without for a week.'

In the event we were so busy that we hardly noticed
the lack of wine. However, Ollie was not very impressed
by the scrupulously healthy vegetarian diet and one day
I did drive into Sheffield to buy some large steaks.
Shopping at the supermarket-sized delicatessen in this
affluent neighbourhood was bewildering, and Rosie
found herself completely dazed by the choice of forty-
five different olive oils.

Back in our Son Rise house everything was blissfully
simple and focused. Ollie stayed in the house all week,
in the playroom from breakfast to supper. First thing on
Monday morning Rosie and I settled him into the room.
Then the door opened and a tall, athletic man called
Sean came in. His entire being glowed with optimistic
energy, and within a moment of entering he had
engaged eye contact and said a huge, warm 'Hello Ollie.
It's *great* to see you!'

As we slipped out of the room, Ollie was already busy
with Sean, playing with the giant bricks. I thought back
to the timid, anxious, withdrawn Ollie of eighteen

months earlier and felt proud: 'Yes, we've come a long way.' But I was also flabbergasted by the skill of the teacher, especially his lightning responses to Ollie and his palpable energy.

Like everything the Option Institute did, this intensive week was highly professional and structured meticulously. For much of the time the Option staff worked with Ollie, while Rosie and I went through a series of training sessions, geared as much to bolstering our *own* confidence as to that of our son's. We did a lot of work on staff training, re-learning how to run meetings and how to give feedback, with tips on how to start each feedback session with a celebration of positive success, before moving on to areas for improvement . . . how to keep meticulous notes . . . how to stick to the specific . . . All common sense, of course, but we needed to be reminded of these things.

As part of the feedback practice, during one session we swapped with the other English family. They each did a fifteen-minute session with Ollie; we worked with their son. I felt quite nervous, going cold into his playroom, scared of rejection. He was completely different from Ollie – quieter and gentler with slow languid movements. At first he barely acknowledged me. Then he climbed up onto the window sill and began traversing around the room, along shelf edges, over cupboards and door architraves. I followed him, offering an occasional guiding hand and acting as a human bridge over holdless sections of wall, watching every move, marvelling at the fluid simian grace of this brilliant climbing virtuoso. Then he reached out and clung to my shoulders and I carried him down to a bench where he just held me silently.

What a contrast to Ollie's mercurial boisterousness! What a salutary reminder that there is no standard autistic type. That afternoon I was videoed in Ollie's room.

I sit at the opposite side of the room from him, impassive as he screams, hands scratching the side of his head in furious brushing movements. Then the screaming dies down and he stretches out his legs. I do the same and begin to hum a Scottish tune. As he becomes totally calm I add words: 'My Ollie lies over the ocean; my Ollie lies over the sea . . .' He suddenly swings his legs underneath his bottom, kneels forward and starts to arrange the pieces of a giant soft jigsaw puzzle into a long line. I join from the other end and attempt to initiate a new game, pulling my end up in the air. He laughs, but then suddenly remonstrates, 'Uh! Uh!'

'Bring it back?

'Unh,' he affirms, and I quickly bring the chain back into position. We continue building. During the previous day's training session, one of the facilitators has suggested that we should be careful not to crowd Ollie – to respect his space and his work, and to consider working in *parallel*. So I start my own complementary chain and only gradually bring it to join his. Then he breaks up his chain. For five minutes he makes and remakes it, and again I work in parallel. There is no talk, no eye contact. Then he suddenly looks up and I exclaim, 'Hello gorgeous – lovely looking!'

Next time it happens I take a chance and go over and sit next to him. He looks up and I stroke his head. Later he stands up and I follow him over to a little platform with hand rails, where I face him, following his rocking movements. Seizing this moment of connection, I get the giant bouncy ball, wedge it between the rails and set Ollie on top. At first he is subdued. He gets down. But then he climbs back up with a shriek of delight and begins bouncing and I celebrate in time to the movement, 'Bouncy! Bouncy! Bouncy!'

Rosie comes in for her session. Ollie resents the transition and tries to push her away, but as I slip out of the room he accepts her and she responds immediately with, 'That's a lovely smile you're giving me, my lovely boy. What a lovely smile!'

He bounces on the platform and on the trampoline. He runs round the room. She follows him, always trying to position herself for eye contact. He has his dummy, so she has one too. At one point he stops and pulls her dummy out of her mouth. She opens wide and he snaps shut her lower jaw with a shout of satisfaction. The game is repeated several times until he spontaneously throws his arms around her neck, hugging her and rocking, head resting on her shoulder.

Later there is an opportunity to request speech. Ollie grabs the mug and straw, holds them up and shouts, 'Uh! Ah!'

'What does "uh" mean?' She acts stupid then asks with encouraging smiles, 'What do you want?' They are now very close, confiding, whispering. 'Can I help you?' she murmurs, 'in here?'

'Uh . . . eh . . . idh.'

'*Drink*!' That correct vowel gets an immediate response. 'You want a *drink*! Let's ask Daddy to get you one.' And Daddy comes in from the other side of the one-way mirror with a mug of juice.

Rosie was faster than me with her responses – bigger, louder, funnier, cuddlier – but the Option professionals were even more theatrical. Bubbly Sean kept up an incredibly enthusiastic commentary, pausing at every opportunity to mouth and accentuate key motivating words like MUSIC and PUZZLE. Imitating Ollie's dismantling of the giant puzzle, he flung off pieces with a flamboyant flick of the wrist, creating theatre out of the mundane. But he never got too close – never imposed. A serene woman with long black hair sat cross-legged on the floor, immediately opposite Ollie but at a respectful distance, picking up each individual puzzle piece to hold it directly in line between his and her eyes, celebrating every single moment of contact: 'You keep looking in my eyes, my friend! So *nice*!' Another woman, joining Ollie rocking on the platform, broke into wild animal whoops, delighting him with her craziness, so that he jumped down, took her hand, and raced her round the room. Then he pulled her towards him and folded up against her, arms held to his chest in anti-tickle pose, as he collapsed in paroxysms of loving laughter.

At the end of the week we had a sample team meeting at which we were given a set of resolutions, divided into three sections. First were ideas on responding to whining and crying (even here Ollie had had moments of frustration). We were reminded to feel comfortable and calm – not to be upset by his crying – and to try and find out the cause, explaining that we are not sure what he wants, that it is easier to understand when he tells us. We were encouraged to respond slowly to crying, but really quickly when he was cheerful – showing him the best way to move people. And we were reminded always to be consistent.

Second, helping Ollie to speak. They told us to focus on key motivating words, such as 'eat', 'drink', 'squeeze' and 'ride'. And to model the sounds for him, for instance showing how with 'squeeze' you first take a breath, then draw your lips wide and press your tongue up against your hard palate, then click back of the tongue against soft palate, then draw lips together to make a 'w' sound, then out again for the 'ee', then finally bring tongue back onto the hard palate for the 'z' – six distinct actions. Above all, we should celebrate every attempt at communication, even if it were just the beginnings of words.

Third, initiating learning once Ollie stopped ritual behaviours – what they called 'isms'. We should go into the room with clear intentions. We might, for instance, take in bubbles with the intention of teaching him the word 'bubbles'. Or arrive dressed as a clown, with a circus theme in mind. But, equally, we had to know when to hold back, when not to push him: 'Sometimes you can just be grateful and *celebrate* Ollie for that moment that he has chosen to reach out to you.'

That sense of celebration was the greatest lesson of the week and when we set off home on the Saturday morning, there was a new hopefulness. It was the first Saturday in September and although the trees were still green there was a dewy smell of autumn, the season I always think of not as an ending but a beginning – the start of the academic year. Eating our picnic lunch in the woods somewhere on the way back to Boston, the three of us sitting together in the dappled light, I felt that we were back on that first holiday in France, all those years earlier, when we were first getting to know this new person; except that now there was the keen anticipation of returning to Edmond and an eagerness to press on with Ollie's home education.

Boston airport held no terrors and soon after we got onto the aeroplane, this time flying at night, Ollie settled down to sleep, only waking as we touched down at Heathrow the next morning. Matthew was there to meet us, the sun was shining, the world was beautiful and we couldn't wait to get back home and down to business.

Chapter Ten

So where did it all go wrong? Why was it that by Christmas we were admitting defeat and contemplating the unthinkable – sending our precious boy away to a residential school, banishing him into the hands of strangers?

The simple answer is that Ollie required full-time adult care, twenty-four hours a day, seven days a week, fifty-two weeks a year, and that was an exhausting job. Siri, who had been with us for over five years, taking Ollie out to run and play every week, was hinting that she was finding him harder to manage, and that at some stage she would have to drop him from her list of clients. In the house, the Son Rise programme gave us a structure, as much philosophical as practical, but it required gigantic energy to run it and most of that work fell on Rosie. Almost every month a helper would leave and she would have to find and train another. The five sixth-formers had now all left for university. Oliver the German music student had finished his year in Britain. Anne Hambrick – dynamic extrovert Anne – would soon be completing her education degree and looking for a full-time job. The turnover was inexorable and during the two and a half years we ran the programme, Rosie trained altogether thirty-four teachers. Most of them were astonishingly devoted; but some left without warning, just as Rosie had finished training them. Or, in a couple of cases – both male – *she* asked them to leave because she did not feel happy about leaving them alone in a room with Ollie.

Even the stars needed inspiration and encouragement, and sometimes this was as much about their own growth as about helping Ollie. One young student, for instance, joining our team before starting an art therapy course, blossomed into a devoted and confident teacher whom Ollie adored, but was very diffident when she first started, requiring regular nurture from Rosie. 'Sometimes I feel as though I'm having to be mother to *everyone*,' she sighed wearily one evening, slumped over a restorative glass of wine. 'And I've still got to do all those wage forms.'

For those helpers who were being paid by the Local Education Authority, she had to fill out detailed time sheets. Because LEA employees could only technically be employed during normal school hours – even though many of their slots actually fell during weekends and school holidays – Rosie had to fit the correct number of hours into notional weekday slots, avoiding any clashes with the other helpers who were paid by Social Services. She knew and they knew what was happening, but due bureaucratic protocol had to be observed.

Then there were endless forms to fill in for our other sources of funding, such as Child Disability Allowance. And the Disabled Parking badge, which had to be renewed each year by filling in a long questionnaire probing painfully the full extent of Ollie's difficulties. And reports to the educational psychologist. And the continuing search for charitable funds to help pay for training and equipment. I seemed to be able to remain fairly detached, but for Rosie every request she made for help was another pained rehearsal of Ollie's difficulties, so distressing that she sometimes wondered whether it would be better to try to manage without the money.

Amidst all this relentless administration, she had to project a cheerful, imaginative, optimistic front, not only to Ollie, but to all the others who worked with him. Occasionally she would accost me – 'Why don't *you* ever take the meetings? Why aren't *you* coming up with ideas?'

'Well you're better at that kind of thing than me.'

'And what kind of excuse is that? He's *your* son too!'

She was right: too often I opted for the easy status quo, leaving creativity to her. But at least, as she always told me, I had stamina: I was able to keep plodding indefinitely, unfazed by crises. Which was just as well, because at the end of October, a few weeks after our return from America, Rosie – that phenomenally tough woman – finally crumpled under the strain. One morning she just stayed in bed, only emerging at midday to immerse herself in a long hot bath before returning to bed, where she stayed for the next few days. Her speech, normally so resolute and articulate, faded to a numb whisper. She needed desperately to escape, so I phoned Shan, who offered immediately to drive over, collect Rosie and take her back to Sussex for some serious pampering.

What a wonderfully practical saint! When I phoned Sussex two nights later I could hear Jake's ebullient laughter in the background. Rosie was still subdued but sounded stronger already. 'I'm having a lovely time,' she said. 'I don't have to do anything at all, and they're spoiling me with lots of champagne.'

She looked much better when she came home two days later, but Shan took me aside. 'She *is* better,' she agreed, 'but I don't think she can go on like this much longer; things are going to have to change.' My father was also exhorting me to accept what he saw as the inevitable: 'You just *can't* go on like this for ever. There are four of you in this family and you've got to think about Edmond.' Again I prickled at the inference, however unintentional, that Ollie was somehow to blame – this innocent boy who tried so hard and who was so completely without malice. Of course my father was not *actually* blaming Ollie, but both our families did feel that we had done all we could for him at home – that the time had come to hand over to the professionals.

David Walker, our GP, was equally pragmatic. We had been with him for three or four years, having left the previous practice after their reluctance to acknowledge initial symptoms of autism and then to react to Ollie's deterioration from leukaemia. David, by contrast, always listened seriously to whatever Rosie had to report. Now when he asked what he could do for her, she just said, 'I'm going bonkers.'

'Well it's not surprising,' he replied, 'you can't go on like this; you *cannot* continue for ever to motivate all these people purely by the power of your own personality.' I nodded sagely, feeling privately rather guilty that my own personality had not been a bit more in evidence, taking a bigger share of the motivating. David typed into his computer a prescription for Prozac, telling Rosie, 'It should help for the time being. But it's not a long-term solution. I think you're going to have to find other people to look after him.'

The relentless stress arose partly from the geography of our house. Sitting down one evening to write one of her characteristically analytical lists, Rosie realised that one of the biggest problems was the sheer physical difficulty of having this noisy, demanding child living at the centre of the house, between floors, visited by a constant stream of helpers tramping up and down the stairs. Opposite 'problems' she then listed 'solutions', and called me over: 'Stephen – I've had an idea.'

'Yes, Rosie,' I groaned, 'what do you want me to do?'

'Are we choosing happiness, my darling?'

'Yes dear.'

'We need to build Ollie an annexe – an extension in the garden . . . beyond the kitchen.'

She was right. As usual. If all Ollie's noise could be shifted out towards the garden, to the far side of the kitchen, the whole running of the household could be much less stressful. We got a surveyor to assess the site, and he agreed that it would be just possible, but expensive, to build a tiny self-contained flat in the available space. Then, shameless as ever, we approached Social Services for a disability home improvement grant but the assessor took one look at our comparatively large house and said, 'Other people manage; why can't you?'

So that idea was squashed. And with it Rosie's hope of making the strain of home education more tolerable. The existing arrangement was simply wearing her down. 'I don't want to do it any more,' she admitted to me one evening. 'I'm getting bored with it. And I think Ollie's getting bored too.' Even with all her colossal energy and all the dedication of our helpers, we were just not exciting enough. The magic was evaporating from the playroom. Ollie needed to move on.

So, saying nothing to the helpers, we set off one November morning to Dorset, to visit a special residential school for autistic children. The head was polite, smartly groomed, professional. Cheerful young staff were cleaning the boarding houses. Peace seemed to reign amongst the uniformed children in their little classrooms. Then we met a boy about Ollie's age, working alone at an exuberantly messy painting, watched by a special carer. The boy had a boisterous gleam in his eye and Rosie said, 'He's just like Ollie.'

'Ah . . . is he?' replied the nervous teacher. 'He's a bit of a handful. In fact he's soon moving to another school'.

Then we visited three schools affiliated to the Rudolf
Steiner movement. I was woefully ignorant about the
Austrian anthroposophist's educational theories, but I
liked what I saw of the schools' gentle, holistic approach.
We liked particularly the Steiner school in Thornbury,
about half an hour's drive north of Bath. Individual houses
were clustered around a slightly crumbling Palladian
mansion set in parkland, with a walled garden providing
fresh fruit and vegetables. Children and teenagers, with
various mild disabilities, wandered amicably in the
gardens at breaktime. We talked to classes in the
carpentry workshop and the bakery, then saw one of the
home houses where seven or eight children sat down
to meals with their house parents at a round dining table.
Then saw the trademark Steiner chapel. The dated, rather
self-conscious, art-nouveauish décor seemed faintly
cranky, but I liked the idea of assemblies combining
music, movement, dance, costume and lighting.

Ollie might be happy here. But how would he fit in?
Most of these children seemed so much more able. How
would he manage to sit still at the dining table? And
how on earth would they stop him escaping over the
fields and off to the M5? We could hear the motorway's
faint roar a couple of miles to the west.

We also saw a Steiner-based school in Bristol and
another one in Hampshire, near the New Forest. We
took Ollie there on a December evening. He tried the
climbing frame then ran joyfully into the woods, fading
into the winter twilight. I caught up with him eventually and we walked hand in hand to one of the boarding
houses for a long 'interview' with the house mother and
the school doctor.

If Ollie came to board here the fees would be
£28,000 a year – nearly three times the cost of his
former local school and perhaps four times the amount

we were currently getting towards home education. That would have to be agreed by the Local Education Authority. It was lobbying time again.

At the November review meeting we submitted a six-page document outlining all the successes of the Son Rise programme – the confidence, the trust, the interaction with other people, the ability again to face the world. We then hammered home some of the *difficulties* of life with Ollie: the constant noise, the endless search for new staff, the neglect of Edmond, the debts which had recently forced us to rent our bedroom to a lodger while we slept in the kitchen; Ollie's impatient obsession with food, causing mayhem whenever he came down to the kitchen; the water play, the random urinating, the perennial smearing of faeces, the dangerous escaping. We then made it clear that, even if there were a suitable local day school for Ollie, it would leave us all these problems during after-school hours, weekends and school holidays. We concluded by requesting a place for Ollie at a residential school.

What kind of an attitoodinal betrayal was this? Whatever happened to our Option philosophy of unconditional love? Why choose whingeing unhappiness?

The answer is that we had to state our case – and Ollie's case – strongly. We wanted the LEA to spend a lot more money on our child and we had to provide good reasons. Most parents seeking residential places for their special needs children ended up going to tribunal. In an exploratory move I telephoned a solicitor experienced in this field and told him that the Steiner schools had quoted £28,000 per year, which seemed a terrifying amount of money. 'Twenty-eight thousand?' he replied derisorily. 'I would be looking for a sum closer to eighty thousand.'

Eighty thousand pounds! That apparently was the going rate, and when the Steiner schools told us that they didn't think they could provide adequately for Ollie's needs (they rely considerably on voluntary help), it became clear that he needed somewhere with higher, much more expensive levels of security and staffing.

Meanwhile our Senior Education Officer telephoned to say that Ollie's needs could be met at a day school in Bath, with additional support at home. Rosie replied the next day, with a long letter restating all the problems of the last two years and insisting that cobbling together some kind of home/day-school package just would not work. She concluded:

> Opting for a residential place for our 8-year-old son is not an easy decision for us to make; in fact it is a heartbreaking one, but we cannot see any other way to meet his very special needs. The holiday periods would continue to be extremely difficult for us, but we do not at this stage seek a 52-week placement because we would miss him too much.

The negotiations rumbled on into the first weeks of the new millennium. At one stage Rosie told Ollie's social worker, Niki, that if the LEA refused to fund a place we would go to tribunal and we would win. The message was forwarded with almost immediate effect, and a few days later the LEA said that it would reconsider our case. I meanwhile was busy promoting my new book, and doing a spate of lectures, including one talk delivered surreally at Puerto Vallarta, on the Pacific coast of Mexico, to the annual convention of the West Canadian Wheat Growers Association. At home, our loyal team of teachers continued to work with Ollie in his playroom. In March 2000 I videoed a typical Monday.

It must be Monday because it is mussels for lunch, a treat only available from Waitrose on a Monday. Wendy arrives at Ollie's door with his lunch tray, comes into the room, locks the door behind her and puts the tray down on the little yellow table which is bolted to the wall. Behind it hangs the rope ladder, which Ollie has bashed repeatedly against the wall, excavating plaster to reveal some rather dodgy late Victorian stonework.

Ollie sits on his little green chair, fingers picking delicately the succulent orange flesh from the blue shells. He is dressed in check trousers (patterns show less dirt), fleece top and his favourite fleece hat – a checked and tasselled Rasta-tartan fusion in brilliant primary colours. Wendy sits on the floor beside him, at his level, talking gently and encouraging him to keep his plate on the table. She is a calm comforting presence.

Later Ollie comes down to the kitchen for his afternoon break. Rosie, in apron, gives him a drink and asks him to sit down at the table, amongst the mussel detritus. 'Good sitting. What a good boy! Lovely sitting.'

Then he is off, heading through the kitchen as she tries to wipe his hands, insisting, 'If you're going outside you have to put *boots* on.' Shrieks of laughter as he runs barefoot into the garden, pursued by Rosie shouting, 'Come on – here they are.'

Later he returns to the kitchen and circles the room, dummy hooked over one finger so that the others can hold an empty mussel shell which he puts in and out of his mouth, enjoying its smooth pearly concavity. He gestures to the fridge and Rosie insists, 'Take that out of your mouth and tell me what you want . . . Ollie, say JUICE.' He continues circling. 'Ollie, say JUICE.'

'Jih.'

'JUICE.'

He does one more procrastinating circle, but then turns to Rosie with a big smiley 'Jee.' That's closer. She rewards him immediately with a glass of fruit juice, which he drains before running back to the garden to play on the swing beneath the pergola, head tipped back to enjoy the flashing pattern of wooden slats against pale sky. After half an hour he runs back inside, just in time for Rosie to take him up for his afternoon session in the room.

At moments like that it seemed heartless even to consider boarding school. We could justify it by re-rehearsing all the difficulties; but it seemed better to turn attitudes upside down and persuade ourselves that a new departure might actually be *good* for Ollie and for us. A new adventure. A new chance, freed from the daily administrative grind, to appreciate Ollie's magical qualities, savouring his weekends at home.

Or something like that. On Tuesday 21st March we set off on an intensive four-day tour of special schools, starting with Sunfield, near Stourbridge. The rhododendrons, thriving on acidic sandstone, were in brilliant crimson bloom. Lawns sloped down to a field full of animals, with spacious views out to the hills beyond Kidderminster. Yes! What a contrast to enclosed, soporific Larkhall. The school looked after several children at the severe end of the autistic spectrum, as well as others with 'profound and severe learning disabilities'. The head, Barry Carpenter, was demonstrably devoted to his school, filled with a genuine pride in the children. Some of them needed constant supervision. Others were able to wander alone around the school. Some, unlike Ollie, had extensive speech and one boy of about fourteen, asked by Barry what he was up to, smiled engagingly and announced, 'I'm making a bomb . . . to blow up the school.'

The headmaster took the announcement cheerfully in his stride and we continued our tour. Suddenly we saw the boy from the Dorset school – the one who looked and behaved like Ollie, whom they had found too difficult – tumbling noisily out of a minibus. Here the staff took his boisterousness in their stride, unfazed. How encouraging. We liked Sunfield, but were put off by the fact that it was geared to fifty-two-week placements. The thought of Ollie living away at school for the entire year was too much to bear. We wanted him home for at least a few weeks each year.

On the Wednesday we headed east to Prior's Court – an old prep school near Newbury, recently sold, gutted and rebuilt into a special school for autistic children. We had first heard about it through a friend of Bridget McCrum – one of many leading sculptors whose work had been bought to adorn the school and its gardens. The idea – and I liked it – was that special needs children and their teachers should live and work in beautiful surroundings. All this was paid for by the school's founder Dame Steve Shirley, one of the richest women in Britain, who had started her software business in her kitchen, whilst looking after her own autistic son, Ben. He had later died, aged thirty-one, and this new school was to be his memorial.

As we headed up the drive we were greeted by a joyful life-size sculpture of a youth riding a horse, his arms held high to release a falcon. There were paintings on every wall, sculptures in the photocopying room, a stunning fountain outside the main classroom block and in the playground a huge friendly bronze by Elisabeth Frink called *Leonardo's Dog*, based on the dogs outside the Renaissance artist's last residence, and placed here to help overcome the canine phobia experienced by so many autistic children. (Ollie was no exception. Imagine the fear of a small hypersensitive child facing a huge, unpredictable, unrestrained creature, with foul-breathed slavering mouth barking loudly, sharp fangs glistening inches away from your face.) Along with several other parents we were given a tour of immaculate, stunningly equipped classrooms and boarding houses. Then we had a talk by the Head of Studies and the Head of Care, both dressed in white polo shirts and navy tracksuit trousers, proclaiming the school's partial adherence to the methods of the famous Higashi School in Boston, which gives autistic children huge amounts of physical exercise. Then the suited head, Robert Hubbard, talked about the school's aspirations.

I liked his quietness and his refusal to espouse evan- gelically any single teaching method. And his admission that this was a new school – so far with just seven chil- dren – which was feeling its way.

How different, the next morning, to arrive at a rather dilapidated establishment in Staffordshire during the morning break, as hordes of huge teenagers milled noisily around the tarmac playground and on the echoing staircase of the main schoolhouse. I couldn't bear the thought of leaving Ollie amongst this loud, jostling crowd. The school had a kind, jolly, friendly atmosphere, but as teachers showed us the tasks their children were doing it all seemed far too advanced for Ollie. When we mentioned this to the head, she rapped our knuckles: 'How do you know? Don't *assume* that he couldn't cope.'

But we were fairly sure our assumptions were correct. In the afternoon we were shown round another school by a man with dodgy eye contact. '*He's* autistic,' Rosie laughed, as we got in the car to leave. 'And what about that dual carriageway, right next to the school! The wall's only five feet high. Ollie'd be over it in a flash.' Emotionally exhausted we found overnight refuge, wine and laughter in Northampton, with Jonathan Dawson – an outrageously funny, successful surgeon friend of my brother Philip – and his equally zany wife Linda.

On Friday morning we saw two more autistic schools in Staffordshire. One we found uninspiring; the other was still being built – a brand new building for teaching the Higashi method. Standing around a half-furnished office, sharing coffee and sandwiches, we chatted with three fantastically enthusiastic tracksuited women who had gone to Higashi School in Boston for special training and returned determined to provide something similar in Britain. Trawling tirelessly through an ocean of educational possibilities, Rosie had been tempted for several years by Higashi. Before leukaemia turned everything upside down we had even considered trying to go with Ollie to Boston. The school challenged autistic children with a rigorous regime of hard exercise, hard lessons and music ensemble, drilling them Suzuki-style to play melodions – hand-held wind instruments with little piano keyboards. The Staffordshire team brought the brand new instruments out of their cases, showed us the huge gym, the embryonic classrooms. We liked their eager optimism and when we got back to Bath and submitted our report on the various schools we had seen, outlining all their different strengths, we made it quite clear that the new Higashi school was top favourite, alongside the other new school, Prior's Court.

The Senior Education Officer had now indicated that the LEA *would* consider joint-funding a residential place with Social Services. However, no sums had been mentioned. We just knew that these schools were both a

lot more expensive than the Steiner schools which had
turned Ollie down. The subject of money was again
discreetly ignored at our meeting the next week, but there
were increasing hints that the necessary amount might
somehow be found. Ollie's social worker, Niki, objected
fairly strenuously to the Staffordshire Higashi school as
being too far away – nearly three hours' drive – for her
to oversee his care. We also baulked ourselves at the idea
of ten to twelve hours' driving on the alternate weekends when we planned to bring Ollie home. We were
also not convinced that Ollie could handle such a rigorous
curriculum. We ended by agreeing that Niki and the
Senior Education officer would both visit Prior's Court
with a view to Ollie starting there later that summer.

That meeting was on 30th March. Two days later, on
April Fool's Day, I set off for Antarctica to join the
world's most famous mountaineer retracing the heroic
hallowed footsteps of Edwardian explorer Sir Ernest
Shackleton.

Exaggeration. Not strictly Antarctica. Like Sir E. in 1915,
we didn't actually set foot on the great white southern
continent: our job was to retrace his steps across the
island of South Georgia, where he and five exhausted
men dragged themselves ashore in 1916, having just
crossed the Southern Ocean in a twenty-three-foot open
boat. They were desperately attempting to seek rescue
for twenty-two other men left marooned on a godforsaken icy beach on Elephant Island, after the expedition
ship, the *Endurance*, had been crushed and sunk by the
pack ice. A gripping tale, re-enacted in this millennial
jaunt for a giant-screen IMAX documentary.

The call from director George Butler had come the
previous Christmas. His big hit had been a documentary on Arnold Schwarzenegger called *Pumping Iron*. A

fascinating study of psychopathy in action, it had launched Schwarzenegger's career. 'I'll make you as famous as Arny,' crooned George over the transatlantic telephone line. I wasn't sure about that, but I was quite sure that I did want to return to that magical island of South Georgia for the first time in eleven years. The fee was adequate to justify a month's absence and the production company agreed to half up front, ensuring that I could pay for extra help while I was away, making life manageable for Rosie. As for the cast . . . it was an honour to be representing Britain, alongside the brilliant American climber Conrad Anker and the celebrated, iconoclastic, South Tyrolean mountaineer, yeti-hunter and MEP Reinhold Messner.

Anxious not to make a complete fool of myself in front of the world's greatest mountaineer, I attempted to put in some pre-expedition training. In February I started rising at five thirty a.m., bicycling in the dark up to the nearby hamlet of Bailbrook, leaving the bike there and continuing on foot, running all the way up Solsbury Hill, reaching the top at sunrise. Then I did a perimeter circuit of the grassy plateau summit, enjoying the sunshine and glancing smugly down into the grey shady frost pocket of the Swainswick valley, before heading back down, lurching through the half-frozen mud crusts of Passchendaele, on down Ollie's cowpat field and back to the bike for a final high-speed pedal down to Larkhall. Then fifteen minutes' yoga on the kitchen floor and a shower. Then the start of the normal daily routine, helping get Edmond ready for school and taking breakfast up to Ollie's room.

I managed this regime about ten times, but by the end of February my ankles, calves and knees had almost packed in, my lungs ached and my back was in spasm. I felt terrible and I was convinced that I had either cancer, or a chronic heart condition, or probably both.

The message was clear: training is bad for you; much better to save your body for the big day. So I spent March recovering from my hypochondria, got thoroughly absorbed in our search for a special school for Ollie and had just about recuperated in time for the flight to Montevideo. Here I met Conrad, Reinhold, George, the production team from Boston, the logistics team from Utah, the IMAX camera crew from Vancouver, the special inflatable-boat driver from Quebec and a large team of hugely experienced British mountaineers sent to stop us falling down any crevasses. We all boarded the *Akademik Shulyekin*, a Russian research vessel turned Antarctic cruiser, and off we sailed for South Georgia, our cabins tended by two delightful Muscovite women – one a piano teacher, the other a marine biologist – who had been reduced to working as cabin maids in post-glasnost Russia.

It was a glorious jaunt. The sun shone, the sea glittered and only after four days did a sudden chill in the air – and the joyful porpoising leap through the waves of the penguins – announce our crossing of the Antarctic Convergence. We made our landfall in proper South Georgian drizzle, turquoise icebergs looming out of the mist, as the captain steered us anxiously into King Haakon Bay to film the very spot where Shackleton and his five exhausted, dehydrated, salt-encrusted, seal-blubber-smeared companions had dragged their lifeboat ashore in 1916.

We came ashore more comfortably, with elaborate safety procedures, in a powerful inflatable Zodiac. The next morning we did some filming; then Conrad, Reinhold and I set off to make the legendary crossing of South Georgia's mountains to the now abandoned whaling station of Stromness. Conrad was nine years younger than me, Reinhold ten years older; both were a great deal fitter. As the world's greatest mountaineer set a cracking pace across the glacier, Californian acolyte trotting jauntily at his side, all my paranoid fears were confirmed. It was a desperate struggle to keep up. My years of domestic entrenchment had taken their toll. Or perhaps I was always a bit too effete for this kind of thing?

The day was saved for me when, leaping across an immense crevasse the following afternoon, the South Tyrolean landed badly and broke his foot. For the man who had made the first and only true solo ascent, without oxygen, of Everest, a mere broken bone was no reason to turn back. No, not a bit of it: we would proceed with our mission; but we would now move, thank God, at a slower pace.

So we continued our journey, Conrad and I marvelling at the stoicism of Reinhold's brisk limp. Although our actual travelling time, fractured Tyrolean foot notwithstanding, was less than Shackleton's thirty-six-hour forced march, our journey was spread comfortably over three days. It was thrilling to see – to immerse oneself in – the contorted glacial landscape which Shackleton, Crean and Worsley had crossed, after leaving their other three companions under the upturned boat on the beach of King Haakon Bay. Moving, almost to tears, to reach the final pass and look down on the now rusted, decaying buildings of Stromness, and imagine the real tears of relief – of redemptive salvation – in 1916.

Re-enacting the Shackleton story, however artificially, induced a state of heightened emotion, accentuated by the fact that Conrad was in the film as a substitute for his best friend Alex Lowe, who had been killed at his side, in an avalanche in Tibet, just six months earlier.

Now Conrad was living with his friend's widow in Utah and helping to raise her three suddenly fatherless children. A sensitive man, familiar with British reserve, he was not the type to pry; he just knew about Ollie's autism and was happy to talk when I felt ready. Which was good, because both Rosie and I liked to talk about Ollie. We didn't want autism and cancer swept under the carpet, kept discreetly in a secret compartment called Disability, to be handled only by professional experts. This was our unique wonderful elder son and we needed to celebrate his huge courageous spirit.

Reinhold's Nietzschean aura made him seem a less obvious confidant. But in fact he proved an increasingly jovial companion and he too was a father, taking regular advantage of the expedition's satellite phone to talk to his children in Bolzano. One luminous afternoon, filming a crevasse sequence on the Nordenskjöld Glacier, engaged in the usual foot-shuffling hanging around drinking cups of coffee that goes with any film, I thought it would be fun to call home too. Edmond picked up the phone eight thousand miles away.

'Hello, Dadda.'

'Hello, Edmond, I'm sitting on a glacier and there are huge icebergs out in the sea.'

'Oh.'

'We've seen lots of penguins and elephant seals.'

'Oh.'

'Are you having a nice time?'

'Yes.'

I tried a different tack. 'Could I speak to Mummy?'

'She's busy with Ollie – he's trying to run away. Granny and Granchie have come to help put up more chicken wire. I must go now. Bye.'

So much for satellite telephones. Our stilted conversation just reminded me how much easier expedition life – particularly the pampered existence of a filming expedition – is than the reality of home.

Better just to immerse myself in the present, soaking up the transcendental beauty of this magical island and enjoying the easy camaraderie as we head back to the ship after a day's pleasurable work, asking our salty Québécois coxswain to stop en route at a berg where I can hack off a lump of ice to grace my gin and tonic that evening, fizzing as it releases bubbles of pristine air trapped for who knows how many thousand years in this ancient floating piece of Antarctica.

The enchanted interlude came to an end and once again I left the southern autumn to fly home to the northern spring. Things had gone well in my absence with a chunk of my IMAX fee paying two of our teachers, Anne and Llinos, to do extra sessions with Ollie, leaving Rosie free to enjoy Edmond's school holidays. Ollie was now spending much more time outside in the garden as we eased out of the Son Rise programme, hugely grateful for the way it had transformed our lives, but also preparing for the big shift to boarding school. There was still no confirmation about funding and we were still awaiting news when I flew to Colorado three weeks later to do a presentation at the Telluride Mountain Film Festival for my occasional employer, Malden Mills, maker of Polartec fabrics.

Another transitory interlude, this time just a weekend in the bright breath-catching air of the Rocky Mountains. On the Sunday afternoon I phoned from the tiny airport near Telluride to tell Rosie that the flights had been changed and I would be returning later than planned to Gatwick. 'That's fine,' she said cheerfully. 'I'll come and meet you with the boys. Ollie will enjoy the drive. Guess what?' she continued, 'The

Education Officer phoned yesterday. They've agreed! Ollie's going to start at Prior's Court in July.'

'That must be a huge relief,' remarked Jeff Bowman, the Malden director who had followed Ollie's journey with sympathetic interest ever since I met him at my first Polartec Challenge meeting in Boston in 1994, a few months after the autism diagnosis.

'Yes . . . I think it's probably the best thing,' I replied hesitantly, half relieved, half embarrassed by a lingering sense of failure. Then I remembered Barry Kaufman, up on his podium, with his microphone, all twinkly and encouraging, telling us, 'Remember – your child is always doing the best he or she can. And so are you.' We just had to embrace this latest adventure whole-heartedly and remember that we had chosen it for good reasons.

A couple of weeks later Ollie helped to remind us of those reasons. Rosie was with him in the kitchen. Someone had accidentally left the street door unlocked. Ollie, always testing, was thrilled to find it open and dashed up the steps towards the street.

'Come back, Ollie,' screamed Rosie above the noise of an approaching car. As she hurtled barefoot after him, the big toe on her left foot crashed into an iron railing and her shriek of pain conflicted with the squeal of rubber on tarmac a few feet away, where Ollie stared with startled innocence at the car shuddering to a halt just in front of his fragile body.

Another visit to the RUH Accident & Emergency Department. Confirmation of another broken big toe. No steel spike this time, thank God, just a month on crutches. A few days later at Gatwick airport, having accepted Julian's and Emmy's generous invitation to return to the Corfu paradise gardens for another week of spoiling, I had to place Rosie on top of our luggage like some beautiful, exotic mascot and wheel her to the check-in desk. At Kanonas sun, rest and soft salt water worked wonders on the broken toe and fortified her heart for the approaching separation. Back at home, we made special arrangements to take Ollie on the least busy morning of the week to the huge John Lewis department store near Bristol, Rosie limping beside me, while I wheeled in our nine-year-old boy in his protective pushchair.

The shop attendant assigned to us was brilliant – quiet, gentle, patient, unflappable. Ollie responded equally brilliantly, gamely trying on tracksuits, polo shirts, games socks, smart black leather shoes, sandals, trainers and – a Prior's Court special – Rollerblades, smiling beatifically and occasionally exclaiming 'gaii-iyeee' as his mother told him how smart he looked.

On Tuesday 4th July I took him on his first visit to the school. He whimpered slightly as we left the M4 at Junction 13, perturbed by the interruption to our smooth eastward movement up the motorway. But when we entered the school's remote-control security gates and headed slowly up the avenue past the equestrian falconer he seemed optimistically curious. He even managed a wary smile when David Heald, the director of studies, met us in the car park in his logoed polo shirt and tracksuit trousers. 'Let's go for a run,' he announced immediately, taking Ollie's hand and jogging towards oak woodland.

It worked! Ollie looked rather bemused, but he was running. With this complete stranger! I ran alongside, encouraging him, occasionally giving him a little nudging prod, as I did at home, guiding him upstairs at bathtime, trying always to keep it good-humoured, sharing the joke: I know you want to run away and do your own thing, but you're coming this way. David opened a gate and we entered the wood, to follow a twisting grass path. Strange objects kept appearing magically in clearings: pillars, heads, animal forms, glittery shiny things. And then a huge swing, its chains suspended from the high branch of an old oak. In the undergrowth fading scilla leaves promised a glorious bluebell shimmer for the following spring.

The woodland circuit took us back to the gate. It was about ten feet high and David remarked how child-proof it was. Ollie eyed up the conveniently spaced horizontal timbers and smiled to himself: you must be joking, mate.

After our run, Ollie visited the boarding house for eight-to-eleven-year-olds. The other children – only four of them so far – were away in their classrooms, so it was a chance for Ollie to explore in peace, meeting one or two of the care staff, including his keyworker, Lynda. He rummaged amongst the shelves, pleased with all the shiny new toys, and then it was time for us to leave.

On 10th July we had another introductory visit. This time it was for three hours, and Rosie came too to meet Ollie's carers and the school chef, to explain about his gluten- and dairy-free diet, and his complicated regime of vitamin and nutrient supplements. We went upstairs to see his bedroom and wondered about the carpeted floor. The school liked children to share, two to a room, but had agreed to Ollie having a room to himself. Rosie was pleased to see the observation window in the door, and the closed-circuit television cameras; carers were vetted scrupulously, but we all knew stories of child abuse in special schools and it was reassuring to see Prior's Court leaving nothing to chance.

On both visits Ollie agreed, at the school's request, to leave his dummy and snuggly in the car. He seemed to manage fine without those familiar props and we dared to hope that he would settle happily when he came actually to live here. But the last week – the final countdown to the big day – was a tremulous time. There was still that lingering sense that we had let Ollie down, that we were passing the buck, that the quest had failed. Time after time we had to remind ourselves that life doesn't necessarily follow the plot. Or, at least, the plot keeps changing. Just because Raun Kaufman learned to talk and went to university, it didn't mean that other autistic children would necessarily do the same. Most people don't ascend steadily, unwaveringly to some hypothetical summit: they falter, or stop for a rest, or traverse off along some meandering ledge, or go back down and try again by a different route. Ollie had done his best. He had found within himself huge reserves of courage, not only to overcome a fatal illness, but also to allow a succession of strangers into his trust. Three years earlier he could not have faced a single day in a strange school. Now he had reached a stage where he could go to live in a completely new community. For his sake we had to treat it as just another exciting new adventure.

Chapter Eleven

The boy followed meekly, uncomprehendingly, as they led him away behind bars. It was for the good of his family. And it was for the good of a society to which he could contribute nothing: he was a freak, a reject, a blot on the landscape of healthy normality. Better to put him away in this sanatorium and, later, discreetly, mercifully, dispose of him.

Terrible irrational images of Nazi euthanasia policy flashed unbidden through my mind as I watched from a high window. The school had offered kindly to let us stay one night in the guest bedroom in the main house. It was early afternoon and Rosie was unpacking our overnight things. I was in the bathroom and could see down to the paved path leading from the boarding house to the gym. High bars – erected for the children's safety – flanked the path down which one of the care staff was leading Ollie. He was wearing his green-striped tee shirt, shorts and sandals. In his hands he carried his shiny new blue Rollerblades. But did he have any idea what they were for – these strange objects? Did he have any idea where he was going? Did he wonder what had happened to his parents? Did he think (in the sense that we 'think' about cause and effect) that he had been abandoned for ever in this strange place – this little boy who looked so forlorn and bewildered?

Of course I knew that actually he was safe amongst kind, caring people. As for the unbidden Nazi visions, they were grotesquely ironic because Dame Steve

Shirley, the school's founder and benefactor, herself escaped Nazi Germany on one of the *kindertransporten*: she was one of the few Jews, far too few, allowed grudgingly to come and enrich the life of Great Britain. Now she had given us this magnificent new school and we had to trust its staff to look after our child.

We arrived in the morning, Rosie leading Ollie by the hand, while I dragged in his enormous suitcase. Lynda took us up to his room, where we unpacked all his new clothes, laying them out in a chest of drawers. Then we hung some framed photos on the wall. On top of his bedside table we left more photos, in an album, of the Himalayan birch gleaming beside the red front door of our house, Ollie playing in the kitchen, Granny and Granchie, Edmond riding his bike, Mummy and Daddy hugging in the garden, Ollie's bedroom . . . reminders, we hoped, that he still had a home to come back to.

Rosie was brave. Very brave. These things are hard enough for a man, but for a mother that instinctive, visceral tug of her own flesh and blood is so much stronger. She kept smiling, talking gently to Ollie as she laid out his clothes. Then we went downstairs and sat in the playroom which opened onto a fenced courtyard garden where Ollie found a watering can and started some serious water play. He made a tentative move towards the fence, appraising the bars with experienced eyes, and as Lynda put out a restraining hand Rosie warned, 'I'm afraid he'll be over them in no time. I hope you can run fast!'

Then, with a casual 'Goodbye Ollie', we slipped away and went to the pub for lunch. Back at Prior's Court after lunch, I couldn't resist that sneaking look through the bathroom window. Later, we drove round the M25 to Surrey, to collect a bike which a cousin was passing on to Edmond, returning in the evening to sleep at the school.

Or rather to lie awake, anguished by thoughts of our son lying in a separate building, only fifty yards away but ignorant of our nearness. We slept falteringly and both woke early, with that same bleak stab of realisation that we had experienced as adolescents waking in strange boarding schools. In my case, that first-day-of-term knot in the stomach had usually slackened quickly as I settled into what was generally a happy productive time; for Rosie, stranded 5,000 miles from home in a dull, petty, bullying, suburban girls' school, it had been a bleak exile. What could it be like for Ollie? How on earth could he make sense of this sudden disruption of his whole world?

Food restored some equanimity when we came down to breakfast in the school dining room, once the children had had theirs. Rosie had another talk about Ollie's diet with the cook, a jolly woman in a zingy patterned chef's hat. Then another young woman, in the school's navy blue uniform, came in and said, 'Hello, I'm Trudi and I'm one of the care staff in Ollie's house. You must be his parents. I thought you'd like to know that he seems to have settled in very well. He had a good night's sleep and ate a good breakfast this morning.' I felt like leaping up from my bacon and eggs to envelop her in a big Option-style hug, but managed to confine myself to a sedate English smile of thanks. Encouraged by this confirmation of Ollie's courageous adaptability, we left after breakfast.

The school suggested waiting one weekend before fetching Ollie home. So for twelve days we fretted in our strangely quiet, empty house. For over two years there had been a constant traffic of staff traipsing up and down the stairs. The kitchen had been filled with the noisy buzz of the intercom, and our saintly neighbour Jill had had to tolerate the endless cacophony of our uncarpeted wooden floors. Outside in the garden the birdsong had been interrupted regularly by Ollie's spontaneous whoops of delight. Now it was all silent and we wondered agonisingly what Ollie might be doing, how he might be feeling.

But we had Edmond, whose school holidays had now begun. Suddenly we were free to come and go, without the constant checking of cover arrangements and dashing back at the allotted hour before the carriage turned into a pumpkin. We were free to spend a glorious summer night camping illegally on Solsbury's grassy plateau, Rosie and I glugging wine in the gloaming while Edmond chattered in the tent with his friend Frank; free to set off spontaneously for a day at the seaside, giving Edmond the attention he had so often been denied during the first seven years of his life.

Then the twelfth day arrived. Today we would see Ollie again! It was a Friday and we arrived in the morning for one of the regular training sessions the school organised to keep parents informed about teaching methods and care policy. It was good to meet another couple we had last spoken to several years earlier when they had been doing a Lovaas ABA home education programme with their daughter – reassuring to hear that they too had decided in the end that they needed the help of a residential school. Today was the official end of term, to be followed by two weeks of special summer holiday activities. In the afternoon we all walked through the playground to a hall for the final assembly.

We sat in a crescent of chairs, towards the back of the hall, leaving the front rows free for the children. And then they arrived – fourteen of them now at the school – dressed in the same white and navy blue as their teachers and carers. Some strode in boisterously; others shuffled diffidently, trying to make sense of the jumbled adult faces. One girl let out sporadic loud shrieks. In any 'normal' environment that noise would induce fear, annoyance or embarrassment; here it was just accepted as her particular thing – her own special way of comforting herself.

Another girl went soundlessly to her father, who picked her up and cradled her against his shoulder. One particularly beautiful boy with lush curls – so many autistic children *are* unusually beautiful – sat in his appointed seat but couldn't resist turning round to shout gleefully at his mother. And then Ollie appeared, holding Lynda's hand, sidling in with his slightly jerky gait, a half-smile playing around his mouth. What did he see when he looked round this room, I wondered? What sense did he make of these random faces? How did this buzz of voices sound in his ears? And when was he going to notice *us*?

It took a while. Only after he had sat down and Lynda got him to turn round did he register the two familiar shapes. There was a flicker of puzzlement – what are they doing *here*? – then a shy smile. He turned away. Then turned round again, checking. Yes – it really was them! The smile widened and he laughed. Then bounced excitedly up and down on the flats of his hand, fingers pressed inward on the chair seat.

There were action songs, awards for some of the children, a prayer from the local vicar and a short speech from the head, Robert Hubbard. The children joined in sporadically, but for much of the time they were busy with their own private agendas. I too found it hard to concentrate – just wanted to hug Ollie and take him home.

Which very soon we did, keeping him at home for

two nights and driving him back to Prior's Court on the Sunday evening. He came home the following weekend as well. During the weekdays he was busy with special holiday activities, visiting theme parks, going to the seaside and riding on toy trains. The school was very good at keeping a record of these activities, sending us an album of photos. In some of the pictures Ollie still seemed rather forlorn, as if wondering what this was all *for*. Who are these people? Why are we rattling along in this funny long segmented car? Why are we traipsing across these boards, past all these noisy shops and stalls and bright colours, amongst this great confusion of people, towards a huge expanse of stones and sand and strange-smelling wavy water?

Three years later, looking again at those photos, I was anguished by that look of forlorn abandonment. But then I concentrated on the *other* images, of a tentatively smiling Ollie, and re-read the narrative. Often the transition from comforting minibus to strange new environment was fearful. But then . . . 'Ollie enjoyed running in and out of the sea . . . Ollie enjoyed pushing a small wheelbarrow round the garden centre . . . Ollie went on a trip to the Natural History Museum and was very interested in a video about water . . . he was particularly pleased when we went into a small garden area and found a large yellow watering can.' Perhaps we had underestimated his adaptability. It was only five years after the event that Lea, one of the carers, told us about the time at Sea World when Ollie outwitted his guards and, quick as an eel, flashed over the wall and into the water, to splash amongst the stingrays. How comforting to know that, right from the start, his adventurous spirit was challenging authority.

Ollie completed four weeks at Prior's Court, two of them technically part of the summer holidays. That left another three weeks' holiday with us. Now that the LEA and Social Services had allocated such a huge chunk of their budget to Ollie's school, there was not much left for home cover. During school holidays we would be on our own. So, I thought, let us roam free. Let us see if, for the first time since our Dordogne jaunt six years ago, we can manage a family holiday. But this time let us go somewhere wild and Celtic. Let us, like the poet Robert Graves, go to those incomparable hills which stand sentinel over Cardigan Bay, framing the coast from Barmouth to Harlech. Let us go to the Rhinogs.

We left early on Saturday morning, stopping for breakfast in a field near Much Wenlock. Then drove on into Wales, to Llangynog, to meet the Freeman-Attwoods for a pub lunch and to see the farmhouse they were renovating in the Berwyn hills. 'Tidy bit of work, eh,' enthused Julian, as we admired Welsh dragons carved on trussed oak beams built to last five hundred years. Then he drove us up a vertiginous track onto the high moor. Ollie loved riding in the pickup and seemed to thrill to the huge open sky. We continued west in our own car to the same cottage we had rented three years earlier.

This time we had to Ollie-proof the house. So, while Edmond and Ollie ran wild amongst the sheep, Rosie and I hid all the glass vases, Derby plates, Welsh china dogs and other breakables, fitted Heath Robinson string locks to the doors and laid a heavy-duty tarpaulin on the floor of Ollie's bedroom, as protection against his wayward bladder. Then I fetched wood and coal to fill the sitting room with glowing warmth.

We stayed for two weeks, hardly bothering to leave the Nantcol valley at all. For me, it was thrilling to be back in the place I had first come to know thirty-four years earlier, when I was only a little older than Ollie was now. Apart from some beautifully engineered improvements to the old cattle-drovers' road – a path which heads west up this valley and over the pass of Bwlch Drws Ardudwy, leading eventually to the distant border market at Oswestry – nothing had changed. Still the same spiky reed clumps and boulders dotted amongst the sheep-cropped grass where, as a boy, I had run bare-foot down to the stream. Still the same slate steps – huge slabs cantilevered out of a wall at the side of the house – where my younger brothers and sisters had sat and played with the toy trolls fashionable in 1966, infuriat-ingly sedentary while I fretted to be away and up onto the titanic tumbled quartz-veined boulders of Rhinog Fawr. Still the same precious remnants of sessile oak forest, bedded in luxuriant moss and leaf mould where, if you were lucky, you might find the half-buried yellow flesh of chanterelle mushrooms. Still the same reek of wild goat. Still the same dithering indecision about which routes to take through this perversely tortuous landscape, with its knee-deep heather, squelching bogs, rock terraces and enchanted fern gardens sprouting at the mouths of long-abandoned manganese mines.

The sun shone and Rosie was content. Edmond, too, loved this wild mountain retreat. And what about Ollie? It was all too easy for me to project my own aesthetic responses onto a boy who could be just as fascinated by a paper bag or a car hubcap or a manhole cover. And yet he seemed to find solace in this place. He loved to sit on the hot smooth slate wall outside the kitchen and time after time he ran up the hillside at the back of the house, racing backwards and forwards between the wind-curved hawthorns, head tilted to the sky. He played with Edmond on a rope swing hanging from the big ash tree; and while Edmond and I built a dam in the stream, although Ollie was not joining us directly, he seemed to be absorbing the atmosphere of contented work, hearing the same joyful gurgle of water on rock, smelling – in his case probably more intensely – the same peaty, mossy, reedy, rocky scents.

In the second week Rosie's sister-in-law Shan and her nephew Charlie came to stay. We were also joined by Edmond's godmother, Maggie, and by Maggie's dog. Much as we loved our sons, we craved adult company and guarded the sanctity of evening 'grown-up time'. Charlie, a professional chef, used every single pan in the kitchen to produce sumptuous dinners, on one occasion driving manically through Llanbedr chasing a fishmonger's van to secure the perfect filets to accompany an exquisitely indulgent Chablis sauce. One evening, to earn our gastronomic reward, Shan, Charlie, Edmond and I walked up to the little tarn of Llyn Hywel, plunging into its icy depths before drying off and heading back down to Nantcol. On another occasion I got up at alone at dawn and walked rapidly up onto the flanks of Rhinog Fach, then changed into rock shoes to climb what appeared to be a new route up a gorgeously textured slab of finest Harlech grit, continuing to the summit, then racing down to the lake for another obligatory swim and heading home for a late breakfast.

The guests left and I had to drive up to Edinburgh to do a talk at the Book Festival. I got back to Nantcol soon after breakfast the next morning, to find Rosie looking slightly harassed. She had woken at sunrise to find no sign of Ollie. The bathroom window had been open, with scuffmarks on the roof where he had slid over the gutter and dropped to the ground. She had run straight down to the farm in her pyjamas. Still no sign of Ollie. So, climbing over drystone walls, she had continued towards the river, several fields away. There she had found him, bent naked over a deep whirling pool, filling a watering can snitched from the farm. On another search, she had been intercepted by Mr Evans, who had asked 'would that be your boy?' and pointed up the mountain to the joyful silhouette of Ollie running naked across the horizon.

That afternoon he lolloped up again to his favourite spot on the hillside above the house. He rarely strayed far from that particular haunt so I didn't bother to check on him for about twenty minutes. But when I did go up to look he had vanished. Not a sign of him anywhere. Not even at the farm. Nor at the river. I ran frantically up and down the hillside, eyes straining myopically to detect a human form amongst the far-flung sheep, brain wondering how soon to summon the mountain rescue people. Rosie called the ever forbearing Evans family at the farm, and the two sons came out on their quad bikes. By now it was starting to rain and we were frantic at the thought of Ollie lost and hypothermic.

He must have been gone for at least forty minutes when a young man, a student, came running up to Nantcol and asked if we had lost a boy. He and his friends had passed a child earlier, as they headed up the main path of the valley. They had said hello, asked him who he was, where he was going, what had happened to his trousers . . . but received no reply. Deciding, very Britishly, not to interfere, they had then continued. But after a few minutes one of the girls had said, hang on . . . boy that age – eight . . . nine? – should he really be wandering around on his own in the mountains, with no trousers? And why can't he talk? Shouldn't we find out?

So, as rain began to glisten on the stone path, they turned round, generously delaying their walk. By the time the messenger had taken us to meet the rest of his party a mildly bewildered, protesting Ollie, wrapped up in an adult-sized woollen jumper, was being carried back down the valley by his equally bewildered rescuers.

Yet another of the countless incidences of the kindness of strangers.

The rain was short-lived and the following day, as Ollie seemed to like the ancient cattle-drovers' road, the four of us all set off on an afternoon walk. It was the last day of our holiday and I wanted to stay for ever. I felt I could never tire of this timeless symbiosis of heather and bilberry and moss and lichen and warm rough stone, its surface etched with the intricate linear scourings of the last ice age. We stopped at a bridge and lay on huge rock slabs, trailing hands in the gurgling peaty water. Ollie slouched contentedly, legs sprawled sideways, Rasta tartan hat perched skewily on top of his head. Then we continued towards a stile where I hoped to cross a wall and head rightwards towards Lyn Hywel, the lake Ollie had still not seen. But we never reached the stile because there were too many bilberries to eat. Ollie foraged happily, mouth and fingers staining purple, tongue savouring the juicy astringency.

Rosie wanted to walk further but Ollie could not be cajoled into moving. So she went on with Edmond, while I stayed behind until Ollie decided to head down to Nantcol. On the way back he got his trousers soaked in wet undergrowth and insisted on taking them off. So for the last part of the journey he walked barelegged and barefoot. Again, perhaps I was imposing on him too many of my own impressions, but he seemed, as he explored the ground's texture with outstretched toes, to be utterly content – this strange, slender, mercurial, Puckish spirit wearing nothing but underpants, stripy tee shirt and tasselled hat, looking ethereally bright against the dark heathery mass of Rhinog Fawr looming

in a slate sky. This wild landscape had no need for words
or explanation. It had no noisy threatening crowds, no
artificial lights, no amplified sound, no incomprehensible
plot to follow. This, not theme parks, was what Ollie
needed!

Purple remembered hills. It was probably not *all* that
perfect and Rosie did more than her fair share of
watching Ollie, terrified that he might damage our
expensively rented holiday house. And, back home
during Ollie's final days of holiday, she had to run the
show completely alone while I flew to Switzerland to
do a job for the BBC.

The job was to climb the Matterhorn in a rather
dapper tweed suit, silly hat and size thirteen hobnailed
boots which had once belonged to Graham Greene's
mountaineering brother, Raymond, to give an impression of the first ascent by Victorian pioneers. I love
dressing up and showing off, especially when I am being
paid to do it. And the Matterhorn, for all its globally
warmed disintegration, is an endlessly beautiful, fascinating phenomenon.

I left England on Sunday morning. On Tuesday we
climbed the mountain and got the summit shots. On
Wednesday we shot some more scenes before descending
in pouring rain to Zermatt, where our hedonistic director
Mick Conefrey insisted on champagne and a gourmet
dinner. Before getting too jolly, I found a call box and
phoned home to tell Rosie that the climb had gone
according to plan, including some stunning aerial summit
shots. 'I'm so glad you're safe,' she replied. 'It's mayhem
here. Some bloody animal has given the boys impetigo.'

'What's impetigo?'

'It's horrible and it's highly infectious, so Ollie
couldn't go back to school today.'

I decided not to mention the champagne. Instead I stressed that we still had several important shots to get and that I would be working hard for the next three days. Which was true. It just happened to be very enjoyable work.

I returned on the Sunday, by which time Ollie's impetigo had cleared up and we could take him back to school. We settled into a fortnightly routine, saying goodbye on a Sunday night and driving back to continue with our lives at home, counting the twelve days to the joyful Friday afternoon when one or both of us would drive back up the M4 to collect Ollie again. One Friday afternoon during that autumn of 2000 the school made a video of a special harvest assembly.

The scene opens with parents arriving in the hall, directed to their seats by David Heald. There is a buzz and chatter of excited voices. Then the children appear, one by one, with their carers. Although many of the children have language, there is also a crescendo of non-verbal sounds. The head teacher addresses parents through the hubbub, unperturbed when a girl bounces up and down shrieking 'eeeee'. Then one of the teachers leads everyone, with piano accompaniment, singing 'Ten Green Apples' – a variation on the more familiar bottles, with selected children brought up to the front to place, and then remove, ten model apples from a cardboard cut-out tree.

Parents and teachers sing gamely as the children join in with varying enthusiasm. One boy keeps trying to leap from his seat. Another, when brought up to the front, flings his apple across the room. But most of them carry out their appointed tasks; some of them smile proudly. The camera's eye pauses on a back view of Rosie's blonde hair. Then two rows in front of her a boy turns round and we see Ollie stealing a delighted glance at his mother. Then, right at the end, it is his turn. 'One red apple, hanging on the tree.' A guiding hand on his white shirt helps him to his feet. He steals another backward glance at Rosie, then goes up to the tree, plucks the apple and puts it in the bag. Then returns obediently to his place and sits down. Then Robert Hubbard gets up to thank all the children and to celebrate that there are now eighteen children in the school, at the end of its first year.

It was all very different from what we had been doing with Ollie at the Option Institute a year earlier. Was this elaborate performance really for the children's benefit, or for ours? And what about the classroom reports, with their references to 'maths' and 'technology' and 'history'? Was it really necessary to give these children 'access' to a National Curriculum dreamed up by tinkering politicians? Did it have any relevance to them at all?

Perhaps I was being cynical. After all, when Ollie first became autistic we tried to integrate him into a mainstream nursery school. And even when we began educating him at home, the hope was always to help him regain the language and understanding which might enable him eventually to join a normal school. Now that hope looked more forlorn, but he still loved, clearly, to succeed at appointed tasks; and many of the other children at Prior's Court had more language than him – more understanding of how to fit into these traditional educational rituals. And perhaps, even for Ollie, after years of one-to-one isolation, this formal socialisation was a necessary way of bringing him closer to the baffling complexities of the life we call normal.

He tried, but found it hard from the start. During the morning 'circle time' in the gym, assembled with the whole school for Higashi-style exercise, he struggled to join in correctly. In the classroom he appeared baffled by the picture symbols and sign language used to aid communication. And, like any schoolchild failing to understand what was going on, he played up. Escape remained his favourite diversion, greatly enhancing the fitness and climbing skills of his keyworker Lynda. He also became obsessed with the fine bosom of his class teacher. She was quite short, so an easy target for a growing nine-year-old with a breast fetish. Unfortunately, taken by surprise on the first occasion, she rewarded Ollie with a dramatic overreaction. So he repeated the game, eventually mauling her so painfully that she resorted to coming to school in full body armour. We apologised profusely, hoping desperately that this bright, vivacious teacher would allow Ollie to stay in her class.

I missed the end of term assembly at Christmas, but Rosie was there. She found it hard to staunch the tears at these assemblies, which, however full of loving care, were such a potent reminder that our son no longer lived at home; but on this occasion the tears mingled with pride as Ollie went up to receive a special award for 'Effort'. Despite his reputation as the naughtiest child in the school − despite the exhausting pursuits over fences; the gradual resigned removal of trashed curtains, carpets and pictures from his bedroom; the endless mopping up of water − the teachers and care staff seemed to appreciate his boisterous personality and were lavish with praise for every little effort to conform.

As always, it was thrilling to have Ollie home. But this was not a weekend: it was a full three-week Christmas holiday. Alison Jones and Wendy Morris, two of his old Son Rise teachers, took turns to help most days for a couple of hours but for the rest of the time we were on our own, trying grimly to Choose

Happiness. Again that schizophrenia: 'We adore you to bits, Ollie, but my God you can be difficult.'

On 9th January 2001 Rosie, Edmond and I took Ollie back to school, waved goodbye, and continued round the M25 to Gatwick. After all the years of confinement in Larkhall, we had taken up foreign holidays with a vengeance. I had also started writing travel pieces for the *Mail on Sunday*, making these holidays a source of income. This first assignment was to Kenya. After twenty years' exile in Sussex, Rosie's brother, Jake, and Shan were now living near Nairobi again, so we used their house on the tea plantation as a base between trips to Lake Naivasha, the Maasai Mara and Jake's new game reserve near Amboseli. We ended with three days on the island of Lamu, feasting on crab and lobster and swimming with dolphins in the Indian Ocean.

A pattern was established. The three of us had a glorious adventure. We wished that Ollie could be with us, but knew that for the moment it would be too difficult. However, the return to damp, grey Britain was always thrilling because Ollie would be there waiting for us. On this occasion we drove straight from Gatwick to Prior's Court. He climbed happily into the back seat next to his sun-bronzed brother and chanted his contented 'Duv-a-duv-a-duv-a-duv' routine (to rhyme with 'love') as we headed west towards Wantage and the snow scudded out of the twilight sky onto cold bare hills.

More snow. This time Scotland. A mad drive, five hundred miles north to a girls' school near Perth, where dear, efficient Maggie Saunders, in between working flat out at schoolteaching and tending her dog, has organised a charity lecture. I arrive in the afternoon, get set up, have a shower, change and deliver my slide show on Shackleton and South Georgia. The girls are wonderful, helping to shift a large pile of my books to a packed audience of the Perthshire great and good, doing their bit to keep the Venables family solvent, alongside the charity. Profuse thanks to Maggie for all her hard work, and then at ten thirty p.m. I head back south, reaching home in time for a quick breakfast, before getting back into the car and driving east to collect Ollie.

It was the March holiday and he was home for sixteen days. During the October holiday I had had to change a flight and return early from Canada, admitting how unrealistic it had been of me to expect Rosie to cope on her own. This time, apart from a one-day event in Chamonix, I stayed entirely at home, generally spending afternoons with Ollie, while Rosie had a break.

I still believed firmly that air and exercise were the best thing in the world for Ollie, and we spent dank winter afternoons touring the familiar landmarks of our local landscape. Solsbury Hill was an old favourite. Later we discovered a longer circuit – a complete circumnavigation of the hill, following ancient paths down Chilcombe Bottom to Northend, then back round the southern flank to Bailbrook – a good two hours' walk.

He had a strong sense of place and several times that week insisted on walking up the path to the house where Andy and Jo's family had recently lived. I tried to explain that they had moved – even took him to their new house – but he returned repeatedly to the old address, startling the new owners when he appeared unannounced in their garden. Faced with these endless diversions I tried to practise what we had preached to the hospital – waiting patiently, never bullying Ollie into compliance. But my patience often failed, or at best I joshed and jollied him along, trying to keep him on task with a guiding hand. When he *did* get into his stride he was a great walker.

For short excursions we had our local Alice Park. Getting Ollie there involved tight surveillance: a moment's negligence and he would be gone, dashing opportunistically down some stranger's suburban garden path – a watering-can-seeking missile homing unerringly on its target. Once we reached the park, though, there were swings, and slides and a large sandpit. And a wide grass expanse to run across. Again, constant vigilance was essential: on one occasion my concentration lapsed and I only just stopped Ollie at the last minute, with an arresting bellow, from opening a gate and running out onto the busy London Road.

As he grew bigger, the discrepancy between his actual and mental ages became more apparent. But he looked completely 'normal', so his eccentricities often took strangers by surprise. Other children ate their crisps, blithely unaware as Ollie stood in front of them smiling; then shouted in startled outrage as an uninvited hand shot into the packet and grabbed a handful of deep-fried potato. On one occasion a little girl screamed tears of dismay as the elfin boy whipped an ice cream out of her hand and crammed it into his mouth. Adults could be equally dismayed. In the big playground at Victoria Park, charging manically through the Saturday crowds, Ollie paused, walked up to a young mother, smiling angelically, then whipped the umbrella out of her hand and ran off with a loud 'Hah!' I pelted after him, grabbed his wrist and dragged him back to the woman, whose umbrella I returned. Ollie giggled and I remonstrated in cheerful mock anger, 'Naughty boy, Ollie!'

'It's not funny, you know,' snapped the woman.

'Sorry, I— oops, off we go. Come back Ollie!' I charged off in hot pursuit, shouting over my shoulder, 'Autism!'

As the incidence of autism spectrum disorders grew

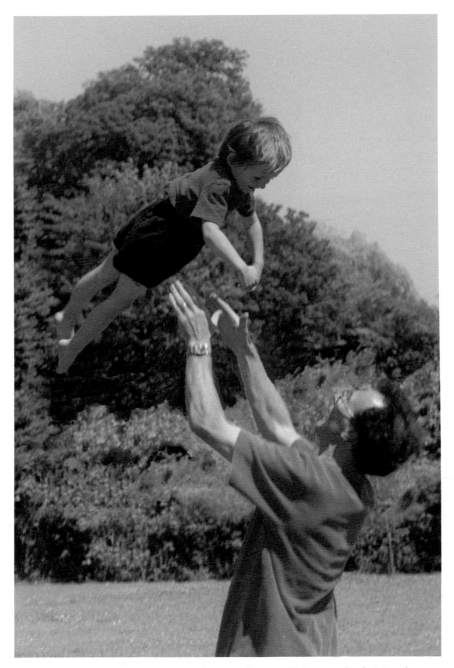

July 1995. Sam Farr took this photograph to publicise our fundraising for Ollie's first home education programme. (© *Bath Evening Chronicle*)

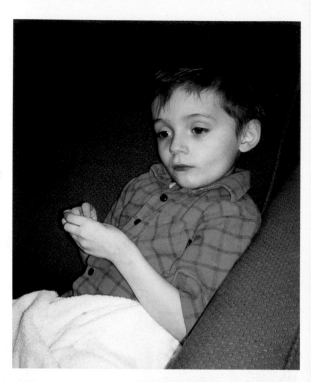

February 1996.
Ollie feeling very
weak just after starting
chemotherapy treatment
for leukaemia.

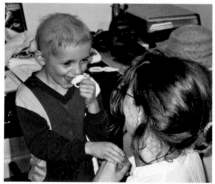

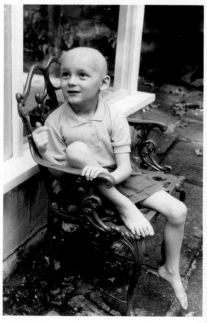

Summer 1997. Soon after the leukaemia
relapse Ollie had to embark on a new
course of intensive chemotherapy, losing
his hair a second time. Here one of his
most gifted helpers, Emma Bird, magics
away his distress.

Two or three weeks later he enjoys
a contemplative moment.

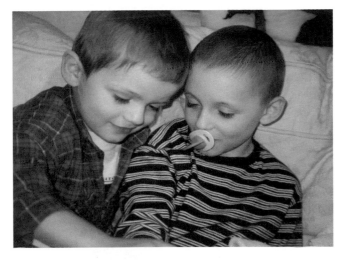

December 1997. At the end of a harrowing year Edmond elicits a hesitant smile from his brother.

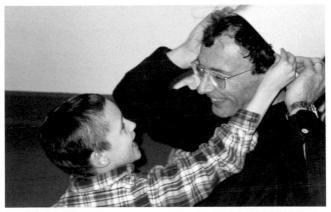

In February 1998 Ollie's life was transformed by starting the Son Rise programme in his special playroom.

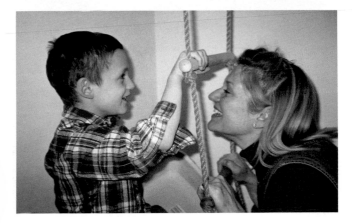

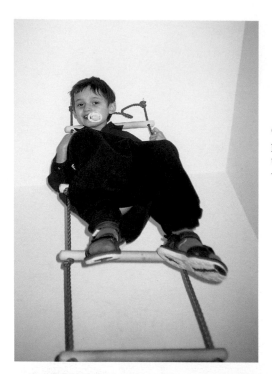

Ollie in his Son Rise
playroom, taking time out on
the rope ladder and working
with Angie Montgomery.

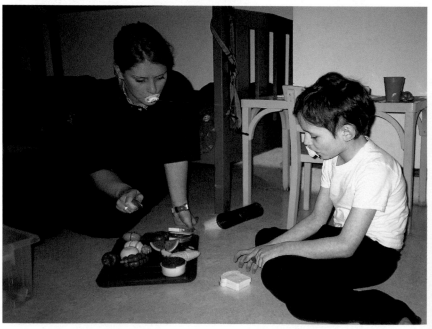

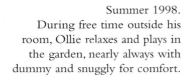

Summer 1998.
During free time outside his
room, Ollie relaxes and plays in
the garden, nearly always with
dummy and snuggly for comfort.

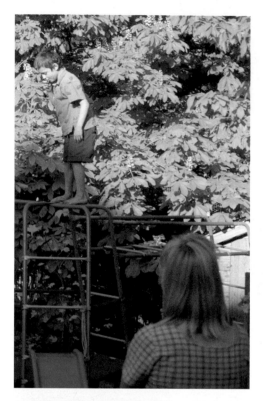

Summer 1998.
The climbing frame has become
too tame; it was later replaced
by a fifteen foot high treehouse.

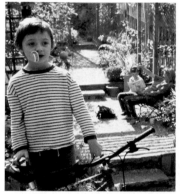

1999. Ollie content with
bike and watering can.

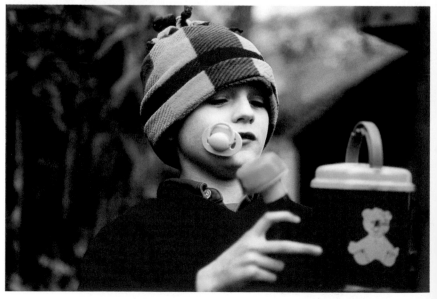

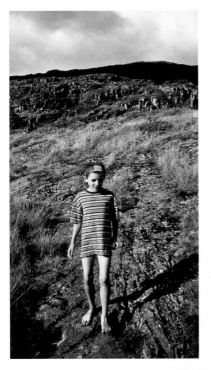

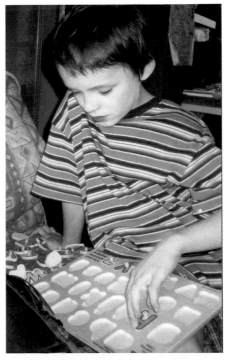

August 2000.
Below Rhinog Fawr.

Summer 2001.
Regaining lost jigsaw skills.

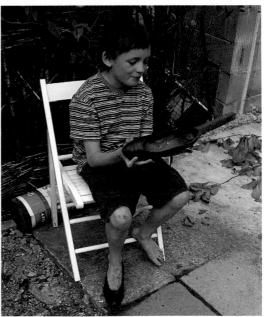

Borrowing his
mother's shoes.

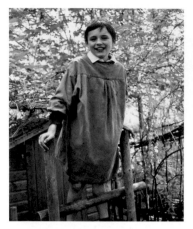

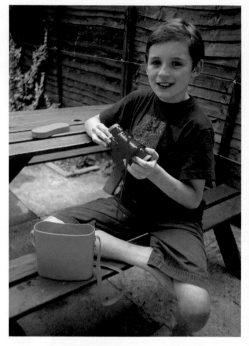

May 2003.
Saturday morning at home on
the trapeze launching platform.

July 2003.
The last photo of Ollie,
with his brother's binoculars.

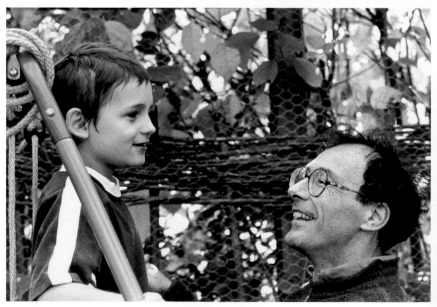

A classic Ollie moment. He is glad of my presence, but looks just past me,
enjoying his own private unfathomable joke. (© *Avery Cunliffe, 1999*)

all over the Western world, people became more familiar with the term, more understanding of these child's peculiarities. Only very, very rarely were they unfriendly. With Ollie we only once experienced downright hostility and even then, it seems to have been the manifestation of a kind of fear.

It was later that year – summer 2000 – and we were having lunch in a pub garden by the river. Edmond helped keep guard, shadowing Ollie and warning us if he got too close to the weir. On past occasions he had climbed up onto the pub roof a couple of times. He had also once sneaked unnoticed through the public bar to find himself in Ollie heaven – an entire room filled to the ceiling with bottles of wine, gin, whisky, vodka, brandy, tonic water, ginger ale, orange juice . . . a dazzling display of liquid delight – a thousand bottles just asking to be emptied.

But today there were other distractions. While we waited for our meal to arrive, Ollie wandered over to a neighbouring table where a large man in a Stetson presided grumpily over his family's steak lunch. I went to fetch Ollie and apologised. Mr Stetson scowled, confounding all our previous experience of American courtesy. A moment later Ollie walked back over to the Texans' table and stood watching them, an innocent smile playing across his face. Mr Stetson shooed him away; wife and daughters stared with embarrassment at their steaks.

'Come on Ollie,' we shouted; but he was too fascinated to move.

'You'd better go over,' suggested Rosie, so I walked over again to take Ollie's hand and explain things to the harassed tourists. 'I'm so sorry Ollie's bothering you,' I said. 'He has autism. We find it best just to be very calm with him.'

But Mr Stetson was beyond calm. Further discussion seemed pointless so I took Ollie away, but a few minutes later he wandered back over to the Texans' table, thrilled and fascinated by their overreaction. He stood watching for a moment, then stretched out an index finger, describing an elegant parabola through the air as he brought the finger down to prod, very gently, the succulent centre of Mr Stetson's steak. The steak remained uneaten and soon afterwards the Texan family drove away; as for our own lunch, we sat it out grimly, but the whole incident left a nasty taste in the mouth.

I think our encounter with Mr Stetson was in late May, at the start of Ollie's sixteen-day midsummer holiday. After that Rosie and Edmond went to Sussex for his half-term holiday, while I stayed at home with Ollie. One afternoon in the kitchen, as he rummaged in one of Rosie's desk drawers, I failed to register the crackling of metal foil and it was only later that I found him at the bottom of the stairs, lolling drunkenly on the floor. As I tried to pick him up, he yawned and flopped back down. Then I found the half-empty packet of tranquillisers – left over from the distant dark days when Rosie had resorted briefly to pills to help her through the staffing crisis.

'Oh Ollie! What have you done? Come on, let's put you to bed.' I carried his floppy body upstairs, then hurried back down to search for further evidence. Most of the foil blisters had been popped open and were empty. I phoned the hospital with the name of the drug and they said they would send an ambulance. I groaned despairingly at the prospect of stomach pumps and continued searching the floor.

Yes – here's one . . . and another . . . and another. Maybe he didn't swallow so many after all! The telephone rang and a very helpful doctor asked me again Ollie's age and weight, and how many pills he might have taken. I re-counted the loose pills on the floor and the empty blisters. Even if the packet had started full, we now realized that he could only have swallowed a maximum of four pills. Ten minutes later she phoned again. 'Hello. I've checked up with the National Poison Centre. Apparently four tablets is just within the safety limit. He'll just sleep very well tonight!'

Hurrah! No hospital! No stomach pumps! You wonderful woman. Thank you so much. And here's the ambulance . . . Thank you so much for coming, Mr Paramedic in your smart green uniform; but it's OK – the boy can sleep it off at home.

The paramedics gave Ollie a quick check and left. The following day we *did* have to go to hospital, but this was just a regular check-up at the oncology clinic in Bristol. It was exciting to take the lift in the brand new Children's Hospital, now completed. Inside, the old familiar faces welcomed Ollie with the usual smiles as I tried to contain him in the play area. Then Tony Oakhill invited us into a treatment room for a blood check. It was now over two years since chemotherapy had stopped, and the portacath had been removed, so blood had now to be taken scarily from an arm vein. The moment the needle appeared Ollie's face puckered and mouthed 'Noo, noo, noo' as he backed away from Tony. I tried reluctantly to hold him. Tony – a large, powerful man – tried also, but Ollie shoved him out of the way, nearly ramming the needle in his face.

'This is dangerous,' announced Tony, 'dangerous for Ollie *and* me. I'm not prepared to do this. He looks absolutely fine and from now onwards we'll only attempt to take blood if he actually shows any symptoms.'

We then realised that we could in any case get some

blood the following week, when Ollie would be unconscious under a general anaesthetic at the Royal Free
Hospital in London. It would also be an opportunity for
a dentist to check his teeth and for someone to check
his eyes for cataracts – a possible side effect of the cranial
radiotherapy he had had four years earlier – in effect a
full maintenance check-up with minimal distress.

On 5th June Ollie settled happily into the car for the
drive to London, only getting agitated when the
soothing smoothness of the M4 was shattered by a decel-
erating left turn onto the North Circular. Half an hour
later we were shown into a private room at the paediatric gastroenterology department of the Royal Free
Hospital.

For Rosie, this visit was just one more step in the
continuing journey to get to the root of Ollie's autism
– to find out what had caused his brain to unravel so
mysteriously and to do everything possible to alleviate
the effects of that unravelling. In 1992 she had noted
Ollie's troubled reaction to the MMR jab – the insult
to his immune system and the exacerbation of bowel
problems, leading, it seemed, to the eventual catastrophic
damage to his brain. After 1994, as she researched autism
tirelessly, talking to researchers like Paul Shattock – and
to other parents – it became clear that this pattern of
'late onset' autism, apparently connected to problems in
the gut, was not unique to Ollie. There seemed to be a
clear genetic predisposition to autism – a fragility, an
inability to cope with toxins – which made these children susceptible to the kind of environmental insults
which most children take in their stride. Thimerasol –
the mercury-based preservative used in many childhood
inoculations – was one possibility. Another, very
different, possibility was that the interaction of live

vaccines (devoid of mercury preservative) in MMR was extremely damaging to the guts of a tiny minority of children.

Right from the day of the vaccination, Rosie had been adamant that MMR had damaged Ollie, so it was grat-ifying to hear about other children who had been affected, more obviously and drastically, in some cases becoming almost immediately autistic; and when a gastroenterological surgeon at the Royal Free, Andrew Wakefield, announced in 1998 that there might be a connection between MMR and bowel problems and autism, it came as no surprise to us. Two years later, while I was filming in South Georgia, Rosie met Dr Wakefield and decided that she would like Ollie to be examined. In February 2001 we took him to the Royal Free clinic to join several other autistic children startling the regular patients in the gastroenterological department with their spinning and finger-flicking and snuggly-stroking and croonings and howlings and bouncings.

Our brave boy managed on this occasion to cope with a blood test and then lie perfectly still for an X-ray. Then we took our turn seeing one of the consultants, who pointed out on the X-ray the impacted stool bulging out of one side of the bowel. 'You see, here – this is the problem . . . nearly the size of a baby's head. It seems to be the same with many of these children.' He asked us about Ollie's history, noting the recurrent alternation between constipation and diarrhoea, and prescribed a powerful laxative, to be repeated when necessary, to remove the blockage. More controversially, we discussed bringing Ollie back for an endoscopy to inspect in detail the entire length of his intestine and to take a biopsy – a tiny sample of the gut wall – for analysis.

So on 5th June we returned for Ollie to have his whole digestive system emptied with the drug Picolax, in preparation for his endoscopy the next morning. 'Poor little lad,' commiserated the nurse who arrived to fit his cannula in the morning, 'what a way to spend his tenth birthday.' But midazolam had helped to calm him, and it felt like old times as I accompanied him through to theatre.

Afterwards we were presented with a delightful movie of Ollie's digestive tract, taken by two miniature remote-controlled cameras, one travelling down from his nose, the other up from his bottom. While Ollie was recovering from the anaesthetic, one of the consultants came in to tell us that he had checked Ollie's eyes and there *did* seem to be a cataract in his right eye, and possibly the beginnings of opacity in his left lens as well – yet another medical challenge for Ollie to deal with. But his teeth were fine. As for his large intestine, as we could see on the video, there were patches of ulceration, although not as severe as in some of the other children.

Later Andrew Wakefield dropped in to state, perhaps more strongly, that Ollie seemed to show a similar pattern to the subgroup of children he had been investigating. He also suggested that Ollie try the drug Pentasa which for some children had proved very beneficial, relieving gut trauma and some of the autistic traits which seemed to derive from that trauma. With Ollie the Pentasa did not seem to help. In fact it seemed to disturb him quite badly. When I telephoned the news to Andrew Wakefield three or four weeks later he sounded surprised, but said immediately, 'If it's not helping, I should take him off it.' Rosie discovered later that Pentasa is the trade name of mesalazine, one of the amino salicylates; in this eternal game of microbiological swings and roundabouts we had come back full circle to early suggestions about the possible exacerbating effects of salicylates on some children's autism.

In August I tried repeatedly to get hold of the other consultant for a follow-up discussion about Ollie's prognosis, at one stage driving all the way to London only to discover that I had been invited to a clinic on his day off. When I did eventually get him to a telephone I asked him if there were any results from Ollie's biopsy: in several children traces of vaccine-specific measles virus had been found in the gut. Although Ollie's whole system had been comprehensively scoured by three years' chemotherapy, making him a very unusual case, we were still curious to know whether he showed any sign of measles vaccine traces. When I mentioned this to the consultant he reacted brusquely: 'That's entirely Andy's business and the samples are not analysed here. If I were to say anything at all about measles I'd risk having my whole department closed down. By the way, I don't know whether you are aware of this, but Andy is about to leave the department.'

Soon after that Andrew Wakefield resigned in a blaze of publicity, vowing to continue his researches in America. In the meantime, Ollie's fragment of gut lining was analysed and – unlike many of the other children's biopsies – showed no sign of measles virus. Given the vagaries of lab results from new experimental techniques – and given the compromised nature of Ollie's gut – we could not be sure that this necessarily proved anything, and we kept him on the list of children in a collective suit against the MMR manufacturers. All along we had known that his was one of the less obvious cases.

What gave Rosie's hunch credence – apart from the evidence of her own eyes – was the stronger, more immediate correlation between MMR and gut-related autism exhibited in the lead cases. With Ollie there may well have been several other factors at work, including, for instance, the early problems with cow's milk and, perhaps, a bad reaction to the thimerasol preservative in his diphtheria, pertussis and tetanus vaccinations at two, three and four months. Nevertheless, MMR had marked the visible beginnings of a significant long-lasting deterioration in his health. If the case were to come to court and if Ollie, along with four hundred other children, were to be awarded damages, it could remove some of the uncertainty hanging over his future. His special care and education, currently costing about £80,000 a year, was being paid by his LEA and Social Services. But at nineteen, when his statutory right to education would stop, who knew what would happen next? And, later, what on earth would happen once Rosie and I were no longer here to fight his corner?

Ollie now spent most of his time at school, but we still had him at home for about twelve weeks a year. Even with all the gates and locks it was hard to control his amiable rampaging round the house. Often in the morning, while we prepared breakfast downstairs, we kept him in his room listening to his favourite Bob Marley or one of the more esoteric tapes sent by my old climbing friend and eclectic reggae collector Steve Razzetti. Sooner or later the mellow Jamaican rhythms were usually punctuated by the sharp clatter of plastic toys raining down from Ollie's window onto the garden paving and announcing that it was time we paid him some attention.

Although our request for an extension had been refused, we *had* now been allocated a disability home improvement grant to adapt Ollie's bedroom – renovating broken plaster, putting in a new waterproof floor and new steel safety bars on the windows, providing him with his own basin, and adding a vandal-proof en suite lavatory – all of which was extremely welcome, and still not cheap. But it didn't remove the problem – a stage-management problem – of getting Ollie to and from his room, via the kitchen, where he ended up spending most of his time, creating havoc.

The two-week holidays, often coinciding with Edmond's, were becoming exhausting and when Prior's Court announced that this year there would be no summer holiday activities, and that children would be coming home for five solid weeks, we realised that something had to change. Ollie was not really coping with the academic expectations of Prior's Court and needed more sustained one-to-one care; nor was he coping with the irregular, stop-start terms and holidays; nor were we coping with his long spells at home.

After much agonising, we countenanced the previously unthinkable: Ollie needed a fifty-two-week placement.

The parents from hell contacted the Senior Education Officer to present yet another request for change: they wanted Ollie to move to an even more expensive school. The initial reaction was a very understandable 'No'. But we persisted, once again lobbying furiously, and she agreed to hear our case at a special review meeting on 18th June. We prepared detailed notes and on the day I went to County Hall to present our case. David Heald and Penny, the keyworker who had now replaced Lynda, came specially from Prior's Court to support us. Ollie's social worker, Niki, came too. Norman Donovan, our ever-sympathetic senior educational psychologist, also dropped in specially to hear what I had to say.

The biggest problem, I stressed, was predictability. When he came home from school, Ollie never knew whether it was for a weekend, or a fortnight, or five weeks. For us, the weekends were a treasured time, but anything much longer than that became a dreaded burden. Again, I had to state the case strongly, hating myself for listing all the problems, including the alienating effect on Edmond, who for the first time in his life was growing resentful of Ollie and writing in his school list of 'how to be good' resolutions – after 'be nice to Mummy when she cries' – 'try not to hit Ollie'. I enumerated painfully the long list of health problems, reminding everyone yet again that Ollie's was a very special case, told them about the incident with the tranquillisers, stressed the safety factor; then pointed out that soon he would be a six-foot teenager. The gist of it was that full-time special schools had rotating teams of people – teachers, carers, cooks and cleaners – to provide efficiently for the needs of children like Ollie, even during school holidays; we were burnt out trying to do all that on our own, so that, instead of looking forward joyfully to Ollie's visits, we were starting to dread them; and then feeling full of remorse after returning him to school. Better that he should come home just for two days at a time, every fortnight, and be loved wholeheartedly.

You can usually tell at a meeting which way the decision is likely to go. The Senior Education Officer tried manfully to keep her cards close to her chest, but without saying as much, she seemed to accept that Ollie needed to move. Soon after the meeting she confirmed that he could start in November at Sunfield, one of the first schools we had looked at, in the Midlands. There he would live for fifty-two weeks a year, but 'home' would still be with us, in Larkhall, and we would fetch him back at least once a fortnight. When we heard that, with special extra cover, this new school place would cost £120,000 a year, I vowed never again to complain about Gordon Brown's punitive taxes.

We still had the summer holidays to get through. My mother, bless her, came up trumps with a generously large cheque – 'it's my money and I can choose how to spend it' – to pay for extra help to tide us over. George, Vikki and Cheryl, care assistants from Prior's Court, came to stay and took turns to play with Ollie, take him on excursions and produce a special scrapbook about his adventures. His devoted keyworker Penny also took time off from her own children to come and spend a day with him. Then Amala, one of his old Option teachers, now at art school, came and spent a week with us at Nantcol, followed by Anne Hambrick during the second week. Unfortunately it rained almost continuously and they found the magic of the Rhinogs elusive. Rosie, too, became thoroughly disenchanted. But we had one or two good walks and some wonderful afternoons on the beach at Harlech, Ollie leaping rapturously through the waves, then escaping, as we tried to dry and dress him, to run naked and laughing, sprinting back down the beach and into the surf.

Then it was time to return for his last session at Prior's Court. The term ended on Wednesday 24th October. Instead of the usual assembly, all the staff and children – over thirty of them now – gathered outside to release helium balloons into the autumn sky. There were a few brief speeches. Then David Heald, shouting above the autistic hubbub, announced, 'Finally, we're saying goodbye today to a very special boy who was one of our first pupils at the school. We'll miss you, Ollie, and we give you all our best wishes for the future.' We said our goodbyes and headed for the car, laden with farewell presents, then drove for the last time down the long avenue, past the joyful falconer and out through the remote-control gates. The following Thursday Ollie started his new life at Sunfield.

Chapter Twelve

We were sitting on the kitchen sofa, putting on shoes ready to go out for a bike ride. At Prior's Court Ollie had learned to cycle and in Wales that summer he had sped a mile along the Nantcol road, a touch wobbly, but coping, mastering the miracle of balance.

Shoelaces were different. 'There we are, Ollie . . . now, let's have your other foot. Then we can go for our ride. Good idea?'

'Yeh.'

'Nice talking! I'll bring your bike through. I wonder where we should go?'

'To the canal.'

What? Surely it wasn't possible? 'Ollie, you can't be—'

'Yes, of course I am. We'll go over the river and up that track—'

'Ollie! I don't believe it. You amazing boy. You could talk all the time!'

'Yes.' He continued fluently, discussing our ride with sophisticated vocabulary; and as he talked a sweet surge of happiness welled up through my body. I tried to shout through the exquisite lump in my throat, calling Rosie, but the words were drowned by tears. And then my eyes opened and I saw her sleeping form beside me. Hovering on the edge of consciousness, I tried to gather the shards of a shattered vision, tried to climb back into the dream; but dawn had broken the spell.

We both often had this dream of Ollie talking –

slipping quietly, naturally, into the conversation, as if autism had never happened. Of course the waking was always a disappointment, but never as bleak as that original sense of loss – of a gift cruelly confiscated – when Ollie first entered his autistic world at the end of 1993. In fact the dreams were rather comforting – a vision of what we still hoped might happen one day. We always felt that he was watching and listening, acutely sensitive, just waiting for the moment when, somehow, the subtle irregularities in his neural wiring would be mended and he would tell us everything.

For the moment though, the practical reality was that he needed to be looked after at a school for children with 'severe and profound learning difficulties'. We took him for his first visit on Friday, 26th October, two days after leaving Prior's Court. Brazen rabbits nibbled the grass amongst the trees surrounding Orchard House, the unit for seven autistic boys, aged between eight and fifteen, with whom Ollie would be living. We arrived at eleven forty-five, when the other boys were away at their classrooms, left Ollie with three of the care staff and then went over to the main school to have lunch with some of the teaching staff in the big dining room. During a brief lull in conversation Rosie looked down at the buttons on her dress, took one between thumb and forefinger, and began to turn it gently, entranced by the dance of light on its shiny surface. Everything went extremely quiet and she suddenly looked up to see several special needs experts watching her with knowing smiles. Given her constant reminders to Edmond and me that all males are to varying degrees innately autistic – in contrast to robust females with their two X chromosomes – I found this little vignette most gratifying.

This first visit was just a brief introduction and after lunch we returned to Orchard House to collect Ollie.

Jenny, one of the care staff, bubbled enthusiastically in a thick Dudley accent, 'Isn't he lovely? He's just *gorgeous*. So responsive.' We clucked proudly. Paul, the deputy team leader, came out of the office with two hot-off-the-press digital photos of Ollie in his red and navy striped polo-neck shirt: one with his head thrown back in abandoned laughter; the other a head-and-shoulders close-up of him looking directly at Jenny with a huge, confident, cheeky smile.

Our second visit, the following Monday, didn't go quite so smoothly. It was our fault for coming into the house – Edmond, Rosie and I – on a non-school day when all the boys were at home. We sat awkwardly in the television room while Ollie wandered around the house. A tall boy of about fifteen stared silently at Rosie and she smiled back. Suddenly, with terrifying precision, he hurled a plastic brick across the room, hitting her smack on the forehead, nearly knocking her out. He was rushed straight out to his bedroom while someone got Rosie a cold compress. After lunch the same thing happened to Edmond. This time the brick hit with less force, thank goodness, but it was still scary to think of our precious Ollie coming to live with these powerful adolescents.

That night I telephoned the head, Barry Carpenter, and explained our fears. He already knew about the incident (the school was meticulous with written reports on every smallest injury or accident) and assured us that it was unusual. As Rosie had concluded herself, the boy was just freaked by the sudden influx of strangers disrupting his routine. A couple of the boys *were* occasionally rough, but they were under constant supervision and in the months to come Ollie grew very adept at avoiding them.

Thursday 1st November was the big day. We arrived

in the morning. While I unpacked all his storage chests full of clothes, toys, books, CDs and cuddly animals, Ollie waited in the car, found a can of touch-up enamel and put some decorative white dabs on the dashboard. We wiped up the mess then left him at Orchard House while we went to the pub for lunch.

The school was very helpful, encouraging us to stay for three nights in the parents' flat while Ollie adapted to his new home. Every few hours we would go and see him briefly in Orchard House, or take him out for a walk, visiting the sheep and donkeys in the big field, and exploring the school's beautiful willow-arched sculpture garden. Edmond had started singing in the Bath Abbey choir so on Friday evening I drove him down for his rehearsal, from which my parents would collect him, then returned to Rosie in the Midlands. On Saturday afternoon we took Ollie for a walk on the Clent Hills above the school, trying not to succumb to the misty melancholy of a November twilight. Then, on Sunday morning, we bade Ollie a brief farewell and drove off. We managed to talk bravely and cheerfully about how well it all seemed to have gone and it was only an hour and a half later, as we approached Bath, driving past the familiar long line of beech trees, russet in the autumn sunlight, that the tears started to flow down Rosie's cheeks.

We never tried again to spend time with Ollie at school. He drew very clear parameters and liked people to remain in context: we belonged at home, not school. At the end of his first week we fetched him for the weekend; thereafter we stuck generally to alternate weekends. By the Monday or Tuesday of his second week back at school we would be saying, 'Oh good, Ollie'll be home in a few days.' And when the Friday afternoon arrived he would be sitting in the window of

Orchard House, looking out for the car then fidgeting impatiently in the entrance hall while one of the care staff unlocked the front door. Usually Rosie did the Friday afternoon pickup. She would wait by the car while Ollie's keyworker, Alan, unlocked the front door. Then Ollie would run down the path and jump into her arms for a quick whirl round, before fretting to be away, into the car, settling on the back seat with a gleeful 'oiyoiyoiyoi' or 'num num num' or 'duv-a-duv-a-duv'.

Arriving home, Ollie often rushed straight past me, ignoring my hellos as he made an immediate tour of inspection, checking all the cupboards and taps, hoping that I might have left a door unlocked or a tap valve open. Sooner or later he usually managed to create mayhem and I tried to take him out at least once a weekend for a good walk. Saturday 22nd December was particularly memorable. Edmond and I took him up the familiar track to the top of Solsbury Hill. The sun shone from a pale sky. Frost crunched underfoot and the orange-pink berries of a spindle tree glowed on the edge of the hill where the two boys ran backwards and forwards, chasing each other amongst the grassy hummocks – remnants of the earthworks which had protected the Iron Age community living here long before the birth of Christ.

Everything seemed to be sparkling with celebratory anticipation; but this year, for the first time, Ollie was not with us on 25th December. Over the last few years Christmas Day had become an increasingly fraught event, with Ollie often confused and upset by the unwrapping of too many presents. This year Rosie and I wanted for once to go to the Abbey together, particularly now that Edmond was singing. So Ollie stayed at school and came home again the following weekend. We took him back on the afternoon of New Year's Eve.

There was snow in the Midlands and we longed to take Ollie tobogganing with us, but fearful of upsetting his firm home–school parameters, we returned him to Orchard House before dragging the sledges up onto the Clent Hills.

2002 started with a big fright. When Ollie came home on 12th January he had lost 5 lb weight in one week. He looked so ill that we kept him home for a week. He had intermittent abdominal pain and looked horribly pale. We were terrified that this was a leukaemia relapse, so on the Wednesday Rosie telephoned Helen Kershaw at the Bristol Children's Hospital. 'Bring him in tomorrow morning and we'll have a check,' she reassured, 'but I'm sure it'll be something quite innocent.'

On this occasion, after an hour of fruitless child-centred coaxing, we had in the end to be brutal and hold Ollie in a firm grip while Dr Kershaw swiftly and skilfully drew blood from his arm. Then he gulped with surprised pride as we told him it was all over.

We started to build up his strength with liquid supplements while we waited anxiously for the verdict. Then, after just two days, the hospital phoned to tell us there was no trace of leukaemia. What Ollie did have was campylobacter – a virulent bacterial infection, possibly picked up by putting some faecally infected object in his mouth. This was a lot better than leukaemia, and antibiotics eventually killed off the infection. Nevertheless it was a vicious bug and it took Ollie a long time to rebuild his weight. In February, still painfully thin, he came home for another week, forcing me to turn down at the last minute an invitation to address the annual meeting of the American Alpine Club at Snowbird, amongst the incomparable powder bowls of Utah. Very reluctantly I returned my skis to the garden shed. Utah would have to wait; Ollie was more important.

Illness notwithstanding, he still took a lot of managing. One afternoon Matthew the cellist and I were standing in the garden, enjoying an after-lunch Golden Virginia roll-up. Rosie and Edmond were in the kitchen, Ollie was playing in his room. Over our nicotine fix we chatted about music, as we usually did. Then I told Matthew about the flood – hadn't he heard about the flood? Oh yes, we did everything on a biblical scale here! One dark stormy night, a year or two after the fire and the house rebuilding, one of the very expensive new smoke alarms went off with a piercing shriek. But it wasn't set off by smoke: it was activated by *water*, pouring out of the piano-room ceiling, straight through the alarm. Then more water started jetting out of the plaster ceiling rose, cascading onto the piano; further tributaries oozed from the newly replaced cornice. Rosie and I rushed round with buckets and mops. I climbed onto the roof, but couldn't find any problem there – just couldn't fathom how this immense volume of water was getting into the house. It was only after many gallons had poured into the piano room that I finally found the source. The builders had left an old waste pipe, open-ended, in the cavity between the piano-room ceiling and Ollie's room, which had once been a bathroom. The other end of the sawn-off pipe was connected to the main waste downpipe from the roof. That had become blocked in the torrential storm and all the water pouring off the roof was backing up into our house.

'It was quite surreal,' I told Matthew, between puffs, 'seeing that waterfall pouring down onto—'

'It's happening now.'

'What do you mean?'

He smiled and took another puff on his roll-up. 'Look.' He pointed to the window above us.

'No – it can't . . . I don't . . . what the hell . . . Ollie!'

The press tap in his room was designed to stop this sort of thing, but he had managed to jam it open, then put the plug in the basin, allowing the water to over-flow onto the floor. I found him splashing merrily in a three-inch-deep lake, now spilling out over the top of the waterproof skirting and pouring down into the room below, onto my late godfather's sorely abused Broadwood.

2002 was the year of campylobacter and the Second Deluge. It was also, more pleasurably, the year of the Tree House. The boys had grown out of their off-the-peg climbing frame and needed something more exciting. I wanted to make a tree house, but we had no suitable tree. So I decided I would have to *build* the tree. Or at least build a house on tall stilts, reaching up into the horse chestnut overhanging the Lambrook – more house-in-the-trees than actual tree house. Later I would add a Himalayan-style rope bridge linking it to the top of the mound.

What fun to get immersed in a building project! All done selflessly, of course, purely for the sake of my children. I drew up plans and ordered a lorryload of timber from the Longleat estate. It arrived in February, filling the path to our front door. The 'approximately 6-7 inch diameter' beams which had seemed so slender in my imagination looked more like telegraph poles, and at twelve feet long were a challenging load to shoulder through the basement and down to the bottom of the garden. That weekend I erected six vertical uprights – four for the main structure and two for an extending platform which would link to the rope bridge – each bedded in eighteen inches of concrete. In May I resumed the job, guiltily abandoning any pretence at real work, as I puzzled out each new stage of the construction. The previous year I had spent my birthday balancing up a gorgeous limestone wall in Austria's Wilder Kaiser mountains; this year I had an equally enjoyable birthday, delighting in this thing – this creation rising so geometrically amongst the burgeoning sappy foliage.

Ollie came home for the weekend and clambered approvingly over the skeletal framework. Then in July, working flat out one week, I finished the floor, fitted side rails, added ladders and bars to swing on, and then nailed roof planks over waterproof felt, adding a final airy ladder onto the roof itself. Here Ollie loved to stand, right on the apex, a bird boy dancing his rocking dance, singing his heart out, balanced masterfully fifteen feet above the ground, while Edmond stayed more warily away from the edge. Later, when I added the rope bridge, Ollie would use it as a trampoline, a steadying hand on each side rope as he bounced vigorously on the single foot rope.

I loved that quirky joy and wondered exactly what he saw as he stared up at the sky; or adopted another favourite position, tilting a chair precariously on the garden steps and perching on it in perfect balance; or dressed up in women's clothing, slipping Rosie's pointy black shoes onto his long feet before removing them and filling them lovingly with gravel; or, on a walk, flung repeated handfuls of leaves into the canal, like the land artist Andy Goldsworthy, relishing the ephemeral flash of dancing colour. A creature of finely tuned senses, he loved to browse amongst the fennel, breaking off soft hairy fronds to suck, so that the plants never grew more than a few inches high. He also loved daisies, reaching through the fence with his toes to pluck them from Jill's garden. And, for all his apparent destructiveness, he had very clear ideas about where things should go. Earlier that year someone gave us a little clump of yellow narcissi in a pot. For a long time the pot loitered forlornly amongst the day lilies, until I chose a suitable home for the narcissi, planting them out in a nice focal point in front of a large euphorbia. They looked good there and I was pleased.

A couple of weeks later I noticed that the yellow flowers had gone. Vanished. I could have sworn I planted them there. Bloody cats from next door! Hang on . . . what's this? Here they are, back in their pot amongst the day lilies. Perhaps I never planted them out after all? Perhaps I'm going mad – early-onset Alzheimer's.

Only a very slight jumbling of stems betrayed the repotting by Ollie Venables.

He showed the same attention to detail one evening as the two of us headed up the long sloping field on the way up Solsbury Hill. His cowpat obsession had, thank God, long since passed, and today he just paused to contemplate my profile against the reddening sky. We stood like that for perhaps a minute, both entranced, until I turned my head to smile at him. He immediately put out his hand and very firmly shoved my head back into the correct position: there – just stay like that, please, until I ask you to move.

I was often away during 2002. Although Utah was cancelled, there were frequent other working trips abroad – to Morocco, Prague, Courmayeur, Geneva, Malta, Philadelphia and Missouri. And, blurring the boundaries between work and play, a spring walk through Tuscany with Edmond and Rosie for a travel article. Then, at the start of June, a week with Henry the Botanist in my favourite place in the whole world – the mountainous coastline of Wester Ross.

We left home on a Sunday afternoon, dropping Ollie off at school on the way, wishing that he were coming with us all the way to Scotland to see his godfather. However devoted his teachers and carers were, we wished he could be with *us*. As Karen, his wonderful class teacher, said at a review meeting when a colleague commented on how well Ollie had settled in, 'Well yes, but he'd really rather be with his mum.' Rosie was still hoping that one day she could 'make him better' so that he could live at home, and travel with us to houses that didn't have alarms and locks and high fences and special anti-flooding taps.

Now that Ollie was at boarding school, even though Rosie was doing part-time teaching, she had more free time to research ways to 'make him better'. She made contact again with the tireless Brenda O'Reilly who recommended special fish oils, obtainable from the Schizophrenia Society. A huge daily dose of nine capsules produced spectacular results soon after Ollie started at Sunfield. At Prior's Court he had become increasingly dispirited by his failure to cope with simple tasks like jigsaws, but early in 2002 he came home one weekend, pulled out a jigsaw, tipped the pieces all over the kitchen table and reassembled them with a triumphant smile.

'Oh my goodness, Ollie– you can *do* it!'

'Yeh,' he grinned proudly.

That mini-miracle encouraged Rosie to continue her researches. On the whole we didn't want to go out and meet other special needs parents socially, for long chatting or whingeing sessions: we didn't want to talk shop; we wanted to laugh and drink and see films and go to concerts. But the Internet groups like gfcfkidsUK (gluten and casein free) were a huge help, allowing Rosie to talk quickly and efficiently with other similarly motivated mothers and to realise that she was not alone in this quest to get at the metabolic causes of our children's disconnectedness.

She also barraged our long-suffering community paediatrician, Simon Lenton, with emails, seeking professional medical support whenever possible. It was he, for instance, who agreed to prescribe melatonin as a harmless, non-toxic way of helping Ollie to settle at night. He too who authorised Ollie's school to administer the special enzymes Rosie ordered from America; although not normally used with autism, enzymes are given to children with cystic fibrosis, so, even if these were different enzymes, there was a precedent of sorts.

Boosting Ollie's deficient digestive enzymes made sense, as did looking again at some of the toxins which seemed to have accumulated in his body. A hair test at the age of three had revealed unusually high levels of aluminium, which some researchers believed was a marker for mercury contamination. The word on the bush telegraph was that some autistic children had a problem with metalothionein – the agent which in a normal healthy body removes unwanted metals. Apparently some children were benefiting significantly from a special treatment, using mainly vitamin B6 and zinc, to stabilise the metal accumulation and compensate for metalothionein deficiency. The treatment had been developed at the Pfeiffer Treatment Center in Chicago. We had to give it a try.

So in June 2002 we set off for America. Once again Ammy from United Airlines smoothed our flight across the Atlantic and on a Saturday evening we checked into the Marriott Hotel, Naperville, Chicago. On Sunday morning we explored Naperville, walking through a silent wasteland of immaculately groomed commercial premises and hotels. Cars passed us, but we saw no other human beings until we reached a public park. Then suddenly there were people – lots of them, getting out of cars to walk. This must be where you come to walk! And you need special equipment for it – special shoes, special tracksuits, special walking caps, special walking CD players and lots of other gadgets to measure speed, pace, distance, calorie consumption and cardiovascular performance.

A serious business, we realised, as we sauntered shambolically along an immaculate gravel path, pushing a rather lethargic eleven-year-old in his pushchair, longing to divert into the woods either side and challenge the notices warning that trespass into this 'wilderness area' was a federal offence carrying a $400 penalty.

We returned to Naperville and while Rosie and Ollie went back to the hotel I searched for a supermarket to buy some supper. All I needed was a friendly person to point the way, but all the people were hidden behind the dark windows of huge motor cars. In the end I had to stride out into the middle of the road and accost an alarmed driver who, once convinced that I was not a homicidal maniac, slid down his window and pointed the way. Mission accomplished I returned with provisions, to find Rosie, very aptly, watching a phone-in cookery programme on the television. A very large woman was teaching the viewers how to make a simple delicious pudding with tinned peaches, when one adventurous proto-chef phoned to ask whether she could use real peaches to do the same thing. Large presenter woman looked totally flummoxed. 'Fresh peaches! Errr . . . we-e-ell yeah . . . yeah, I guess you could.'

Into this surreal world we tried unsuccessfully to imprison ourselves. The problem with hotel rooms is that their locks are designed by non-autistic people, for non-autistic people, to stop other people, of whatever neurotype, from getting *in*; there is no way of stopping the occupants getting *out*.

So Ollie escaped. Repeatedly. And I had to tear myself away from televisual gastronomy to race down the corridors. The hotel was built on a plan of several interconnected H's so there were lots of right-angle bends and T-junctions – endless possibilities for an athletic eleven-year-old to outwit his middle-aged, orthopaedically challenged father. I would arrive breathless at a junction, stare left and right and see nothing – just two identical corridors, as spookily empty as the corridors in *The Shining*. But sooner or later there would be a distant shriek of laughter and I would race off towards it, and as I came round a corner bewildered chambermaids would stare at the toeless barefoot Jack Nicholson figure charging past them, even more demented than the crazy child who had just run off with their mop.

It was all good exercise and we slept well that night, rising fresh on Monday morning to walk the half-mile to the Pfeiffer Center, where everything was reassuringly bright, brisk and efficient. Once Ollie had submitted bravely to a blood test, Rosie had a long meeting with one of the clinic nurses. I played with Ollie, while she discussed his medical history. The nurse outlined a protocol for a very gradual build-up of supplements, mainly vitamin B6 and zinc, intended gradually to stabilise the heavy metals in his system. The exact schedule would be fine-tuned once they had results from the blood tests, and the nurse promised that we could phone for further consultations whenever we needed to.

And that was that. We flew back to England that night and on Wednesday Ollie was back at school. Summer holidays came. Edmond, Rosie and I house-sat for my old climbing sculptor friend, Dick Renshaw, in the Black

Mountains, where I worked on the picture-captioning for a big new illustrated Everest book. Then we spent ten days camping in Brittany, returning just in time to fetch Ollie from school for another medical examination.

A new hospital this time – the Bristol *Eye* Hospital, where a consultant surgeon would investigate the extent of Ollie's radiotherapy-induced cataracts under general anaesthetic. The surgeon was very helpful – agreeing to have a dentist run an opportunistic check over Ollie's teeth at the same time – but his bedside manner was a little on the brusque side and, for an optical specialist, he seemed to have remarkably little eye contact. While Ollie was still in recovery he came to see us and without any preamble, staring at a point somewhere just to the side of Rosie's shoulder, announced cheerfully, 'Yes, well as we suspected, the cataracts are quite advanced. Reasonable visibility in the left eye, but that may well get worse; and he's almost completely blind in his right eye.'

Rosie gulped. The surgeon asked how we would like to proceed. We said we would like to think about it, but that, yes, probably it would be best for Ollie to have a new artificial lens in his right eye and leave the left one to see how it developed. We would put Ollie on the waiting list for the operation; in the meantime he would continue to squint and sight sideways out of his left eye. We wondered how much difference this new blindness actually made. Ever since he became autistic, his sight seemed to have been quite distorted and, for all we knew, his whole visual experience of the world had been quite different from ours for many years; he seemed to have taken this latest optical challenge in his stride.

In August we extended our hospital repertoire further. Orchard House telephoned to say that Ollie had fallen over and cut his forehead. They had rushed him to Kidderminster, only to be reminded that this was the marginal parliamentary seat New Labour had recently lost because of the closing of the hospital's Accident & Emergency department. So, onward to Worcester, where Ollie was now waiting to see a doctor. I raced up the M5, and found my way to A&E. Ollie was sitting in a chair, flanked by two Orchard care staff, with a dark gash just above his left eye. As I came round the corner and saw him I was rewarded with a huge smile of delighted surprise.

We spent two hours in a treatment room, while attempts were made to inject a local anaesthetic and stitch the one-inch cut, but Ollie would have none of it. I suggested midazolam but he was given an insufficient dose which, far from sedating him, gave him a manic fit of the giggles. In the end we just had to leave the wound to heal itself, resulting in a small scar. The following year Rosie booked Ollie into Bristol for an operation to reduce the scar. People might question the ethics of that purely cosmetic operation; we felt that Ollie's beauty was a potent weapon in his struggle to face a difficult world, and that we should do everything to preserve his good looks.

The days began to shorten. In a beautiful grand house near Caernarfon rented for the weekend, with beaches, mountains and famous gardens nearby, my parents celebrated their golden wedding anniversary with all their children, children-in-law and grandchildren – apart from Ollie, whose enigmatic smile had later to be pasted digitally into the group photo. We collected him on the way back south for a surprise weekday break at home. Then at the end of September my parents had their official party in a marquee on their lawn near Bath and I, as

eldest son, made a lunchtime speech. Wendy Morris –
wonderful trampolining Wendy – had agreed kindly to
look after Ollie, who was home that weekend; but
halfway through my speech there was a phone call and
Rosie had to slip out. Down in Larkhall, Ollie had
managed to climb out of the garden and go on the
rampage amongst the neighbours, leaving Wendy,
unequal to his climbing skill despite her expertise on
the trampoline, locked *in* the garden.

That babysitting by Wendy was a rare delegation
allowing us to attend a special event. The only regular
respite was provided by Irene Weller, who had known
Ollie since she looked after him in the Abbey crèche
when he was one year old. Later, despite being in her
eighties, she had helped with the Son Rise programme
and now she still phoned frequently, when she wasn't
away surfing on the Atlantic coast, to ask when she could
come and see Ollie, who adored her. We were also
helped enormously by Tom and Alice Craigmyle. Alice
would phone every week and ask, 'How can I help you,
Rosie?' Nearly every weekend when Ollie was home,
requiring all our attention, Tom or Alice would quietly
come to collect Edmond and drive him over to the St
Catherine valley, where he could ramble freely with their
four sons in a large house and garden, relishing some
normality away from the Venables madhouse.

Rosie and I blocked out Ollie weekends and both
stayed at home with him, Rosie usually drawing up a
timetable detailing which of us would be on duty at
which times. Sometimes the duty seemed irksome. Or
attempts at creativity backfired. On one occasion I got
out the easel and poster paints and lost myself in a
vibrantly coloured abstract, hoping to inspire Ollie to
join in. He *did* join in, but on his own terms, with both
hands gloved to the wrist in glistening black. When I

looked up from the easel I found him on the stairs decorating the yellow wall with bold Picassoesque hand
strokes. But at other times he was enchantingly co-
operative. Saturday 12th October 2002 was a good day,
almost sedate in its early stages, which I recorded on video.

At breakfast Ollie eats several gram flour pancakes. I can
now make them almost as thin and crisp as the masala
dosas I tasted in the Greater Kailash market on my first
ever visit to Delhi in 1979. Ollie, addicted to strong
flavours, has his dosas spread with Marmite and Patak's
lime pickle. Today he eats three; and then another. And
then I ask, 'Another pancake, Ollie?' and he affirms, 'Yeh.'
   'Well, sit down – no . . . sit down – and I'll bring it
to you.'
   Edmond meanwhile is ready in purple-belted judo
suit, and after breakfast we set off to walk up to the
community hall for his class. Last time we took Ollie
with us, but he objected to the unfamiliar route, so today
we leave him behind. It is a gorgeous morning with
yellow leaves underfoot and huge juicy red berries overhead. On the way back down Dafford Street I pause to
admire Barbara Cartland Pink nerines, the last blousy
brilliance of some massed dahlias and Celia's cosmos in
their final defiant efflorescence, brilliant beneath a *Don't
Attack Iraq* poster in the window. Across the street our
pale Chinese rowan berries are pinkening to make a
winter feast for the blackbirds.
   As I walk back into the kitchen Rosie is in her
dressing gown at the computer, busy as usual with
gfcfkidsUk correspondence. Some Baroque trio sonata
plays on the radio and Ollie dances with the violin,
cello and harpsichord, running up and down the
kitchen.
   We go outside, sauntering past the huge crinkly

green-yellow-orange-scarlet-crimson-purple leaves of the vine, under the arch and down to the tree house, where Ollie looks up at me with a questioning smile, face straining to plead 'O?' (pronounced as the 'o' in 'hot'). 'O . . . unhh?'

'OK – off you go.' I give him a helping hand as he hooks first one leg then the other onto the trapeze, then swings his whole body, propelling himself into a wild arc, shouting joyfully, gutturally, 'Yoh . . . vehyahh . . . aiyeearghh.'

He runs back up to the house. Then back down the garden and onto the mound and up the ramp to the twin vertical posts supporting the rope bridge, where he lifts his left foot high onto the left post and tries to get his right foot onto the other one. But he hasn't quite mastered this balancing feat yet, so with a resigned laugh, he settles for a more straightforward bounce on the foot rope, all done in heel-less slip-on shoes, to the accompaniment of chattering rooks high above us in the oak tree.

Edmond returns from judo. After lunch we settle into a lazy domestic afternoon, Rosie playing patience on her computer, Edmond reading on the sofa. Ollie circles contentedly with the centrifugal salad dryer. He tries to make Edmond join in. Overcome with enthusiasm he bangs his palms down on Edmond's knees, shouting, 'Arghh . . . unghaiyeearghh,' then presses his forehead against Edmond's.

All three of us are now laughing with Ollie, sharing his pantomime moment. He chases Edmond up off the sofa – 'No, Ollie, I'm trying to read!' – then back to the sofa. Then leaves Edmond, to continue circling the room with the magic salad dryer.

I put on a CD of Bruch's *Kol Nidrei*. Over the cello's plaintive Hebrew prayer Rosie asks, 'Has he weed in it, darling?'

'Probably.' Ollie is tipping something down the sink with a laugh.

'*Ollie*, bring it to me. We're going to wash it.'

'Unh. Ah.' But these normally affirmative noises are accompanied by negative headshakes.

'Yes we are. Bring it here.' He brings it over. 'Put it in the sink.' But he insists instead on putting lid, bowl and spinner back together, unwashed, and returning the whole unit to its shelf, tidying it away. That is where it belongs – on the shelf, not in the sink.

Sunday afternoon and Rosie is helping Edmond with his homework. 'What's the sink?'

'Um . . . er . . . the sink . . . the sink . . . ummhh.'

'Come on, you've done it lots of times. The sink? It's *l'évier. L'évier, l'évier, l'évier, l'évier!* Now write it out ten times. And say it as you write it.'

Ollie twirls past, rotating a large cooking spoon on the rim of a half-filled glass of water – half whirling dervish, half Buddhist musician.

Later he settles on the sofa with his flip-over photo album. With a look of rapt contentment, he holds the pictures nine inches from his clouded eyes, examining Daddy in suit and Malmaison buttonhole at Julian and Emmy's wedding, Bruno and Rosie on the sofa looking at the book of Andrew Wyeth paintings, Ali the cheerful blonde CLIC nurse, Edmond in stripy shirt on his first little bike, Ollie in his Rasta tartan hat and dummy examining a toy watering can, Edmond and Mummy laughing on the garden bench. He flicks the images backwards and forwards, their shiny plastic sleeves reflecting light onto his face, illuminating his hands.

One might conclude that Ollie is delighted purely by the shiny reflections, rather than the familiar images of his life. But later with Edmond he looks through his non-reflective children's encyclopaedia – the present

Granny and Granchie gave him for his first birthday – and holds Edmond's hand to point at individual pictures. These two-dimensional images *do* resonate with him, and at school they tell us how he likes to sit in his room and look at pictures of home.

Enough studiousness. Edmond lifts up his elder brother to give him a piggyback, holds him for a moment, then buckles under the weight and the laughter. Then gives him crawling horse rides round the floor. Ollie laughs and bounces on Edmond's back. Then jumps up without warning, grabs a chopping board from the sink, runs over to the window, grabs a chair to stand on and—

'Ollie,' intercepts Rosie's mock-angry voice, 'what are you doing?'

'He's throwing the chopping board out of the window of course,' pipes up Edmond. Whereupon Ollie rushes back and gives him a spontaneous Ollie kiss, mouth pursed into a little dry O, which he presses jerkily on his brother's cheek.

By six o'clock that evening we were exhausted, as we always were at the end of an Ollie weekend. After an early supper, Edmond and Rosie came out to the car to wave us off, trying to get Ollie's attention from the pavement. But once he had belted himself onto the back seat he was already in a different dimension, fixed on the return to school.

Those melancholic Sunday night drives – a four-hour round trip to Sunfield and back – became inseparable from the Radio 4 schedule, with the British history series *This Sceptred Isle* usually coinciding with the moment we left the M5 at Junction 4, Anna Massey's gravelly narration an unwitting accompaniment to sad farewells, Michael Rosen's gloriously eclectic language programme, *Word of Mouth,* helping me back south. *The Westminster Hour* was usually just starting as I drove back into Larkhall and started on the final chore – tidying, sweeping and mopping away the mayhem in our kitchen in readiness for the new week, wishing that our wonderful cleaner, Mandy, would come back. But on this Sunday, 13th October, the car broke down on the motorway soon after Ollie and I set off. As the AA man drove us back to Larkhall in a glow of schadenfreude – well if you'd replaced that toothed belt none of this would have happened . . . even if it's only two or three valves gone it's gonna cost you . . . ooohh . . . seven hundred quid? – all I cared was that we had had a special reprieve. Ollie could have another night at home! And go back to school in the other car on Monday morning.

Edmond's boys' choir at the Abbey alternated morning and afternoon duties with the girls' choir. The weekends when he was singing at morning Communion and Matins ruled out going away, so we tended to have Ollie home on those weekends. Rosie or I would go with Edmond to Communion at nine fifteen, then the other, having first got the Sunday joint in the oven, would drive with Ollie to meet outside the Abbey and swap for Matins, bringing Edmond home in the other pre-parked car at twelve fifteen.

But one weekend that autumn Ollie was home on an Evensong Sunday. Rosie was busy, so I took Ollie with me to fetch Edmond at the end of the service. I dared not leave Ollie in the car so I took him with me into the Abbey. As we walked in through the west door I realised that it was nearly ten years since he had last come to a service here. I held his hand and we walked slowly up the south aisle. The choir was in the vestry, disrobing, but the organ was still playing. I wondered whether Ollie would be frightened, but he seemed eagerly curious. He looked up at the soaring clustered shafts of limestone and at Gilbert Scott's magnificently restored fan vaulting, and smiled. Perhaps it was just my fanciful imagination, but there seemed to be a flicker of remembrance – a faint stirring of memories of being happy in this place long, long ago.

The moment passed as Ollie's bladder suddenly played up and I had to rush him into the vestry, much to Edmond's embarrassment, to use the lavatory. 'Nevertheless,' I thought, 'we must try and bring Ollie back here again, even if it is just for five minutes to listen to the music.'

Edmond had now been in the choir for over a year and had begun, through a mysterious process of musical osmosis, to absorb an ever-expanding repertoire. This time at the big Advent service in December, instead of fiddling abstractedly with the strings of his cassock, he sang robustly, giving everything. Starting from pitch darkness, with childhood memories of 'Once in Royal David's City' and 'O Come, O Come, Emmanuel', processing eastward, to culminate in the blazing light of a thousand candles – as boys, girls, men and orchestra performed Bach's *Wachet Auf* from the steps of the high altar before processing back down the nave with a thousand people joining 'Lo, he comes with clouds descending' – it was the great set piece of the Abbey year.

That sense of shared ritual memory was uplifting, but it was also painful to think that we had once hoped for this for Ollie. A month later, on Christmas Eve, in the Abbey again for the final carol service before bleary-eyed last-minute stocking filling, the bittersweet poignancy of it all was too much. Surrounded by happy families, while Ollie was separated from us, a hundred and thirty miles away, Rosie couldn't hold the tears from rolling down her cheeks and blurring the candlelight.

Saddest of all was my favourite carol, Tchaikovsky's 'Crown of Roses', in which the child Jesus has a garden which is plundered by a gang of cruel children, who make a crown of thorns. In the final stanza, with searing dissonances the choir sings, 'And with rough fingers pressed it down; Till on his forehead fair and young; Red drops of blood like roses sprung.'

Christmas, with all its resonance of suffering deferred, never lent itself wholly to facile joy. However, it was very touching to hear later from Saranne, the care worker on duty at Orchard House on Christmas Day 2002. She had given up a 'good job' in a bank to work with special needs children, which she found far more rewarding. She wrote to us:

'I was working 7 a.m. until 3 p.m. There was Ollie and one other student at Orchard House. I didn't feel too well, but Ollie brightened my day up for me. He was making lots and lots of his happy sounds and every time he made one, I copied. Ollie loved it and in the end we were chasing each other around the house copying each other laughing.'

He probably had no idea that this day was different from any other and he loved the one-to-one attention. Nevertheless, we decided that in future, despite all the fraught chaos we remembered from earlier Christmases, we would have to have Ollie at home, if only for our own sakes. Even though he was being cared for by loving people – and even though this was what we had asked and fought for – the separation was too painful. The relentless emotional tug of the fortnightly routine – like a compressed lunar tidal sequence – was wearing Rosie down. She was tired of having to spend a whole Saturday getting Ollie readapted to family life, then preparing on the Sunday to say goodbye again. She was sick of lying in bed at night worrying about him, wishing that she could go and kiss him goodnight. And she was tired of the endless phone calls to care staff who, however devoted, were never going to be as finely attuned as she to the nuances of Ollie's fluctuating metabolism.

'I've had an idea,' she said early in 2003.

'Yes?' I answered warily.

'I think we should move: we should go and live near Ollie.'

For once I managed to respond positively. She was right. Things were going quite well at Sunfield and if this continued Ollie wouldn't have to leave until he was nineteen – not for another eight years. He could continue to live at the school, with all those teams of dedicated people providing the constant care and education he needed. But if we lived nearby we could see him far more often: even if he just came home for an hour at tea time, we could see him every day.

Chapter Thirteen

2003 was for me a year of mountains. It was the fiftieth anniversary of the first ascent of Everest and there were parties, launches, films, festivals and television and radio programmes to get involved in. Celebration was in the air. Work took me to Germany, Austria, Switzerland, Hungary and Spain. And we also flew as a family three times to the Alps, determined to give Edmond the adventure – aesthetic and physical – which most English schools ignore with their slavish devotion to team ball games.

So my memories of Ollie that year are like precious jewels glinting amongst luminous summits and indulgent celebrations. We were busy and contented and the summer was suffused with hopefulness as we prepared to move to the Midlands to be closer to Ollie, knowing that Sunfield was the right place for him to be. That confidence in the school was based on all sorts of observations, but one particular incident clinched it. Rosie had taken Irene, our octogenarian surfer, with her to collect Ollie one Friday afternoon. They arrived early, so Sue, one of the Orchard care workers, took them over to Ollie's classroom to see him at work. As Sue entered the room ahead of them Ollie rushed joyfully up to her and flung his arms around her waist. Only then did he notice Rosie and Irene hovering unscheduled in the classroom doorway, and come over all confused before giving them hugs too. 'He loves them, doesn't he?' said an approving Irene.

Rosie choked back the tears. 'Yes, I think he's happy here.'

He was continuing to make tiny incremental advances in the classroom, still with the same infinitely patient teacher Karen. In the gym he began to learn how to throw and catch a ball; he climbed wall bars and whirled across the floor in a magnificent inverted cone like a giant spinning top, eyes shining gleefully. We were at first disappointed when his large, gentle, Buddhist keyworker, Alan, was promoted; but his replacement, Chris, proved equally devoted and was punctilious about keeping in touch with parents. He spent hours diverting Ollie's watering passion into raising seedlings in the Sunfield garden. He set him new domestic targets – such as clearing the table at the end of meals – and had ambitious plans to keep extending the repertoire of useful activities. Ollie loved to arrange and tidy, even if that meant throwing everything out of the window; when he succeeded in channelling that passion for order into more traditional chores, rewarded with lavish praise, it was thrilling to see his pride.

Perhaps we were just manipulating him – trying to mould him into a compliant automaton for our own convenience. But I don't think so. For one thing, I don't think he ever would have let us do that. He was fiercely independent and had a gigantic personality. As Rosie often said, he was the sort of person who lights up a room when he comes into it – his flame seemed inextinguishable. At all three schools he attended he was notoriously 'difficult'; but that cussedness also carried immense charm, so that people's occasional exasperation was tempered by huge affection: he seems to have been loved by almost everyone. Although he treasured his independence – and needed sometimes to be alone – he also needed to engage with other people. He never

conformed to some mythical autistic stereotype, withdrawn completely from human society. In his own batty,
charming, baffling, eccentric way, he seemed to be trying
constantly to join the rest of us. So I felt we were right
to attempt a bit of gentle moulding – teaching him some
of the tricks and conventions of neurotypical society,
watching his pleasure as he mastered those tricks.

By the summer of 2003 he had been over four years
in remission. A few more months and he would be officially all clear from leukaemia. Despite the gloomy prognosis when he had had the relapse back in 1997, it now
looked as though the gamble of treatment had paid off.
True, his torso did look noticeably short in comparison
to his long limbs, and the cataracts were yet another trial
to face: the radiotherapy had left its scars; but at least he
was going to live. We had to cherish our survivor –
treasure the little boy who would soon become an adult.

That summer of hope now seems, in retrospect, an
enchanted interlude when nagging fears were
temporarily ignored. Earlier, on 17th March, Ollie had
a fit. This had happened twice before: first in 1996 when
he reacted to ketamine, and then again in 1998, when
the oncologists thought the seizure might have been a
reaction to intrathecal methotrexate. But this time, five
years later, there was no obvious cause. Ollie was in the
school playground, feet apart, rocking his familiar sideways dance, eyes to the sky. Then his teacher Karen saw
him lying on the ground but did not worry as this was
a standard routine in his playground repertoire. But a
few moments later she noticed that his whole body was
twitching violently. She rushed over to find him unconscious with his face turning blue and called frantically
for help. Then she rolled him quickly into the recovery
position, he started to breathe again and after about a
minute he came round. A few minutes later he stood

up and started to walk about, but was wobbly and disorientated. When the ambulance arrived after twenty-five minutes he was still a little unco-ordinated.

In April he had four more fits, three at school and one at home. Each time there was the same pattern of violent convulsion and brief unconsciousness, followed by dazed confusion. I telephoned Bristol Children's Hospital and spoke to one of the oncology consultants who had treated Ollie's leukaemia. We all knew that epilepsy was a common development in autistic children, but could these fits be a signal of some more sinister damage to Ollie's brain? The consultant said something like this: 'The fits could be induced by some kind of scarring of the brain tissue caused by cranial radiotherapy. It's a possibility. Knowing Ollie's unusual history I think it would be wise to arrange a brain scan, just to check.' Somehow that scan never happened. It seems to have been partly a reluctance by the physicians to subject Ollie to yet another general anaesthetic; partly a shelving of the problem when the fits stopped at the end of April.

In the meantime, the week after the first fit, Ollie *did* have to endure a general anaesthetic; but this was for the dreaded cataract operation. Dreaded, because we were terrified about what would happen when Ollie woke to the sudden soreness in his right eye. How on earth would we stop him ripping the miniature stitches from his sliced cornea?

Rosie contacted two delightful men from the medical technology department, who arrived at our house like James Bond's Q, with a plethora of gadgets to try out: arm splints to keep Ollie's hands away from his face, helmets and a range of industrial goggles. But they underestimated Ollie's wilful strength and in the end

Rosie had to develop their ideas further, ending up with tight-fitting goggles sewn onto a rugby helmet.

Ollie came home the night before the operation and tried on the helmet. Rosie told him he looked fantastic in his Spiderman outfit and he smiled. The next morning, 26th March we took him to the eye hospital. Going through the usual pre-operative checks, one of the nurses commented, 'That's strange: he still weighs the same as he did last July.'

'Yes,' Rosie replied, 'he has been looking a bit peaky. He's become rather small for his age.'

'Well, these things go in phases – it's probably just a temporary blip.'

'Yes, probably.'

As usual, I went through with him to theatre, then returned to Rosie in the ward. Another patient, a young girl, was wheeled in from her operation. Waking to find both eyes temporarily blind, she screamed with pain and terror. We smiled sympathetically at her parents and braced ourselves for Ollie's return. Thank God he was only having one eye done.

He arrived writhing and moaning, struggling to pull his arms out of the splints and straighten them, longing to get at the bulbous object encasing his head. A large wad of bandage was jammed beneath the right side of the goggles, taped around his eye. For an hour he screamed and fought, eventually ripping off the splints, so that I had to wrestle his arms to his side, holding down his wrists, smothering him with brutal tenderness, trying to talk gently, soothingly, willing him to compre-hend the future: 'Ollie, it will soon be better . . . just be brave . . . we just have to do this for a short time . . . *soon* your eye will be better . . . I know it's horrible . . . you brave, brave boy.'

The pain and confusion subsided and we drove home

to spend a long week on guard duty. All of that afternoon and night we had to force Ollie to keep on the hot itchy Spiderman outfit, but the next morning we could bear it no longer and took it off. Now he had to be shadowed even more closely, bullying hands alert to pull his arms down if he looked like scratching at the eye dressing.

His social worker, Niki, had kindly organised carers to share the work, but they were mostly agency staff with no experience of Ollie. One woman sat rather ineffectually in the kitchen, distracting Rosie and irritating Edmond with well-intentioned chatter, so that Rosie ended up looking after Ollie *and* Ollie's carer. Later that afternoon the carer whimpered tentatively, 'Should you be doing that, Ollie?' as he manhandled the boys' see-saw rocker over a ten-foot-high fence into the next garden, prompting the neighbours' boy, Dublin, to observe, 'He's jolly strong, isn't he!'

Jolly strong and proudly obstinate. Poor agency staff – they were out of their depth. Ollie was supposed to avoid strenuous exercise and on no account was he supposed to touch the bloodshot eye for several days. Some of the staff from Sunfield came down in relays to beef up the respite care, but there were long gaps when Rosie struggled to cope. When Ollie finally returned to school after a week of mayhem, she was so frazzled that she and Edmond missed their flight from Heathrow and arrived late at Geneva.

I was there waiting for them, having deserted Rosie for the last four days to help launch the German edition of a sumptuous new anniversary Everest book. It was the old story: wife struggling with the children while husband goes off to earn money. Except that this wife was at her wits' end trying to stop a severely autistic boy ripping open the stitches on his cornea; while the husband's work was a hugely enjoyable lecture tour of Bavaria, Austria and Switzerland, complete with sacher-torte in Vienna and, in Zurich, a sumptuous lunch amongst the original Monets and Chagalls at the delectable Kronenhalle. All to flog a book.

A week in Argentière, staying at the chalet of our famously generous friend Mich Sogio, soothed Mrs Venables's frazzled nerves. And while she recovered, Edmond and I slalomed amongst the pine trees of Le Tour or took to the wide, powdery slopes of the Grand Lognan. He skied well, with a nice sense of adventure, always keen to seek out the steeper, unpisted slopes, away from the crowd. Ollie would love this, I thought. If only, if only, if only . . . if he could just make those connections, cope with all the sensory assaults of travel, focus all that energy and masterful balance . . . he too could be skimming down this slope, breathing this crystal air, seeing these glittering mountains – Verte, Chardonnet, Drus, Charmoz, Midi – which for me were so redolent with personal memory.

Too much projection, perhaps, but it seemed right to aim high – never to underestimate Ollie's potential. Soon after that holiday a mountain guide from Verbier, Marie Hiroz, sent me a film of her disabled brother skiing the famous Alpine Haute Route, travelling from hut to hut. He had Down Syndrome – very different from autism – but the joy and fulfilment radiating from the film was an inspiration. Even if for the moment Ollie's only immediate 'advance' was to help clear the table after meals, we had to keep raising our aspirations for him.

We returned refreshed to Larkhall on a Friday and I dashed off that night to Canterbury, to do a corporate talk first thing on the Saturday morning, racing back in the afternoon to get home just as Rosie and Edmond arrived from the Midlands with Ollie. His right eye was no longer bloodshot and, as far as we could tell, he was seeing properly through its new artificial lens. We had discussed it carefully with the surgeon, who had explained that, unlike our own miraculous human lens, which in a healthy eye can change shape to focus from three inches to infinity, an artificial lens has a fixed focal length. In Ollie's case we decided that it should be fixed close to infinity and that we would try to persuade him to wear glasses for close-up work.

He was a bit thin, but otherwise he looked well. But he was still having intermittent unpredictable fits, so I removed the ladder leading to the top of the tree house – just in case. It was a gorgeous spring and life was good. On Good Friday we were treated to one of the most moving experiences of my life when the Monteverdi Choir came to Bath Abbey to perform Bach's *St John Passion*, complete with a translation of one of Luther's Good Friday homilies, delivered from the pulpit during the interval. For the rest of the performance the pulpit was occupied by the tenor Mark Padmore, as the Evangelist, bringing a new, intense passion and lucidity to the familiar, anguished story as he wove his narration around a succession of sublime solos and choruses. I wanted it to go on for ever and far too soon we reached the final chorus, with its glorious sweeping arpeggios accompanying a message of redemptive hope: *Ruht wohl, ihr feiligen Geheine, die ich nun wieter nich beweine* – Rest in peace thy sacred limbs, no more will I bewail thee.

And then we celebrated Easter with Ollie, Edmond helping him search for the dairy-free eggs I had hidden around the garden. He came home again a fortnight later and then a fortnight after that, on 16th May, at which stage there had been no fit for over three weeks. On the Sunday evening I dropped him back at Sunfield and continued north to the Lake District to spend three contented days making a video commentary for a new Everest exhibition.

Then back south for Edmond's half-term. Indulgent days staying with his friend Frank and with our Cary cousins. Brahms's clarinet quintet, achingly beautiful, at the Bath Festival. Then off to London to stay with brother Mark while I took part in a big 50th anniversary Everest celebration at the Odeon Leicester Square, thrilled to be sharing a platform with the elderly veterans of the 1953 expedition and our gracious compère Sir David Attenborough, brought in to give the climbers some extra media clout. Then, to round it all off, a champagne party, with a confused Edmond failing to say hello to the Queen, because his mouth was stuffed embarrassingly full of canapé.

Celebration still hovered in the air the next morning, Friday, as we drove north past creamy fountains of May blossom to fetch Ollie. He had been told we were coming and when we arrived at midday there he was, watching from the window. Edmond and I reached the entrance hall first and he rushed up to throw his arms around our waists, gurgling gleeful 'gaiyee' noises, then settling into a contented 'duv-a-duv-a-duv' as he belted himself into the car.

The celebratory busyness continued. On Saturday I dropped Ollie back at Sunfield, before driving into Birmingham to host a showing of Everest films at the IMAX cinema, thrilled to be meeting again Tenzing Norgay's daughter Pem Pem and his famous nephew Nawang Gombu, after whom our friends Harish and Geeta Kapadia had named their second son – the Nawang who had given me holy flower petals from an ashram in Pondicherri to take on my own journey to the top of Everest. Thirteen years later, as an idealistic young officer serving in a Gurkha regiment, caught in an ambush on the Kashmir line of control, at eleven o'clock on the eleventh day of the eleventh month, 2001, rushing to the aid of a wounded comrade, Nawang had been shot dead.

Onward, to Hay on Wye, for the literary festival. Then home. Then back to London where Harish was being awarded a gold medal at the Royal Geographical Society. Then a book-signing in Stanfords, en route for Henley, to collect Ollie's birthday present from god-father Lucius – one of his unique Lucius-patented wooden swing seats. Then a morning corporate pres-entation at Marlow, followed by a drive back north to the Lake District, for an evening show at the new Rheged Centre. Thursday, and it was time to do some real climbing, with ex-*Independent* parliamentary corre-spondent turned outdoor freelance, Stephen Goodwin. On the Friday morning there was just time to fit in a couple more rock climbs in Borrowdale before driving south to collect Ollie.

I reached the M5 turn-off a little early, so I did a short detour up onto the Clent Hills and went for a walk amongst the shimmering beech trees. It was 6th June. Midsummer was approaching fast, but the fresh, sappy translucence of spring had not yet dulled to prosaic green uniformity. Looking out over the plain towards the Shropshire hills I thought, yes, we will be happy living here. Perhaps we can find somewhere in the country, which Edmond will love. And we'll see Ollie every day.

On this Friday, Ollie's twelfth birthday, he had had a special lunch complete with gaudy pink fizzy drink, normally forbidden because of all its neuro-toxic addi-tives. Later we saw photos of him admiring the twelve glowing candles on his cake. And pictures of him in the classroom, elbows resting on the table, unwrapping presents with fleeting expressions of tentative curiosity, excitement, delight . . .

The birthday celebrations continued at home that weekend and he loved the new swing. Two weeks later he came home again, on this occasion doing a sudden runner as we walked out to the car from Orchard House; after mobilising all the care staff for a search and rescue operation I eventually found him amongst the rhododendrons close to the house, an elusive Puck flitting through dappled light beneath the trees. Or perhaps an Ariel? At home that summer Edmond was singing Thomas Arne's effervescent setting of Ariel's song, which could have been Ollie's theme tune:

> Where the bee sucks, there suck I
> In a cowslip's bell I lie;
> There I couch when owls do cry.
> On the bat's back I do fly
> After summer merrily:
> Merrily, merrily shall I live now
> Under the blossom that hangs on the bough.

He came home again for 4th and 5th July. The following Thursday his keyworker Chris phoned with the immensely gratifying news that Ollie, normally indifferent to television, had been thrilled to see me on the screen, taking part in a special Everest edition of the *Tomorrow's World Roadshow*. Ten days later he had another weekend at home, when I took what would prove to be the last still photo of him.

He sits in the warm sunshine at the table outside the kitchen, dressed in shorts and the Jambo elephant tee shirt from Kenya which his Auntie Shan gave him. His long fingers hold a pair of bright red binoculars. He loves these binoculars, loves taking them out of their blue case, fingering their plastic smoothness, removing and replacing the lens guards. And he loves particularly the fact that they are Edmond's – he has stolen them and the stealing elicits a pleasing reaction. So as he looks up at the camera there is a hint of pleasurable guilt in his smile. He looks very handsome, despite the little scar above his left eye still awaiting plastic surgery, but his hair has lost some of its lustre and his limbs look fragile. And his face which used, like that of many autistic children, to have an unearthly symmetry, has become slightly lopsided, the left corner of his mouth drawn up in a slight snarl.

The fits had now stopped for two months but Rosie still sensed that something was wrong. Although hospital tests revealed adequate sight in his new cataract-free right eye, it seemed weak, as though he were squinting to look through the left, supposedly deteriorating, eye – hence this new asymmetry in his face. 'He looks so fragile,' said Rosie. 'And he hasn't grown now for a year. I think there's something wrong: he looks the way he looked when he was getting leukaemia.'

Anxiety was assuaged by the knowledge that soon she would be living close to Ollie, able to keep a check on his health. We had always assumed that, having persuaded BANES (Bath & North East Somerset) to pay for Ollie's residential care, we dared not move to another county and risk having that funding removed. But, after several letters and telephone calls, it now seemed that we probably *could* move to one of the counties whose borders met near Sunfield. Worcestershire had made the most encouraging noises and we were set on moving there the following summer, 2004, when Edmond would be eleven and ready to start at secondary school.

So – only one more year of those long commutes up

and down the M5. The bigger Ollie got, the more testing these drives became. Paying for petrol at the service station, I dared not leave him in the car, now that he knew how to work the locks. So I had to take him into the shop, one hand locked round both his wrists to stop him laying waste amongst the sweet counters, while I fumbled debit cards and receipts with the other hand, apologising cheerfully when Ollie slipped my grasp to ransack the shelves. On the move, he was usually a paragon of idle contentment. But occasionally he liked to unclip his seat belt and try to climb into the front. So we would stop, dangerously, on the hard shoulder. 'Ollie, put your belt on. Ollie, we're not going until you sit down.' He would clip himself back in. But then there might be a provocative giggle as I accelerated down the hard shoulder, seeking a gap between the thundering lorries, and a pair of hands would grasp the front seat beside me. So, back onto the hard shoulder, trying to sound utterly bored as I intoned again, 'Ollie, we're not going until you sit down.'

It was summer holidays now, so often the three of us went with him, making the drives much easier. On 23rd July he came home for a check-up at the eye hospital, and the next morning we took him back to Sunfield, continuing ourselves to North Wales for an indulgent stay at the Pen y Gwryd – the hotel beneath Snowdon from which John Hunt's team planned their Everest expedition in 1953, and over which Jane Pullee exerts a firm maternal grasp, warmly proprietorial towards her Everesters and their memorabilia, which hang on all the walls. At her suggestion we escaped the rainy mountains and went to Anglesey to swim in the bracing surf on Newborough Warren.

'It's like the beach we took Ollie to, isn't it Mumma,' shivered Edmond.

'Yes – Harlech. When was that . . . two years ago? But this is even better. He'd love it here.'

'We should bring him,' I suggested. 'It's only three or four hours from Sunfield.' I was daring to dream again of expanding Ollie's horizons, allowing myself bigger aspirations for him.

Ollie came home again the following week for a final interlude before we left for France to house-sit for our friends the Amys, near Grenoble. It was the hottest summer for years and in Paris the old-age pensioners were dying like flies. Down south, at Bernard's and Noëlle's house in the deep valley of the Isère, the temperature rose to 42 degrees centigrade and Rosie spent hours with her feet in a bucket of water. Inured by numerous Indian trips, I found the sweltering heat easier. And by rising early, it was just possible to climb in the Chartreuse, in a Chinese landscape of gnarled trees clinging to pale rock. One morning we got up in the dark to explore the other side of the valley – the Massif de Belledonne. We drove up before dawn, looking back to huge forest fires, blazing orange in the dark like some sinister medieval procession, then walked up to high alpine meadows where we dived into the cobalt waters of the Lac de Crop, icy beneath cliffs of lichenous gneiss.

Every couple of days Rosie telephoned Orchard House. It was hot there too, but Ollie, as far as we could tell, was content and was still having no further fits. We were impatient to see him again but first, after two weeks in France, we had to fly up to Edinburgh where I was doing a talk at the book festival. We remained for three days of musical indulgence, staying with Henry the Botanist at his flat, now sadly bereft of its rabbit.

At last, after twenty-two days' separation – our longest ever – we returned south and collected Ollie for the weekend. We took him to the Botanic Gardens for our annual browsing of a lusciously fruited mulberry tree. Then, for the first time in years, we climbed – illegally and irresponsibly – the civic garden's magnificent cut-leaf beech tree. Ollie was unusually hesitant and Edmond had to show him the awkward balancy moves up the huge branches which swept almost to the ground, but once he had mastered the moves he glowed with renewed pride.

The long hot summer metamorphosed almost imperceptibly into a radiant autumn, and during the first week of September we had another treat – looking after the beautiful house of Anthony and Charlotte Rowe, a mile from Larkhall, while they were on holiday. Edmond swam every day in the icy pool and I spent happy hours in Anthony's piano room, learning a new intermezzo by Brahms – one of the very last pieces he wrote – immersing myself in its elegiac chromaticism.

At the end of that week, on 5th September, Rosie and I took Ollie to Hampshire to see Dr Tettenborn, an expert on yeast in the gut. Many autistic children seemed to suffer from candida or gut disbiosis and this was one microbiological avenue which Rosie still wished to investigate. She discussed with Dr Tettenborn the protocol she had been following from the Pfeiffer Center, with its large doses of vitamin B6, then mentioned the sudden outbreak of convulsions in March. Dr Tettenborn looked concerned and said, 'In this country very few doctors would recommend such a large dose.'

'None of the other children seem to have had any trouble,' replied Rosie, 'but, come to think of it, Ollie's fits did start in March, when he first took the full dose.'

We drove home gloomily, Rosie agonising about how to proceed. Already in March she had reduced Ollie's dose of evening primrose oil, wondering if that might have had something to do with the fits. Now she wondered about the B6 and other supplements recommended in Chicago. 'Maybe we should pack in the whole Pfeiffer business,' she sighed. 'What do you think?'

'I just don't know. I'm sorry – I just don't know what to think. This is highly complex biochemistry which even the experts can't agree about. I don't know *what* we should do.'

We decided to cut back on the supplements for a while and see what happened. In the meantime we had a weekend to enjoy. My parents phoned to say they would drop in on Sunday morning with a bucketful of their wonderful autumn raspberries. First, immediately after breakfast, we went to the Botanic Gardens. Again we ate mulberries and climbed in the spreading beech. Then we walked over to the pond, where Edmond spotted fat carp while Ollie made feinting movements to climb over the fence and get in amongst them. Then the two boys chased each other up and down the big dell and climbed the tempting pedestal of the stone monument to William Shakespeare. We finished at the old redwood tree. Its top had died and fallen off in a recent storm, but the parks authorities had imaginatively left its ancient stump to be sculpted into a stylised god figure – a giant, jolly, heathen deity clutching chiselled sheaves of corn. The sculptor had left irresistible incut edges to his carving, which just cried to be climbed. Edmond led the way while Ollie followed, spiralling round the carved trunk as I pointed out little foot ledges and sidepulls.

We missed my parents by five minutes, but they had left on the doorstep a magnificent offering of raspberries, on which we feasted, after a first course of roast lamb which Ollie devoured with his usual carnivorous enthusiasm. After lunch I took what would prove to be the last video of him, playing with Edmond.

The two boys see-saw on the rocker outside the back door. Ollie laughs with pleasure but then suddenly gets off, without warning, to leave an uncounterweighted Edmond crashing backwards to the ground. Edmond laughs and Ollie grabs the rocker, climbs up onto a table and tries to manoeuvre it into the garden next door.

Then he runs, smiling, towards the house. Suddenly there is a flicker – an infinitesimal hiccup or nauseousness, a shadow flitting across his face – a momentary absence, which at the time I did not notice. The instant passes and he rushes cheerfully into the kitchen, chuckling to himself as he grabs sheaves of Sunday newspaper, holding the pictures close to his face, examining them with an intense smile. Then he goes through the doorway to the stairs, where he laughs at his luck, finding one of Edmond's misplaced possessions. There is a shout from Rosie at the kitchen sink: 'Edmond – he's got your gumshield. I should rescue it if I were you. It's your own fault for leaving it lying around.' Ollie laughs at the general air of consternation; then, as Edmond rescues his rugby equipment, goes back outside to lift the rocker up again. 'Ollie – are you thinking of posting that?'

And there the precious clip ends.

While Rosie took Edmond to Evensong, I tried taking Ollie for a bike ride. But he seemed lethargic and at the bottom of the road he stopped to investigate the still-red blackberries before dropping his bike on the playing field. We went into the toddlers' enclosure where he climbed briefly on the familiar climbing frame. The surrounding ashes had been puny saplings when he first came here; now they were thirty-foot trees. After a while he left the enclosure and sat down on the grass, looking dizzy, weak and abstracted. As he stared at the sky I wondered if he was going to have a fit. Clouds were blackening, so we ran home, racing the rain; and as soon as we got into the kitchen Ollie gestured upstairs – 'Unhh.'

'You want go to your room?'

'Yeh.'

He put himself straight to bed and I locked the door, coming back down to do the washing-up. About fifteen minutes later I returned to find the bedroom spattered with raspberry-coloured vomit and Ollie looking green. As I mopped up he was twice more violently sick. When Rosie and Edmond returned we decided to keep him at home until Monday morning, but by tea time he had perked up. As he embarked on a manic re-sorting of the kitchen Rosie announced, 'I think it's time Ollie went back to school.'

He seemed quite content returning to Orchard House but the following Thursday they phoned to say that the fits had started again – two small ones, followed by vomiting. They wondered whether he would be well enough to travel in the car for the home visit sched-uled for that Saturday. I said I would come anyway.

I left early for a reconnaissance of Worcestershire, driving contentedly along narrow lanes, deep beneath red earth fields and big skies. On the radio the film director Anthony Minghella was enthusing eloquently about his favourite music, which was mainly Bach. I thought how lucky we were to have all of this. Life was inexpressibly beautiful and I was growing more and more excited about the prospect of moving to this new county. I did a little detour west towards Kidderminster to investigate a tempting tract of forest country, before closing in on Sunfield and arriving at the appointed hour to collect Ollie.

That afternoon we went again to the Botanic

Gardens. We found a perfect hornbeam to climb, then returned to the sculpted redwood where Ollie tried again to complete the complete circuit of its trunk. Then, childishly, I had my own barefoot turn on the trunk, interrupted by a shout from Rosie, 'He's escaped!'

So much for fits and sickness! He still seemed to have huge energy reserves and only just missed being run over. Again he returned calmly to school on Sunday evening.

The following Thursday I was at a meeting in Cambridge and phoned home to hear continuing reports of Ollie not being very well. We asked Sunfield to keep us informed and stuck with the plan for that weekend – more mulberries, this time with Pru and Keith Cartwright at their house in Herefordshire which, as well as mulberries, sports a glorious wine cellar. On the Saturday, while Keith scored godfatherly points taking Edmond fishing, Rosie and I went groggily to visit a potential school for Edmond in Stourbridge, a few miles from Sunfield. Once the tour was over we drove around some of the villages, prospecting, and stopped to have lunch in a pub. It felt strange sitting there, just two miles from Ollie, wishing we could drop in and see him but knowing that, until we had a proper new routine established, an unscheduled visit would just unsettle him.

For the first three days of that week I was in London, staying with Anna Black. Rosie phoned on the Monday morning to tell me that at school Ollie was still unwell. He was being sick a lot, he was weak and he was not eating. On Wednesday he was to be taken to the local GP for a blood test and she was dreading his potential fear and pain.

In the event he coped bravely and there was no horrible struggle. By Thursday I was back at home and

Rosie was in bed, ill with anxiety. 'Why haven't they phoned? Can't they see that I'm desperate to know whether or not my son is going to die of leukaemia?'

'I'll give them a ring.' I got Chris, Ollie's keyworker, but he said no result was due until the afternoon. After lunch I pestered him with more abortive calls. Then at last he phoned back to say that the lab had found no sign of leukaemia.

'No leukaemia. Thank God for that. But did they find anything else?' I persisted. 'Any infection?'

No-one was quite sure. But they did tell us that Ollie was being sick again and was refusing fluids. Rosie was now desperate and persuaded me to keep up a barrage of phone calls, trying to track down the medical team, all of whom were busy on a course. Then I tried the headmaster and the head of care, but both were away. Then I tried the local surgery, but it was closed on a Thursday. So I tried the roving duty GP, but only raised a secretary, who said she would try to get hold of him.

'We are very anxious,' I told her. 'As far as we can tell he has been repeatedly sick and is eating and drinking virtually nothing. He could be very dehydrated and it sounds to me as though he should be in hospital, on a drip.'

'I'll pass that on to the doctor,' she reassured. Ten minutes later she phoned back to say that the doctor had spoken to the school and was satisfied that Ollie was OK where he was.

Perhaps I should have gone immediately to see Ollie. But as always, reluctant to interfere, knowing that his carers were following doctors' orders, I decided to leave it until Saturday when he was due to come home. I had to prepare a lecture for an engagement on Friday, which had been booked for nearly a year, at the King's School,

Worcester. The plan was to stay there on Friday night and continue to Sunfield on Saturday morning.

I arrived in Worcester in the middle of the afternoon to be shown round the school by the headmaster, Tim Keys. King's was top of our list of potential schools for Edmond and, as the head took me round, I was very impressed. The director of music had virtually offered Edmond a place in the cathedral choir – a scholarship which would pay half the school fees – and, after getting my slide projection set up in the school lecture theatre, I walked across the close to the cathedral to hear the boys do Evensong. Sitting in that immense, complex Gothic space, its dark sandstone so different from Bath's brightly renovated limestone, I was excited at the thought of Edmond joining these talented singers, absorbing all that spiritual ritual and unending music.

My talk that night was on the ill-fated Panch Chuli expedition and a lump swelled in my throat as I brought up the slide of Ollie, aged one, swinging amongst the roses in Larkhall Terrace – a brief flashing image of what I had nearly lost in the fall. The Keys family kindly put me up for the night and I left after breakfast, timing the drive to Sunfield as a reference for the daily journeys we would probably start making with Edmond in eleven months' time. Yet again it was a beautiful morning, with golden stubble gleaming under a luminous sky. Again that autumnal sense of new beginnings, banishing all thought of Ollie's mystery illness. The drive took under half an hour. This was going to work – this new life in Worcestershire!

I drew up the familiar drive, past the donkeys and the sheep, and parked in the usual slot outside Orchard House. I walked up the tarmac path, past the lolloping rabbits, and there was a rattle of keys on the other side of the glass door. I hadn't seen Ollie for a fortnight and as soon as I walked through the door the deterioration was obvious. He stood barefoot in the entrance hall, his green sweatshirt hanging loosely over a yellow polo shirt, trousers draped on stick legs. As I put a hand around his frail bony shoulders I couldn't resist murmuring, 'Ollie, my darling poor boy – what's wrong with you?' His hair was dull and dry, his face pale, with shiny plates of dry skin stuck to cracked lips. The left side of his mouth was now drawn up into a more distorted snarl, revealing a superfluity of new sharp teeth puncturing sore gums.

As we left I said cheerily, 'See you on Sunday evening,' but as soon as we drove away I realised that Ollie would probably be staying at home for a while: however caring his school staff, this was no time for parents to delegate. After half an hour's drive, I stopped at a service station to telephone Rosie and just as I drove off again Ollie was sick. I cursed my stupidity for not bringing spare clothes and mopped him up as best I could, stroking his head and whispering words of comfort. We drove on through the gleaming autumn landscape and as we left the M4 to head down into Bath, the Baroque music specialist William Christie came on the radio to introduce his new recording of Couperin's exquisitely sad *Tenebrae*. Yet again our microcosmic drama with Ollie was played to the accompaniment of timeless sacred music.

At home I bathed Ollie, put him in clean clothes, then tried very gently to clean his teeth. Then I brought him down to the kitchen and persuaded him to drink some Polycal – a fruit-flavoured calorie concentrate. I cooked lunch. Rosie and Edmond came back from picking raspberries at my parents' house. Rosie bent lovingly over Ollie, stroked him and inspected his mouth. 'Look at all these new teeth! Is that what's making you so ill? We'll have to take you to the dentist, won't we? Perhaps they'll have to take some of these teeth out: we don't want you growing up with bad teeth, *do* we?' She reminded me about the old mouthcare routine, using Difflam to numb the soreness, then sent me to the chemist to buy some of that and some large syringes, with which we could gently persuade Ollie to take whimpering mouthfuls of water, fruit juice and Polycal.

'Do you think we should take him to hospital straight away?' Rosie asked.

'Let's leave it until Monday,' I suggested, reluctant as always to drag Ollie off to hospital unless it was absolutely necessary.

'Whatever happens, Ollie,' Rosie insisted, 'we're keeping you with us until you're better.'

We drew a chart and kept a record of fluids, rehydrating him and continuing his mouthcare over the weekend. On Monday morning I got up at seven to take Edmond to school. A year earlier we had moved him to a new establishment and now we could bicycle to school along the canal. Ducks and moorhens paddled with their adolescent broods on the steaming surface; overhead white sunlight was starting to burn through the swirling mist, promising another glorious day. On the way home I diverted into town to drop off some film for processing, and order that Couperin disc. I bumped into one of Ollie's old helpers, Angie, who was now training to be a nurse, and told her that Ollie was not very well – perhaps she might be able to drop in and see him? There was no urgency about it. This was just another of the many challenges sent to test the stoicism of our son.

When I got home at ten Rosie was on the telephone making an emergency appointment to see our GP,

David Walker. Fifteen minutes later, as I walked Ollie up to the surgery door she chided anxiously, 'Careful – you must *hold* him; he might fall over.' She was right: his legs were wobbly and wayward.

He sat quietly next to us in the waiting room and when we went through to the consulting room he didn't even attempt to ransack drawers or play with medical equipment. We discussed possibilities – could this be appendicitis? Or a complication from Ollie's perennial constipation? Or an infection spreading from his sore mouth? – but we all knew that we were skirting around the issue. Rosie pointed out the asymmetry in Ollie's face. 'Do you see,' she said, 'how the left side is distorted, because the right side seems to be paralysed – droopy. We wondered whether he might have had a stroke . . . And his right leg is dragging. And, look – he's not using his right arm . . . he's doing everything with his left hand.'

There was no skirting now. David agreed that something might be seriously wrong, possibly some neurological problem. He telephoned the oncology department in Bristol, and very calmly jogged the memory of one of the consultants – 'Ollie Venables, a boy with autism . . . treated for acute lymphoblastic leukaemia, starting in – hang on a moment – yes, 1995 . . . recent episodes of fits . . . it was decided not to do a scan, but now the fits have started again . . . vomiting . . . apparent weakness on the right side . . . wondering if this could be a glioma' – for the first time I heard that unfamiliar label, pronounced gl-eye-ohma, for a brain tumour – 'would it be sensible for him to have a scan? Even if surgery were not possible, a clear diagnosis could help with decisions about any possible palliative treatment . . .'

So, yet again, all Rosie's anxieties were probably justified. How wonderful to have someone listening and acting on them so decisively. And sympathetically. He said that he could not at this stage refer us to Bristol, and with one more phone call booked us in to the Royal United Hospital, Bath.

The children's ward had now been moved into a gleaming brand new wing. Arriving with just one hour's notice, we had to make do with an open ward, but Ollie settled amiably on his bed in a curtained bay, too weak to wander . . . until a very young doctor came to take blood. I felt sorry for her as she confessed that it was her first day on the ward. Ollie led her a merry dance, staggering repeatedly in and out of the lavatory to avoid the inevitable. Then he sat on a chair in the corridor, where the young woman tried unsuccessfully to take blood, and I dithered ineffectually. It took Rosie, returning from buying some snacks, to take charge of the situation. 'Come on Ollie. Don't be silly. Get back on the bed. You've just got to do it, I'm afraid.' Within moments the lidocaine cream had been wiped from an arm and we were all whispering congratulations as the doctor pricked a vein and drew out the required blood.

Ollie was now eating a little solid food, so I went into Weston to buy more supplies, including some vital stress-relieving wine for our own dinner that night. In the afternoon I bicycled up to Edmond's school, took him home and drove him to Bradford-on-Avon for his piano lesson, returning to the hospital just as Rosie and Ollie came out to the car park. 'We can go home,' she said, 'but we've got to come back soon. I met the registrar, who was very nice and said he wants to do a brain scan, preferably an MRI. He thinks it's very urgent and will book one as soon as he can get a slot.'

The four of us went home together. On Tuesday we

continued to give Ollie liquids and as much food as he could take, but he was again violently sick in the afternoon. The hospital phoned to say that he was booked in for an MRI scan first thing the next morning,

So we all left at eight thirty on Wednesday morning, dropping Edmond at school on the way to the hospital. Ollie looked happier, and Rosie said, 'You're looking a bit better today, aren't you Ollie?' It was 1st October, exactly thirteen years from the day I had returned from Switzerland to learn that Rosie was pregnant – that this unknown person had begun to exist.

Warned, perhaps, about the notorious parents from hell, everyone at the RUH was extremely helpful. We rehearsed the old routines carefully with a very helpful anaesthetist and I went with Ollie to the X-ray department to be with him as he sank into unconsciousness – again that little death – ready for sliding into the cylindrical scanning machine. While his brain was scanned Rosie and I walked down to the smart new reception area – a white atrium decorated with three huge oil paintings of luminous green and gold Wiltshire landscapes under spacious skies. We drank coffee nervously, then returned to the ward to wait for Ollie.

We were sitting on his still-empty bed when his old Bath oncology consultant came in. We hadn't met since the rows in the old John Apley ward over five years earlier and I immediately put out my hand with a crass cheery 'hello', failing to register the import of his sombre look. He took my hand reluctantly and said to both of us, 'I think we should go and find somewhere else to talk.'

Like guilty pupils following the headmaster, we shuffled off down the corridor, opening successive doors, only to find each room occupied by doctors, managers at computers, nurses dressing wounds, cleaners hoovering . . . We continued our awkward journey, until at last the headmaster found an empty room. 'This will do,' he said, pulling up chairs for me and Rosie and sitting himself protectively behind a desk.

'We've got the scan back and there *is* a tumour – quite a large one, on the left side of the brain. I'm afraid that this is probably very serious: things could now move very fast. We can't be sure that it's malignant, but I think that Ollie should go over to Frenchay Hospital. I'm going to speak to Mr Pople, the neurosurgeon on duty, and he'll probably recommend operating straight away.' He continued with more practical details, then changed key. 'I'm so sorry . . . Ollie has been through so much already. I know that we had some disagreements in the past, but I hope that you will accept that I am sorry about that and that we will try to do everything that we can to help you now.'

It was a courageous speech, moving in its humility, and Rosie smiled redly at him as he asked whether we would like some time alone in the room. He left, and we just sat there, holding hands, saying nothing. Then we walked in a trance back down the corridor towards the ward. In a few minutes Ollie would return from Recovery, conscious again, but completely unaware of the devastating news we had just been given.

Chapter Fourteen

There was no time for tears. And in any case they would have been no help to Ollie. If anything, we were more brightly cheerful . . . but also more tender, acutely aware of the need to treasure every moment. And, like most people in these situations, we sought refuge in practicality. Ollie was given an anti-inflammatory corticosteroid called dexamethasone. I knew the name well as it is often used as emergency treatment for cerebral oedema at high altitude. He began very quickly to look better. Meanwhile we began a series of phone calls to make arrangements for Edmond with the ultra helpful, mini-compact-driving, mothers at his new school. While Rosie sorted out the hospital paperwork I went home to gather overnight things, check emails, open the post, glance at a gloomy letter from the solicitors to say that the judge was throwing out the MMR case – what immaculate timing! – and collect Rosie's car from the MOT garage. Life had 'to go on'. Mandy, our dynamic cleaner, now back with us again, asked what news I had of Ollie. 'Not good, I'm afraid,' was all I could manage.

Frenchay. Yet another new hospital. Another adventure. A relic of the Second World War, its sprawling grid of squat brick blocks beside the M32 exudes military utilitarianism; but they now house one of the top neurological units in the country. And plastic surgery: as we wheeled Ollie's pushchair into the Barbara Russell children's ward, the receptionist said, 'Isn't he booked in for next week . . . for a scar reduction on his face?'

So this was where he had been due to come for that minor cosmetic surgery. What horrible irony. Never mind . . . we were pleased to discover a bright modern wing, with small dormitories and single rooms radiating from a central oval. Outside Ollie's room was a courtyard where he played in the sunshine and sipped fruit juice while an Australian nurse, older than us and hugely experienced, took his notes. Like all the staff here, she had a palpable air of competence. She twigged immediately that our son was called Ollie – not Oliver as in his notes – and got it right from the word go. That sensitive attention to detail was typical of the place.

It was the same with the surgeon, Mr Pople, who came to see us while we were sitting Ollie down to supper at a table in the communal area. He spoke carefully, unsure how much Ollie would understand, avoiding punctiliously any hint of dangerous drama or gloom. He asked us when Ollie had stopped speaking and we told him it had happened when he was two and a half. He mentioned that the tumour was on the left side of the brain, pressing on the speech centre, exacerbating any problems with talking. 'You've seen the scan, have you?' he asked.

We hadn't, so he pulled the huge celluloid sheet out of its envelope, and showed us the pale globe – an alien planet sitting brazenly in the left hemisphere, just above the ear, nearly the size of a tennis ball. If left, it would continue to grow rapidly, increasing the pressure on the rest of the brain. The loss of appetite and nausea would get worse; the paralysis would intensify; soon he would go blind. But this was an easy part of the brain to get at, so he felt that he should definitely operate. The craniotomy would relieve the pressure; it was also the only way to determine what type of tumour Ollie had.

Ollie continued eating his supper. Mr Pople said that

the tumour might prove benign, but he implied clearly that malignancy was more probable. He explained that the bulk of the alien globe was cystic, liquid – that was what was causing most of the pressure – and that final outcomes would depend on how clearly defined were the demarcation lines between the actual solid tumour and the surrounding brain cells. If we agreed, he would put Ollie first on the operating list next morning.

Afterwards Rosie said, 'It doesn't sound quite so bad as I thought. Perhaps he might even recover.' She kissed Ollie goodnight and returned to collect Edmond from a schoolfriend's parents who, bless them, invited her in for supper and a welcome drink. I stayed with Ollie, sleeping in the room beside him.

Thursday. Like the day he was born. And the day his leukaemia was discovered. This particular Thursday was October the second. I woke early to discover Ollie already sitting at the table in the main area where he had had his supper, arm raised to gesture expectantly at the ward kitchen.

'Sorry, Ollie. Not now, later. *Later* you can have food.' He had to remain 'nil by mouth', and I had to try and wash his hair with medicated shampoo in preparation for the craniotomy. I coaxed him into a bathroom and filled the tub, but he was having none of it, so I filled a basin instead with warm water and he agreed eventually to let me wash his hair in that. 'Well done. Good boy. Let's get your hair lovely and clean.' I ran my fingers through the wet soapy hair, letting it ripple in the rinsing water like fronds in a stream, then dabbed it gently dry, cradling the still childish skull in my hands.

Rosie arrived at eight thirty to help get him ready for theatre and at nine I set off with him and the porters, down the long, sloping yellow corridor. I suddenly remembered Tumbledown Lane at the RAF base in the Falkland Islands – reputedly the longest corridor in the world – with its same coded uniforms, the same inscrutable jargon, the same busy, purposeful human traffic, maintaining a huge complex machine. But here that traffic was so much *more* complex, the specialities more varied, the coded language more obtuse, the vast network of interdependencies keeping this huge organism functioning so much more miraculous.

And all to repair the failings and injuries of the other traffic – the pale, sick withered bodies on their crutches and Zimmer frames and castored beds and wheelchairs. How wonderful that all this expensive complexity was devoted simply to making patients better, or at least to making their lives more tolerable. How wonderful that these experts had the knowledge and skill to cut open my son's skull and remove the alien presence lurking beneath.

It was a long operation and Ollie would be unconscious for about three hours, so Rosie and I drove fifteen miles back to Larkhall. There were 'things to do', and we craved the therapy of mundane practicalities. We returned to Frenchay at midday to find Ollie propped up on pillows in the ward's High Dependency Unit. He was plugged into several drips and monitors, with nurses constantly checking blood pressure, heart rate, oxygenation, temperature . . . Sedated with fentanyl, he lay very quietly, a serene smile playing in his unnaturally bright eyes. I had expected to see a huge shaven patch on his head, but no: these brilliant craftsmen had simply folded back a flap of skin, with its unshaven hair, to saw open a small panel of skull, afterwards fixing the panel back in place and laying the skin, like lawn turf, back over the top. All there was to show for it was a neat line of stitches and an elastic bandage, like a little turban.

The paralysis had vanished instantly. His face was no longer lopsided and he was holding his left hand in front of it, manipulating thumb and fingers before smiling eyes, as if delighting in this rediscovered dexterity.

Later that afternoon Mr Pople came to see us. 'It all went very well, but I'm afraid the demarcation was not as clearly defined as I had hoped it might be.' A craniotomy is often a compromise between trying to remove every trace of tumour and trying not to slice too drastically into the surrounding healthy brain tissue. In Ollie's case there were still tumorous tentacles spreading into his brain. The surgeon went on to say that the tumour *did* seem malignant: 'We won't know exactly what it is until Pathology has looked at the biopsy, but some of the cells did look as they might be quite leukaemic.' He then told us that we would meet the following Wednesday, in six days' time, to hear the full prognosis.

In the evening Edmond came to see Ollie, leaving shoes at the door, putting on a sterile overall and washing hands thoroughly in disinfectant, before entering the High Dependency Unit. Ollie was propped on his pillow, still smiling serenely, drinking occasionally from a carton of fruit juice and sampling the most delicious gluten-free biscuits and snacks Rosie could find. She and Edmond went home for the night; later I kissed Ollie goodnight and went up to the parents' centre for wine, sandwiches, bath and bed.

When I went back down at seven thirty on Friday morning they said that Ollie had been awake, but happy, all night. There was a bright young nurse called Nix on duty, joking, laughing, flirting and throwing up her hands in mock shock – 'Oh, spare my tender eyes!' – as an increasingly giggly Ollie flung off sheets to reveal a little naked penis. Later that morning we removed all the clips and tubes from his body and took him back to his room.

At lunchtime Rosie said, 'You really ought to tell your parents, you know.' I had not wanted to spoil their annual week by the sea with one of my father's sisters, but I couldn't protect them for ever. So, armed with the mobile phone I had finally, reluctantly, bought that summer – and which was now being put to such constant unwelcome use – I walked outside the hospital to ring Cornwall. 'Hello, Stephen . . . yes, it's Anne here. We're sitting outside having lunch. October! Isn't it marvellous . . . yes, they're here. I'll get your mother.'

I didn't tell her that Ollie was going to die; we didn't even know for sure that he *was* going to die – or at least not for quite a long time. I just said that I had bad news . . . that Ollie had a brain tumour . . . that, yes, it had already been removed – amazing, isn't it? – just twenty-four hours after the diagnosis, and that he was doing very well . . . But it still seemed to hit her like a falling rock. She said they would come and see us when they got home on Sunday.

That night I slept again in the parents' centre, but was woken at one o'clock in the morning by a nurse telephoning to say that Ollie was making a terrible racket, disturbing all the other children. He had now been awake non-stop for thirty-six hours since the operation and as soon as I went down to the ward I heard the familiar percussive rattle of plastic coming from his room, where he was hard at work, lost in a timeless ritual, filling, emptying, filling, emptying . . . repeatedly scooping up handfuls of bricks into a bucket, punctiliously collecting every single brick before tipping the whole lot back onto the floor. The only difference from the usual routine was that this Lego (the original definitive mother of all bricks, circa 1960) had a slightly higher, brighter note than the big modern Duplo bricks at home.

'Come on, Ollie, let's put it all away. That's right . . . in the bucket . . . yes, and that piece . . . and that one . . . good boy – oh, all right, one more time –' CRASH '– now all away. Finished. Good. Well done. No – finish! Now, back to bed . . . Night night.'

At last he settled and fell asleep. In the morning, having collected painkillers and further doses of dexamethasone from Pharmacy, we set off home, Ollie walking unaided between the two of us, as we headed out to the car park. It was hard to believe that just two days earlier he had had his skull cut open. That afternoon, looking like a little Sikh in his turban bandage, he was back in the garden, dancing his old joyful dance on the wooden pier supporting the rope bridge.

On Sunday my parents came to see him and told us that the Rector had included his name in the Abbey prayers that morning. At the moment painkillers seemed to be keeping his post-operative headaches under control and he was looking healthier than he had done for ages. Prompted by Rosie, he was pronouncing whole words, saying 'Mummy' and 'Daddy' with a clarity he had not managed for years. 'I wonder,' pondered Rosie, 'if it's been lurking there for several years. It would explain why he kept losing bits of learning, never managing to hold onto new words. Perhaps it started as soon as he had the radiotherapy . . . perhaps it caused all that head-banging . . . do you remember – at Prior's Court, when no-one could understand why he seemed to have those sudden rages?'

We had expected *some* cognitive damage from the radiotherapy, but with Ollie the lapses had seemed particularly disheartening, as if he had been struggling hopelessly up an interminable scree slope, continually sliding back down. If the tumour *had* been lurking – albeit in a smaller, embryonic form – for several years, it might explain some of those difficulties.

But now we had to enjoy his brief renaissance. And, 'to cheer ourselves up', knowing that this *was* probably just a short interlude, we were hiring lots of comedy videos. That evening Ollie hovered happily in the kitchen, coming over occasionally to join us watching *Blackadder*, laughing with us at Stephen Fry's fruity buffooning moustachioed First World War general.

After the recent days of Ollie's illness we had become blasé about locking doors. On Monday I was at the surgery, collecting Edmond's asthma prescription, when Rosie phoned frantically: 'You left the door open – he's escaped.' She had come downstairs to find the kitchen deserted. No Ollie! For fifteen minutes she ran desperately up and down the streets, telephoned the police, accosted passers-by, rushed into the greengrocers . . . until someone shouted, 'We've found him!' One of the assistants from the local school had seen the turbaned boy running along the road, had remembered hearing about Ollie and, assuming this must be him, had grabbed him by the wrist.

Friends and family were fantastic, sending flowers and cards. My astute brother Mark sent a cheque with a card instructing us to go and buy some nice wine. Meanwhile, I continued with sporadic bursts of work, driving up to London on the Monday evening to stay with the Blacks, ready for a *Sunday Times* job on the Tuesday. Rosie phoned in the morning to say that Ollie had been awake all night, apparently in pain. I promised to get back early in the afternoon. First I drove round to Willesden to do my planned interview with a cellist friend of Bruno's – Anita Lasker-Wallfisch, who had survived Auschwitz by playing in the infamous women's camp orchestra and had then been deported back west to Belsen, where she was still just clinging to life when the liberating British troops arrived. Sixty years on from that unimaginable horror her calm meticulous objectivity – and total absence of self-pity – was deeply impressive. Interview finished, we had coffee in her kitchen and talked about our respective families. I told her about Ollie's autism. Then said I had to get back to Bath because he was unwell: he had just had a brain tumour operation. Announced publicly like that, to someone I had only just met, it sounded surreal.

That night it was my turn to sit up with Ollie, but he managed to get to sleep soon after midnight. The following morning, Wednesday, just one week after the tumour had been discovered, he came with us back to Frenchay to hear the verdict.

Three senior medics hovered uncomfortably while we took some time to get Ollie settled with a nurse in the playroom. Then we slipped away to talk privately. As with the Bath consultant a week earlier, we played out a little farce, searching for just the right spot, finally dragging chairs into a corner of the main oval area and sitting round in an expectant circle.

Everyone smiled calmly. Rosie and I waited for the pronouncement. Then Mr Pople started: 'Well, it isn't the *most* malignant kind of tumour, so the news is not as bad as it might have been. Ollie has an anaplastic oligodendroglioma . . . normally quite fast-growing, but possible that it could have been there in smaller form for some time . . . no traces of leukaemia [so this was a completely new cancer after all] . . . not usually seen in children . . .' – good old Ollie, I thought, you never were a standard off-the-peg case, were you? – 'not normally associated with radiotherapy, but still conceivable that

that could have been the cause . . . oligodendro can respond quite well to treatment . . .'

Then a soft-spoken consultant oncologist we remembered well from leukaemia days, took over. Rosie and I leaned forward, straining to catch words, lip-reading, as he discussed options. There *was* a treatment for oligodendro tumours which was proving quite successful. About thirty per cent of patients, with a particular genetic marker, were responding well to a regime of procarbazine, CCNU and vincristine, with many of them surviving five years or more, *but* it would pose problems in this case — yes, we knew: alopecia, myelosuppression, nausea, the trauma of repeated monitoring blood tests etc etc — *and* it was probably only effective in conjunction with aggressive cranial radiotherapy, which Ollie, having already received high radiation doses in 1997, could not tolerate again.

That just left t e m a z o — we leaned further forward, straining to hear, watching his lips intently . . . what was that drug? He repeated the word: temazolomide . . . oral doses . . . only minor side effects . . . was proving moderately successful . . . tolerated by children . . . but he would have to have regular blood tests to check for neutropenia . . . Before any decisions were made Ollie needed first to have a follow-up MRI scan to assess the results of the operation.

That, more or less, was that. The third man said nothing. No-one spoke of death; but, in their careful, sensitive, elliptical way, the doctors implied gently that any treatment we decided on would only be buying time. Afterwards we waited to discuss pain relief with the excellent pain nurse, then collected drugs from Pharmacy and drove Ollie home.

Desperate for another opinion, that evening I telephoned our London neurologist friend, Charlie Clarke, to ask him about the oligodendroglioma. He was as urbane and charming as ever. But not totally inscrutable. When I told him that the surgeon had not managed to remove every trace of the tumour, he said, 'They never do.' I asked him what he thought about temazolomide, and he said something like this: 'Oncologists tend always to recommend treatment because that's their job – that's what they do. But for all we know Ollie may be fine for quite a while. I'd just leave it – see what happens. And then, if he does become ill again, *try* temazolomide: it's quite a good drug; it might help.'

We had been here before. Several times after the leukaemia relapse, when Ollie was flattened by chemicals and radiation, Rosie had said, 'It's not fair on him: if he has another relapse we mustn't put him through this again.' Now we had been caught unawares by another cancer. And despite everything we had said before, desperate now to hold onto Ollie, Rosie seemed to be considering the possibility of some kind of treatment – was still wondering whether he might continue at Sunfield, with us moving nearby – whereas I was now reluctant to drag out any inconclusive treatment. I almost felt it would be easier if someone said bluntly, 'He's going to die,' and gave me a date.

As soon as we returned from the consultation, Frenchay phoned to say an MRI slot had suddenly become vacant for the next day. So in the morning we returned to the Barbara Russell ward for the follow-up brain scan. It was Thursday again, 9th October.

Ollie was a model of sweet-tempered co-operation as we settled him in his room, unpacking toys and cassette player, applying lidocaine cream to both hands and arms for multiple cannula possibilities, then giving him his midazolam pre-med. Then we set off down the great sloping highway, this time to the X-ray department. Rosie waited in Reception while I followed the porters through to the anaesthetic room. How many times – thirty, forty, fifty? – had we been through this routine? Putting on the tape of Byrd – or was it Palestrina? – allying sixteenth-century polyphony to modern medicine, soothing Ollie as I helped take off his shirt and stroked his hair, telling him how brave he was, while the anaesthetist found the vein and slipped in the needle. Yet again the thick white juice flowed into his vein; again I felt his head grow suddenly heavy and he dropped away, as if in rehearsal for the real thing.

After the scan Ollie was kept in Frenchay for observation while we tried a new painkiller, a synthetic opioid called tramadol, which we hoped would have fewer side effects than natural morphine derivatives (Ollie had reacted very badly to morphine during his leukaemia relapse in 1997, as had his grandfather when he got lung cancer at the same time). Most of the afternoon Ollie dozed off the anaesthetic, but by the evening he perked up and I tried to persuade him to have a shower. He just shook his head. So, *pour encourager l'enfant*, I had one instead and he laughed rapturously at the sight of his naked father sluicing himself with hot water. I was tired and tried lying down on the camp bed but Ollie was in high spirits, refusing to let me go to sleep until long after midnight.

Sunfield, determined to help, had promised to send some of Ollie's regular care staff all the way down to Bristol to give us some respite for four hours at a time; it was a characteristically generous offer, which, with nearly four hours' return drive, removed duty staff from the school for eight hours. On Friday afternoon keyworker Chris arrived with a bag of Ollie's clothes from Orchard House. Rosie came at the same time to

give Ollie a dose of Picolax to clear his perennial constipation, exacerbated probably by painkillers. Then we both
drove home, leaving Chris to cope heroically with the
results.

By the time I returned at the end of Chris's four-
hour shift the worst of the evacuation was over. Bowels
clear, Ollie settled earlier that night and was lying peace-
fully in bed at about ten o'clock when an agency nurse
appeared smiling at the door. She looked very familiar
but it took me a few seconds before I twigged – yes,
of course, it's Elaine! She was one of the two CLIC
nurses who had treated Ollie's leukaemia. From the security of his bed, he gave her a shy smile, clearly remembering her after four and a half years. Half an hour later,
as if to prove that he was still the same old Ollie, he
escaped into the main area and had us all running round
the oval, chasing him for several minutes before
cornering him in a broom cupboard. A couple more
escapes and then he went to sleep.

I was woken at about three in the morning by metallic
banging. Fumbling for glasses, I looked blearily over at
the other bed, where Ollie's head was thumping up and
down. For a moment I thought he was having a tantrum,
then with an electric jolt I realised what was happening.

It was the first time I had witnessed a fit. His back
was arched and twitching unnaturally, his eyes rolled up
in a white stare, his head crashing rhythmically against
steel. I pulled him away from the bed frame and rolled
him into the recovery position, yanking the alarm cord
at the same time. Elaine arrived just as he was coming
round. She checked his skull and we were relieved to
see that he had been banging the other side from the
operation wound. The fit was noted and Ollie settled
back to sleep.

On Saturday morning the pain nurse came in specially

to discuss how the new medication was working. The general feeling, as I understood it, seemed to be that the fit during the night was not a direct reaction to tramadol. As for the headbanging, which I was terrified might have damaged the operation site, a doctor assured me that the human cranium was extremely resilient. Although they had been intending to observe Ollie longer, the hospital staff said I could take him home if I wanted to. He was getting restless, so I did. Mark, one of the Orchard care staff, who had just arrived for a session, came home with us, watching Ollie while I checked neglected emails then cooked lunch. Then Rosie arrived back from Worcester with Edmond, who had been doing his audition for the cathedral choir.

It all seemed horribly ironic, now that there would probably be no time to be with Ollie in Worcestershire. We knew that soon, probably, the tumour would start to grow again. In one anguished moment Rosie asked, 'Why can't they just do more operations – just keep removing it?' But we knew that indefinite surgery was not an option. Nor was a radical chemical and radiological cure. Instead we were going sooner or later to have to watch Ollie become progressively more paralysed, then blind, then . . . For some reason we were beginning to think that the end might come around Christmas time, so there was an urgency to enjoy the precious moments while they lasted.

That Sunday, 12th October, was a day of enchantment and I hoped that there would be others like it before Ollie was taken away from us. Rosie went to Matins and collected Edmond, while I kept an eye on Ollie and cooked lunch. When she returned, Ollie's godmother, Fiona, and one of his Son Rise teachers, Caroline Sharp, dropped in to see him. He smiled with pleasure as they told him how well he was looking, then ran several times up to the sofa to kiss Rosie, pressing little pursed Os on her forehead. Then posted some cutlery out of the kitchen window, delighting the two little girls who had moved recently into Number Four.

After lunch James, the team leader from Orchard House, came to do a session and, as Ollie was behaving impeccably, not requiring much supervision, James rolled up his sleeves to do the ironing: 'I didn't do many useful things in the army but I did learn how to iron.' Then Rosie set him cleaning with the bleach, insisting that our macho team leader wear a protective pair of turquoise rubber gloves.

What a treat to have all my shirts ironed by someone else! But I still regretted my inefficiency and wished that I did not have to spend the whole afternoon on a last-minute rejigging of a presentation for the following day, when I would be leaving before dawn for Hungary. Every half-hour or so I stole away from the study to join the others downstairs and get another glimpse of Ollie, who was rocking contentedly to a Sixties Seekers album, then another retro relic of Rosie's childhood, The Mamas and the Papas.

'Listen to this,' beamed Rosie, distracting Ollie from his dancing. 'Ollie – say "Mummy".'

His face strained briefly with the effort, then he produced a perfect 'Mu-mmy', then, on a prompt from Rosie, did a perfect 'Da-ddy'.

'Well done, Ollie!' we all applauded as he rushed off into the garden, overcome by embarrassed pride.

In the evening my youngest sister Lizzie dropped in from Yorkshire with her husband Rob. As we drank a glass of wine in the sitting room, Ollie appeared quietly beside us, smiling beatifically, then disappeared again. Later someone asked suddenly, 'Where's Ollie?' jolting me into search-and-rescue mode, but he was just sitting quietly in the kitchen eating crisps. He had spent most of the day foraging and was at last looking plumper again.

After Lizzie and Rob had left I gave Ollie his shower. Two years earlier he had still been terrified of getting his head wet, but this was another little phobia he had mastered, with help from school. He stayed in for ages, soaking up the heat and steam. Then, eventually, I switched off the water and wrapped a towel round him, manoeuvring him out to the kitchen sofa for the familiar weekend routine, rubbing and patting him dry, planting a kiss on the old radiotherapy tattoo mark on the back of his neck, getting him to put on his pyjamas – 'No, Ollie, you're quite capable of doing it yourself' – then returning to the shower room to clean teeth – 'Say, "ah . . . aaahhh" . . . open wide' – then taking him upstairs to his room.

I wanted to stay with him for a few minutes in his bedroom, but with a polite smile he shut the door firmly in my face. He had important work to do with his toys and he wanted some time alone in his room before going to sleep.

Fourteen hours later I was being driven through the suburbs of Budapest, trying to feel businesslike. I called Rosie, who said that Ollie was still in bed. Then the phone rang and I spoke to someone from Bloomsbury asking if everything was OK for this morning's talk at the Cheltenham Festival. 'Well actually I'm in Hungary. But don't worry – we arranged for someone else to take my place.'

My place in Hungary was a converted schloss in the Magyar forest where I talked that evening to a group of East European brewery managers, temporarily shelving all thoughts of Ollie as I tried to project a dynamic professional front. On Tuesday I decided to abandon my planned tour of Budapest: I just couldn't get enthused about sightseeing. Instead I got up late and went for a walk in the forest, where the wistful smell of autumn was stronger than at home, the leaves already crackling beneath dappled grey trunks of alder and beech.

Straight after lunch I took a taxi back to the airport, impatient to see whether I could change to an earlier flight. But everything was booked up, so I had to wait another three hours, eking out some spare euros on beer and sandwiches, trying to concentrate on a book. I thought about telephoning Rosie, but decided not to bother her. It was only later, back in Britain at 9.57 p.m., when the Heathrow bus put me down in the car park, that I pressed 1, then #, then the green button, and put the phone to my ear.

'How are things?' I asked cheerfully, hoping to lift the dejected tone of her dull 'hello'.

'Ollie's terrible. He didn't sleep at all last night. He's been crying all day: he's in terrible pain and no-one seems to know what's wrong. I don't think he's going to survive the night.'

Chapter Fifteen

Rosie outlined very quickly what had happened over the last two days. When Ollie woke on Monday morning, after my phone call from Budapest, he came into Rosie's bed, seeking comfort. He seemed unwell all day and by the evening was clearly ill. He lay awake all Monday night, clutching his abdomen and refusing to drink water. On Tuesday his old keyworker, Alan, came down from Sunfield and sat with him, a calm presence, for four hours. Ollie stayed in bed all day, refusing food and barely drinking.

'I phoned Frenchay,' Rosie sobbed, 'but they say they can't have him because we discharged him voluntarily on Saturday. They say we'll have to go to the RUH.'

'Maybe there's nothing they can do,' I suggested bleakly. 'Just try and hang on, and I'll be back before midnight.'

I raced out onto the perimeter road and headed for the M4 as *The World Tonight* announced that the Conservative leader, Ian Duncan Smith, was being investigated for reputedly paying excessive tax-deductible secretarial fees to his wife (an allegation subsequently refuted). 'For God's sake leave the poor bugger alone,' I shouted at the radio. 'So what! Can't you find anything better to talk about? Don't you realise my son is mortally ill!' Then I groaned at the spanking new digital notice-board near Slough triumphantly announcing traffic delays. That was all I needed.

But the god of motorways was merciful that night.

The jam eased quickly and soon I was racing at 100 mph, desperate to get back. I kept my foot hard on the floor and by eleven thirty I was parking the car in Larkhall, just as Karen the new CLIC nurse arrived.

Rosie was sitting on the side of the bed, where Ollie lay wide awake, his face gaunt with pain. As Karen came into the room his mouth turned down at the corners, as if in terror, and emitted a piteous wail.

'Oh, I'm sorry, Ollie. Did I frighten you?' she murmured.

'No, it's not fear,' I reassured her, 'it's not *you* – that's pain.' He clutched at his stomach, then struggled over to the lavatory, where he sat straining and coughing.

Karen had spoken to the neurologists in Bristol, who had assured her that Ollie's current crisis did not seem to be caused by anything happening in his head: as far as they were concerned this was not related directly to the tumour. Seeing him clutching and straining, I suggested that perhaps this was just an extreme form of Ollie's old, old problem – constipation. What about all that food he had eaten on Sunday, when we praised him so fulsomely for building up his strength? Had he done a pooh since then? He hadn't, so Karen had brought a sachet of Picolax for him to take. She also tried, without much success, to give him an enema.

I went down to the kitchen to have some food, then dragged a mattress and sleeping bag onto the floor of Ollie's room, hoping naïvely that Rosie would get some sleep in the other room. First I lay on Ollie's bed, curled around him, rubbing his back. He seemed to like it and when I paused motioned to me to continue. Later I went to lie on my own mattress. Through a semi-conscious haze I heard Rosie telephoning the RUH to ask if they had another sachet of Picolax. She drove over to Weston and returned at about three o'clock in the morning to give Ollie the medicine. I lay with him again, then returned to my mattress, getting up every ten minutes to help Ollie over to the lavatory for more fruitless straining. At about six in the morning I heard Rosie telephoning the hospital to say that nothing had happened. They suggested that we bring him in at eight thirty.

At seven forty-five Rosie settled Edmond in the car, while I carried Ollie down and put him beside his brother. He *had* survived the night, but he looked very sick. We dropped Edmond off at school then turned west along Cleveland Walk. 'Look at the tulip tree,' I exclaimed, 'isn't it wonderful!' Its huge smooth leaves were blazing gold in a blue sky, effulgent, defying winter.

At the children's ward we were lucky: there was a private room available with adjoining bathroom and family room. Chris, the registrar whom we hadn't seen for nearly five years, came in to look at Ollie and said to Rosie, 'We need soon to have a talk about what kind of pain relief we can organise . . . something that isn't morphine-based. They make fentanyl patches for adults . . . I'm wondering whether it might be possible to cut them in half, to make child doses.'

I was encouraged by this advance planning: this frank admission that at some stage we would need to help Ollie through his final struggle. But for the moment we had to deal with the immediate crisis. I think that at this stage we had already noticed some tiny red pimples on his back, like minuscule blood blisters. Rosie certainly pointed out the eczema on his lower left eyelid, which had cleared up the previous week but was now looking red again and starting to become inflamed. Then Chris left to continue a busy ward round. A nurse promised to get paracetamol but was diverted by all the other frantic calls for attention. After half an hour Rosie muttered angrily, 'I bet she would hurry if it were *her* child in pain.' Then the consultant came in, apologising to Ollie for the indignity as he did a rectal examination. He could find no blockage and suggested, 'The only other possibility is an examination under anaesthetic, to see if something is blocked higher up. I'll book him into theatre and he'll have to be nil by mouth.'

At ten o'clock I telephoned a travel PR consultant to say I might not be able to come on the planned press trip to the Majorcan mountains the next day. At eleven I telephoned Sunfield to leave a message for Ollie's teacher Karen, who had offered generously to come and visit him today, to tell her that he was too ill for visitors. A few moments later I went back out into the sunshine to take a call from the Apter training company: the feedback from Budapest was excellent and would I be free for a London event on 20th January? I remained brightly cheerful, detached from the suffering, still blithely confident that Ollie would weather this latest crisis. The final scene was scheduled for several weeks or months ahead.

I returned to the room to find Joanna Cary, who had planned for some time to visit Rosie that day, sitting quietly in a corner, calm, neutral, knowing exactly what was needed. Rosie looked at me tentatively. 'Joanna's offered to take me out to lunch. Would you mind very much if I go? Perhaps you could join us later?'

'That's very kind, but I'll stay with Ollie. Just let me go and get some sandwiches.' I walked down to the reception area, past the three Wiltshire landscapes, green and bright above all the old battered people sipping their cups at the Atrium coffee bar, bought some sandwiches and returned to the ward.

Ollie and I waited all afternoon, but there was no theatre slot available. Every fifteen minutes or so I helped him into the adjoining bathroom, where he strained unsuccessfully. On one occasion he leaned over to the basin and turned on the tap; but he needed to remain nil by mouth so I pulled his face away from the tap, accidentally cutting his mouth on a rough calcite encrustation. 'Sorry, Ollie; I'm so sorry. No drink now. *Later.*' He was too tired to protest and I helped him back to his bed.

I was still hoping that Ollie's apparent blockage was going to be cleared, averting the crisis. But Rosie seemed better attuned to the situation and that afternoon, collecting Edmond from school, she told him for the first time that his brother might die. The two of them arrived at quarter to five and sat either side of Ollie. Rosie pointed out that the eczema around his eye was now swollen and bleeding. Then she noticed the blood in his mouth and I explained about the tap. 'Naughty Dadda,' reprimanded Edmond.

'He didn't do it on purpose, darling.'

I went out to telephone Julia, my PR person, to confirm cancellation of my Majorcan walking trip. 'Do you mind, darling?' apologised Rosie. How naïve of me to have imagined, so late in the day, that I might still be going on a press trip.

There was still no news from theatre. Nor had there been an X-ray. Nor had anyone organised serious pain relief. Perhaps they needed to hold back with analgesia while Ollie was still waiting for a general anaesthetic; perhaps they didn't want to exacerbate the constipation; but both of us felt frustrated by the medical profession's prevailing tendency to be conservative with pain relief, and when a doctor came to check on Ollie, Rosie asked, 'Why isn't anything being done about his pain? It's intolerable that he should suffer like this.' The doctor had no immediate answer but said she would ask again when a slot was likely to be available in theatre.

'Bad people,' was Edmond's gloss on the situation. 'They're not looking after him properly.'

'No darling,' insisted Rosie, 'they're doing what they can. It's not their fault: no-one knows exactly what's wrong. They're doing their best; we're all doing our best. Now, will you kiss Ollie goodnight?'

Edmond leaned over, kissed Ollie's forehead, stroking his hair and piping gently, 'Goodnight Ollie.'

Then Rosie kissed him and turned to me: 'Will you be all right, darling? I'm sorry to leave you on your own, but I think I need to be with Edmond.'

'Of course it's all right. You had two days all on *your* own: now it's my turn.'

The long night started. Every fifteen minutes or so Ollie would sit on the lavatory then gesture towards the chain, too weak to stand up, imploring me to pull it. 'All right, Ollie, but you haven't done anything.' But that was irrelevant: flushing the loo, that predictable, comforting ritual, was even more important than usual in this hour of need. In between sessions I sneaked off to the parents' room to munch a sustaining sandwich and have a few nerve-soothing swigs of the sumptuous Rioja we had bought with Mark's generous cheque. Then, suddenly, back in the bathroom at about quarter to ten that evening, Ollie reached down and pulled out a turd. As the floodgates opened and I washed his hands with lashings of disinfectant soap, my eyes stung with tears of relief and I whispered, 'Well done, Ollie, well done . . . that's wonderful . . . you're going to feel better.'

As soon as he got back into bed I telephoned Rosie with the good news: 'Ollie's done a pooh!' so that she could at last stop worrying and get some sleep.

Poor boy – so many problems had revolved, with such indignity, around his erratic bowel. So much mopping up. So much protective scatological humour. So much visceral business to deal with. But thank God this latest blockage had finally cleared.

It had cleared, but the diarrhoea continued, at ever more frequent intervals. And Ollie did not look any less ill. If anything he was looking worse, still clutching his abdomen and groaning. After fourteen hours, there was now, at last, a possible theatre slot appearing on the night-time horizon. But to have any clue what to look for, the surgeon would need first to see an X-ray. The X-ray had been ordered but we waited in vain for a porter to arrive. Eventually, at ten forty-five, I went out to Ollie's night nurse and pleaded, 'This is absurd – can't we just take him ourselves?' She was a sympathetic young woman and agreed to bend rules, so the two of us set off, wheeling Ollie's bed out into the corridor, past the now deserted Atrium coffee bar, past the luminous land-scapes, then into the old wing, trundling down memory lane, passing the X-ray department where Ollie had had his first MRI scan . . . then the ward where I came to have toes amputated all those years ago . . . then, here we are, this must be Accident & Emergency, where I checked in after the Panch Chuli episode, and where Rosie brought Edmond when he drank the aromatherapy oils and they told her what an irrespon-sible mother she was . . . and here we are in the dear old A&E X-ray room.

I put on a lead apron and lifted Ollie onto the X-ray bench. The radiographer asked if he could sit up and I said, 'Ollie, can you sit up?'

He looked weakly at me, so I helped him into posi-tion, whispering, 'What a *brave* boy,' as the man held the cold film plate to his chest. 'Well done, Ollie, nice and still . . . you're amazing.' Then I lifted him onto another bench to lie flat for the second photo. Then said, 'Well done, all finished,' and we wheeled him back to the ward.

There were more visits to the bathroom. In between Ollie rested in bed and I switched on the television to watch the film *Carrington*. I had seen it before, but it was good to see again the gorgeously reconstructed painted interiors of Dora Carrington's house. And to see Jonathan Pryce as a provocatively camp Lytton Strachey, carefully placing his plump cushion on the hard wooden chair before seating himself in front of the First World War Conscientious Objectors' panel and declaring, 'I am a martyr to the piles.'

More visceral stuff. I help Ollie to the bathroom, then return to see Strachey curmudgeonly on his deathbed: 'If this is dying, I don't think much of it.' He fades away and Emma Thompson's Carrington remains alone in the empty house. She comes down at dawn and loads the shotgun. The camera shifts to the summer garden and pans with agonising slowness across the dewy lawn, lingering on the house exterior with its one lit window, and the slow movement of Schubert's string quintet is suddenly shattered by a vicious bang.

A junior surgeon came to tell me that theatre was now clogged up with road accidents. Later the duty surgical registrar came in. He showed me the X-rays and pointed to cloudy areas of what seemed to be gas, but said he could see no actual blockage or injury: our constipation theory had been a complete red herring. I wondered about appendicitis, but that would have showed up. 'But what's causing all this pain?' I asked. He couldn't tell me and he didn't think that cutting Ollie open would necessarily reveal anything. His beeper went off and he said he had to go.

'But, what —?'

'I'm sorry, I have a patient waiting under anaesthetic. I have to go.'

Our vigil continued. Some time after midnight the

trips to the bathroom became more frequent and the diarrhoea became a reddish colour. Ollie became progressively weaker and on one occasion slipped on the tiled floor, banging his hip. He was in a terrible mess and I asked him if he would be prepared to get under the shower, but he shook his head, so I just showered around his legs as he sat there.

Then things became calmer. Now that surgery seemed improbable I asked the nurse if we could start giving Ollie fluids. We got a routine going, giving him glass after glass of Dioralyte and recording fluid intake. A doctor came in and I pointed out how dramatically Ollie's hip had bruised, and how the old cannula hole on his hand had turned gun-metal blue, like the eczema blister on his eyelid. 'And what about this bleeding in his mouth,' I asked, 'why doesn't it stop?' She told me it would soon stop if I pressed a swab against it, but I was unconvinced. His face was growing pale and his lips blue. His whole vascular system seemed chronically impaired and whenever Ollie would allow it, the nurse was checking pulse, blood pressure and oxygenation.

It was now Thursday and Ollie had not slept since Monday morning. I was in my second night without sleep and I lay across the end of the bed, holding Ollie's cold feet in my hands. 'Is that nice, Ollie?'

'Hunh.'

'What an amazing boy you are. You try and get some sleep.'

I stared at his feet. The right one was a miniature version of my own still-complete right foot, the same narrow heel and long foot widening at the toes. And the toes themselves – identical! The same unusually long second toe, as long as its big neighbour. And the same kink in the fourth toe. I had always assumed mine must have been bent by wearing too tight shoes as a child, but Ollie had never had shoes too small: it was just genetic freakery. Then I remembered a recent walk along the canal . . . Edmond and Rosie behind, laughing at Ollie and me – two slopy-shouldered slender bottles shuffling along with exactly the same gait, heads in the sky.

Flesh of my flesh, lying peacefully beside me in the dead of night. He couldn't sleep but, with his meditative ability to create his own island of calm, he seemed to subdue the pain and achieve a kind of composure, lying curled on his side, very still, apart from when he reached up every few minutes for the glass of Dioralyte, taking a sip through the straw, then replacing it on the cupboard top, adjusting it until he was completely satisfied with the rightness of its position. Or he placed it on the mattress beside him, for more frequent sips on the straw. Or balanced it, with infinite precision, on the bony curve of his upturned hip. Despite the bleeding and the bruising and the gauntness, he still looked beautiful, peaceful, serene.

Soon, too soon, the bathroom visits resumed and the nurse joined me full-time, mopping, wiping and running relays to the washing machine. She found some spare clothes, including some socks to warm his icy feet. At ten to five Ollie's body suddenly arched back and his eyes stared with what seemed a look of piteous terror. For a ghastly instant I thought he was dying, then realised it was just another fit. I pulled the alarm and the doctor returned. She fired questions to which I tried to give precise answers. The diarrhoea continued and now that Ollie was too weak to stand I carried him backwards and forwards between bed and bathroom.

The darkness faded and sunlight began to illuminate some abandoned fridges in the tiny courtyard garden outside our window. In search of more exciting stimulation while Ollie rested, I switched on the television. A chatty blonde weather woman with a huge, wide, smiley mouth was standing under a radiant sky telling us that it was going to be another beautiful day.

It was Thursday.

At eight o'clock I telephoned Rosie and left a message asking her to bring lots of spare clothes and some food: the poor boy must be starving. But then, looking at him again, in the full light of day, I left another message: 'Rosie, darling, I should forget about the food and just get here as quickly as you can. He looks very ill.'

The morning ward round started and a tall suit appeared with a cluster of white-coated acolytes. There was no introduction or explanation, but I surmised that he must be the consultant surgeon when he mentioned the night-time X-ray and cancelled operation. He examined Ollie breezily, trying perhaps to protect me from the truth. I pointed out the tiny red pimples – the petechiae, which had now increased – and the bruises and the bleeding, and wondered whether there might be some problem with platelets. He agreed cheerily and said he would talk to the medical registrar about getting some bloods. Then he swept out with his entourage.

Now the morning shift had started a new nurse came into the room. Infinitely compassionate and experienced, Gill remembered Ollie from the leukaemia days and, seeing his name on the ward list that morning, had requested to look after him. She got straight on with the job, fetching clean sheets and stacks of absorbent pads. While she mopped and wiped, I cradled Ollie in my arms, trying always to lay him gently back on the bed.

Rosie arrived at eight forty. Almost immediately she said, 'Hasn't Chris seen him? I think you should go and get her.'

I went out to the doctor's station where Chris was preparing for another long day on the ward. 'Has the consultant surgeon spoken to you?' I asked.

'No, not yet.'

'Please would you come and see Ollie. He looks very, very ill.'

She came immediately and, despite obvious alarm, managed brilliantly to remain utterly dispassionate with Ollie as she examined him. Unable to stand back passively, we pointed out the huge green hip bruise, the petechiae and the bleeding in his left eye. She suggested optimistically, trying to shield us, that the blood seemed to be coming from the eczema wounds, but I insisted, 'Look, I think it's actually coming from under the eyelid.' Then Rosie said, very, very quietly, 'Oh no, look – the operation wound!' Blood was seeping between the stitches.

Things now swung very quickly into action. Chris announced that she would get bloods for the lab immediately. Rosie looked at me and said, 'You must be exhausted. Why don't you go and get some sleep?' I agreed that I might be more use after a rest and said I would go home. I was still imagining idiotically that this crisis would somehow be resolved, that our indestructible son would pull through once more, deferring the final scene to some still undecided future date. But Rosie insisted, 'I think it would be better if you slept here,' and Chris agreed. 'Yes – better to stay close.'

At ten past nine I went into the family room, pulled out the bed, drew the curtains, took off shoes, socks and trousers, and lay down. Inchoate images of brain haemorrhages and other half-imagined disasters swirled briefly through my consciousness, but were quickly swamped by random dreams with no obvious connection to Ollie. They faded almost instantly when Rosie's voice cut urgently through my sleep: 'Stephen . . . Stephen, wake up. You have to get up.'

'What's the time?'

'Eleven o'clock. You must get up quickly.'

'What's happening?'

'The consultant —' her lips quivered, and tears gushed as she completed the sentence — 'he's got to talk to us.'

My heart was thudding and I was desperate for a pee. As I headed for the door, Rosie burst into tears. 'Put your trousers on — the room's full of doctors.'

I fumbled with belt and flies, then started searching for socks and shoes, until Rosie urged, 'Just go barefoot. Hurry!' I caught a glimpse of Ollie, chalk-pale amongst a blur of white coats, as I padded through to the bathroom. Then I returned to the family room and stood barefoot beside Rosie, arm around her waist, as Chris and the consultant came in. The latter directed his words at me. 'I'm afraid Ollie's situation has deteriorated very rapidly during the last two hours. He has a condition called DIC — disseminated intravascular coagulation — which means, basically, that all the blood-clotting mechanisms stop working.' I stared intently at him, wondering what terrible new decisions we would have to make over the next few days. Then came the awful realisation as he continued, 'We *could* try to give him platelets' — a slight pause and pained look — 'but we would have to put a line into his *groin*' — then the punchline — 'and at the very best, it would only give him a few hours.'

Hours!

So this was it. Now. Today. This very Thursday. No more deferrals. No slow, careful, controlled decisions about how to ease Ollie's future death. It was happening right now.

I knew exactly what we wanted to say, but let Rosie speak first. 'No,' she said, quavering just slightly, 'please

– no more needles. I don't want to make him suffer any more.'

The consultant looked relieved and promised, 'We'll get out of the room straight away. It'll be very quick now and we'll make sure that you can be alone with him, as peaceful as possible. And I'll give him some fentanyl to make him as comfortable as possible.'

Rosie was only able to tell me later about the misery of those hundred minutes while I lay dreaming in the family room: the desperate struggle to find a vein on Ollie's wan little hand; his anguish at the needle; her resisting the desperate longing to hold and hug him, because he wouldn't like that, so that instead she just held his hand and told him over and over again how brave he was and how much she loved him, as his eyes slid in and out of focus, recognising his mother then withdrawing behind the mist; and his last request, to do a pooh, too weak to get to the bathroom, but still determined to do things properly, reaching out for a cardboard bedpan, placing it on the bed and trying to muster the strength to sit on it, because he knew that that was what he should do.

We went through to Ollie's room. His Gregorian Chant collection – a Christmas present from adored Irene – was playing softly on the CD machine. And there, propped up on pillows, was an Ollie quite different from the Ollie I had last seen properly two hours earlier. His face was completely white, puffed slightly with oedema, blue lips parted just enough to breathe. He tried for a moment to sit up, made a weak cry and gestured to the consultant to go away. The consultant said, 'It's all right, Ollie, I'm going to leave you alone now.' He slipped some fentanyl into Ollie's vein, then left the room. Gill, the nurse, pulled the bed away from the wall and brought over two chairs, so that we could sit side by side, facing Ollie. Then she too left the room.

For the first time since the discovery of the tumour, a huge involuntary sob burst from my body. Rosie held my head to her chest and said, 'It's all right – you can cry.' The tears stopped after a minute or two and I turned again to Ollie. I was forty-nine and although I knew many people who had died in the mountains, I had never been there myself when it had happened. Unlike Rosie, I had no direct experience of death. I had rehearsed in my mind so often what Ollie's death might be like, but I had never really known what to expect.

After the sleepless struggle of the last three days he was now, thank God, free from pain. He lay on his side, eyes closed, hands clasped in front of his chest, just under his chin. We wanted to pick him up in our arms, but even in his drugged state he would have hated it, so we just sat and gazed. Gill came back into the room and stood on the far side of the bed, silent and discreet, occasionally putting a stethoscope very gently to the skin of his back. She handed us tissues to wipe the blood trickling from his nose. That was the most useful thing we could do – keeping him clean and beautiful.

It all happened very quickly – far too quickly. Just after midday his breathing became faster and even fainter – tiny, hurried little whispers. Then there was a little cough followed by silence. As we dabbed his face, Rosie said, 'I think he's gone.' Gill slid her stethoscope under his stripy pyjama jacket, listened intently and said, 'Yes – it's very faint now.' Then she moved away and stood by the window, leaving us to gaze alone at our dead son.

'Isn't it extraordinary,' said Rosie, 'that total stillness.' She stroked his hair and murmured, 'Still warm . . . so beautiful, isn't he? Do you remember how rude we were when he was born?' It seemed unbelievable that almost twelve and half years had passed since that moment when we first met him, just two hundred yards from this room, and stared at his squashed little ugly-duckling face. I stroked our handsome swan and said what a beautiful nose he had and Rosie laughed, 'Well you would say that – it's exactly like *your* nose.'

The consultant came in, apologising for the intrusion, and swiftly, deftly performed his task of confirming death. A few moments later Chris, the registrar, came in, sat beside the bed and said how dreadfully sorry she was. As she left the room, Rosie said, 'This must happen so often. It must be so terrible for them. What a desperate job.'

Even though she had witnessed both her parents' deaths, Rosie had no previous experience of a child's death: she was an ingénue, like me. We were new to this business and not sure exactly what to do. I asked Jill how long we could sit with Ollie and she told us we could stay as long as we liked. There were no rules. But would we like her to telephone anyone?

'Oh thank you, so much,' replied Rosie. 'Would you ring Ollie's school, please. And the Abbey. And Edmond's school; we'll come and collect him after the afternoon break and take him quietly out of class. What about your parents, Stephen?'

'I can phone them,' I replied.

'Are you sure?'

'Well, perhaps not. No – perhaps it would be easier if Gill did it.'

We stayed for an hour, then left to tell Edmond. I wanted to stay and help clean Ollie, but it would have been too hard for Rosie to go on her own. We said nothing to Edmond until we had walked right out of the school building and got into the car. He said afterwards that he knew perfectly well the reason for this sudden interruption to his day, but he still had to ask, 'What's happened, Mumma?'

'What's happened is that Ollie has died.' She asked if he would like to go and see his brother. He didn't have to if he didn't want to. But he said he would like to, so we headed back towards Weston and as we drove along Cleveland Walk there it was again, the tulip tree, still as brilliantly golden as it had been when we had passed it with Ollie thirty hours earlier.

Perhaps it was a mistake to go back to the hospital. I had not realised how drastically rigor mortis would change the body before it resumed a more lifelike form. The thing which lay on the bed was no longer Ollie. As Edmond said afterwards, it looked as though it was made of plasticine. It was like a waxwork: all the correct features were there, but the luminosity – the subtle subcutaneous radiance of the real person – had gone.

Despite that, Gill had laid him out beautifully in a clean pair of his trademark stripy pyjamas, hands still clasped in front of his chest. The three of us sat beside him for a while, then Gill asked whether we would like a cup of tea and Rosie said that that would be lovely.

'And what about something to eat?' asked Gill.

'Actually, I'm *starving*,' Rosie laughed. 'Any chance of some toast and marmalade?'

And so the three of us ate our buttered toast and marmalade, standing in the room with Ollie, close yet separate as we had been so often in the past, when he couldn't join our casein- and gluten-laden feast. Edmond grew bored and went into the next room to watch television, starting guiltily when Rosie went in and blurting, 'Am I being disrespectful to Ollie?' He seemed unsure what to do, embarrassed that the tears would not flow; but Rosie assured him that there was no correct procedure: we would just have to make things up as we went along. Some of the time we would be very, very sad, but that didn't preclude happiness and laughter.

My mother came to join us and said that someone was still trying to contact my father on a golf course. He arrived about fifteen minutes later and seemed the most stricken, remembering probably his child sister who died from peritonitis before the days of antibiotics, but also feeling deeply for the grief of his son. The CLIC nurse Karen came to see us and said that the Rector would be coming to our house the next day to discuss the funeral. She and my parents left. Soon after that we left too. We felt, wrongly perhaps, that we would not want to see Ollie's body again before the burial and so, as we each bent down to kiss his cold cheek, it was a kind of farewell.

Then, delegating to the professionals, we walked out, touched by the kind words of nurses, doctors and secretaries, as we left the ward for the last time. As we walked across to the car Edmond asked if we could hire a video on the way home, 'to cheer ourselves up', and Rosie answered, 'Not today, darling. We will soon, but today Daddy and I just need time to be quiet and think about Ollie.' In the car park rowan berries were plumped up, fruitfully mellow to order, scarlet against the intense blue sky. Probably the gathering swallows were also twittering obediently. The whole world seemed to glow with an intense beauty and as we drove off Edmond said he felt that Ollie was there, all around us.

Amidst all that autumnal glory the mundane still made its demands. In Larkhall I stopped to get milk from the supermarket, incredulous that all the other shoppers were continuing about their daily business, untouched by this momentous event. Only later did Tony the greengrocer tell me that two other Larkhall people had died that day. Back at home we ate some supper, then put Edmond to bed. Rosie ran herself a steaming therapeutic bath. I glanced into Ollie's room, at the sheets still ruffled from two nights earlier, then went back downstairs. I poured myself some wine then opened the cupboard to choose a CD. I needed music – something to express the inexpressible – and it didn't take long to make my choice: Beethoven's C sharp minor quartet, written in the last year of his life, recorded on this disc by the Allegri Quartet. How many times had I listened to that opening phrase on the first violin? The rising third, then the semitone, reaching up to the tonic C #, hinting tenuously at resolution before plummeting to that plangent sforzando, which dissipates in the onward flow – calm, mellifluous, seamless – as the second violin echoes the opening four-bar phrase; and then, four bars later, the viola, adding darker richness; and then Bruno on his cello, in the last recording he made before retirement – 'not bad, eh, for an old man of seventy' – pouring a lifetime's humanity into this yearning lament.

I sat utterly still, letting each of the seven continuous movements soak into me, allowing the tears to flow, reaching out to the unknowable, wanting to know where our son was, longing to bring him back and tell him everything, desperate to ask him so many questions. But all I could do was lament over and over again, 'Oh, Ollie . . . Oh, Ollie.' We came to the penultimate movement – the tantalisingly brief adagio, with its repeated falling phrase, like a supplication – then plunged into the final allegro: restless, frenetic, anguished, but also soothingly complete and whole as it alluded insistently to the quartet's opening, bringing the journey full circle and ending in a defiant blaze of major chords. Afterwards I sat silently for a few minutes longer, then went up to join Rosie in bed; and soon, very quickly, the two of us cried ourselves to sleep.

Chapter Sixteen

No-one was quite sure why Ollie had died so suddenly – what had caused his whole system to go into meltdown. He had often been in the kind of perilous condition known to trigger disseminated intravascular coagulation. Leukaemia, tumours, post-operative trauma, immunosuppression resulting from chemotherapy . . . all these were familiar causes of DIC. But Ollie had been in remission from leukaemia for over four years. And as for the brain tumour operation, he had recovered well from that and, apart from cortico-steroids, was taking no immunosuppressive drugs when the illness struck so unexpectedly. In many ways the suddenness was a blessing, sparing him and us the slow, languishing death for which we were bracing ourselves. But the shock of it still left us wanting to know 'Why?'

So we asked to have his body sent to Bristol for an autopsy. And I thought how lucky we were, in this rich country of ours, that after all the hundreds of thousands of pounds which had been spent treating our son, no-one quibbled about this additional expense. It was only several weeks later, some time after Ollie had been buried, that we finally saw the autopsy report. It had taken some serious sleuthing to discover exactly what had killed him.

Professor Seth Love, the neuropathologist at Frenchay, examining a microscope slide of brain tissue from the operation site, noticed several rogue cells with a familiar pattern – a nucleus that contained dark reddish material with a surrounding 'halo' – the characteristic insignia of a virus. He did antigen tests on the tissue, and came up eventually with a positive result for VZV, short for varicella zoster virus – the shingles/chickenpox virus.

There had been no trace of the live virus in the biopsy taken from Ollie's brain two weeks before he died: it had flared up since the operation. Curious as to whether this was just an isolated incident in the brain, Professor Love asked to see samples of the main internal organs and found nearly all of them – spleen, liver, lungs – riddled with VZV. Nearly all of us have the virus lying dormant in our bodies, a remnant of childhood chickenpox, and occasionally, usually in late middle or old age, it can flare up painfully in the form of shingles. But it can also activate internally, rampaging through the body as disseminated VZV.

In Ollie's case the virus probably originated with the chickenpox scare he had during leukaemia treatment in the summer of 1997. For some reason the virus was activated six years later, several days after the craniotomy. Professor Love stressed categorically that there was no indication of any fault with the actual surgery: this sudden eruption of an unexpected complication was just sheer bad luck. Like DIC, disseminated VZV was often associated with the immediate aftermath of chemotherapy or severe trauma; but again, Ollie's case did not fit that pattern – he had survived those threats. Nor did his case fit the textbook pattern of internal dissemination being accompanied by an obvious, easily identifiable, skin rash. Good old Ollie – even in this last fatal illness, he was a one-off, defiantly different from everyone else!

We were naturally curious about the possibility of measles, but no trace of measles virus was found in any of the histological samples. So if Ollie's early problems were initiated by his MMR vaccination, with him, unlike some other autistic children, there was no clear indication of association. That did not alter our belief that the vaccination had been one important factor, amongst others, in his becoming autistic. And it seems conceivable that that initial insult to his immune system could have led, through a very indirect and convoluted series of compounding insults – leaky gut, neurological damage, leukaemia, chemotherapy, radiotherapy, brain tumour – to his death. Perhaps. The only thing we know with any degree of certainty – and even here the precise sequence of cause and effect is not definitive – is that at the end a sudden outbreak of shingles made him extremely ill. That vicious attack on his internal organs was probably the cause of the mysterious abdominal pain. The resulting infection and trauma probably sparked off the disseminated intravascular coagulation. Once the vascular system packed up, even Ollie's robust little body could take no more.

We buried him on the thirty-first day of October, fifteen days after he died. During the intervening fortnight we lived in a kind of limbo, finding it hard to believe that he really was dead. Edmond had some time off school and stayed at home. Rosie was for the first few days extremely ill in bed and at one point she wondered if she had caught Ollie's still undiagnosed fatal illness, but hers proved to be just a particularly virulent flu, which subsided mercifully.

We sustained ourselves with the therapy of busyness, writing letters and emails, organising the autopsy, looking at graveyards, preparing the memorial service, organising a coffin, registering the death. I spent happy hours going through all the photos from the last twelve years, ordering reprints and transparency conversions, then preparing three huge collages of Ollie images for framing behind glass, plus one single large print to display, at brother Philip's suggestion, during the memorial service.

All that activity helped. But far, far more important was the surge tide of love and affection pouring in from the hundreds of people who had known Ollie. Perhaps most touching of all, for the parents from hell, was to receive a handwritten letter from Ollie's Bath oncology consultant. And messages from the other climbers – Harish Kapadia, Jim Fotheringham, Stephen Reid, Jim Curran, Chris Bonington – who had lost children. The house was filled with gorgeous bouquets of flowers, from local friends, from all Ollie's schools, from Edmond's school, from Rosie's teaching colleagues, from the Option Institute, from the solicitors, from Ammy at United Airlines and from Jake and Shan, who arranged specially to fly over from Kenya. It felt like Christmas, with cards and letters – including personal messages from every single one of the Option Institute teachers who had worked with Ollie – pouring through the letter box every morning. And they *did* make a difference – a huge difference – along with the line-jamming rush of emails.

We were enveloped by generosity. Rosie's sister, Nonie, drove straight over to Bath to live with us for a few days and take care of all the cooking and shopping, making sure that, as well as food, we had plentiful stocks of therapeutic wine. On a more spiritual note, the Rector came round to pray for us and for Ollie, and to promise that we could have a memorial service – a service of thanksgiving for Ollie's life – in the Abbey. Determined not to lay our son in an off-the-shelf coffin, I asked my old cabinet-making companion from the Panch Chuli expedition, Stephen Sustad, if he would make something simple and beautiful and to tell me how much it would cost. He emailed back to say that it would cost nothing and that Julian Freeman-Attwood was donating some of his finest quarter-sawn oak. Dick Renshaw was going to carve the nameplate to go on the lid. We asked him to put: 'Ollie Venables, 1991–2003, A Brave Boy'.

And so one fine morning Rosie and I drove up the old familiar route to Shropshire, meeting Sustad for a pub lunch near Bridgnorth. He hugged us both, and described how he had adapted a recent wardrobe design. Said this had been the saddest job of his life, but what an enjoyable time he had spent chatting in the workshop with Dick, who had stayed up all night carving his meticulous V-cut Roman script. We transferred the coffin, which was beautiful, to our car and headed back south. On the way home Rosie had to buy some new boots from John Lewis – she was determined to look good at the service – so we stopped at the giant shopping centre, laughing at the sight of the car parked outside with its coffin, like something in a gangster movie.

My father persuaded his amenable Parish Council that, although Ollie himself had not lived in the village, his family was associated closely enough to justify a discretionary burial in the tiny village cemetery where every spring the ground was spangled densely with flowers like a Botticelli painting, and where there was always the sound – so quintessentially Ollie – of water splashing in a fountain nearby. Although I acknowledged the illogicality of placing so much importance on the lifeless body – that caricature waxwork we had already kissed goodbye – I was discovering the importance of mourning ritual and of having a special place for the body to rest. I began to understand the agony of friends who had lost sons, daughters, lovers and spouses in the

Himalaya and been denied a body to grieve over; realised why it was so necessary for so many of them to go to the place where their loved one had died.

Jake and Shan flew in from Africa the day before the burial and drove over to Larkhall with their daughter Robyn. We feasted and toasted Ollie with champagne, bracing ourselves for the morning's trial. In the morning godfather Henry arrived from Edinburgh. Lucius's wife, Joanna, and godmother Fiona met us at the graveyard, with my parents and most of my brothers and sisters. We arrived at the last possible moment, flowers clutched in nervous hands, panting as we walked up the steep lane, hearts jolting as we saw the coffin resting on its trestles beside the pale stony cavity.

The weather had finally broken and the grass was sodden underfoot. But for the moment the rain abated, confined accommodatingly to a dark bruised sky which accentuated the amber intensity of the huge beech tree standing sentinel over the grave. A few more days and the leaves would be gone.

The Rector did his job perfectly, leading us with a few short simple prayers, crystallising Ollie's special spirit by telling us how he was now 'free as a bird'. He knew that for all of us this grim interment was the hardest bit: tomorrow we could celebrate joyously in the Abbey. Nevertheless it was hugely comforting to have immediate family there, acknowledging. And to see the flowers. The floral watering can from Sunfield was a touching stroke of genius – pure Shakespearean comic relief after the awful finality of throwing our own handful of yellow freesias into the grave. Then we looked more closely at the other flowers beside the still-gaping chasm: a gorgeous autumn arrangement of cream roses, scarlet hips, steel-blue viburnum berries and silvery wild clematis from Fiona, little bouquets from Ollie's cousins, cyclamen from my parents and a bouquet from Edmond with a handwritten note: 'Dear Ollie, I will always remember you.'

I stayed for lunch with my family then returned to Larkhall, and that night we had a consoling pub dinner with all the godparents. Then, on Saturday morning, All Saints' Day, we were blessed again with brilliant sunshine and I thought, as I strode in my suit up the gracious wide pavement of Great Pulteney Street, with Shan, Rosie and Robyn all looking incredibly stylish, 'How lucky I am to be accompanied by these beautiful women!'

We had made a detailed seating plan for the Abbey, trying to put all Ollie's closest family, friends and carers near the front. It was thrilling to see so many Sunfield staff, all dressed formally in their smartest clothes, over-flowing their allotted space and filling three whole pews on the north side. Rosie, Edmond and I sat in the front pew on the south side, with my parents. As midday approached my father looked back down the nave, aghast, and whispered melodramatically, 'How on earth will we feed them all?'

'Don't worry,' I laughed, 'they haven't come for the sandwiches: it's not important. As long as everyone gets a drink . . . that's the main thing.' He had generously booked a large hotel reception room and refreshments so that people didn't have to melt away immediately after the service, but had underestimated the numbers. As far as I was concerned it was just wonderful to see the pews filling with aunts, cousins, friends, neighbours, teachers, carers, nurses, doctors – even members of the Alpine Club! – all giving up their precious Saturday morning to acknowledge Ollie. The Abbey choir also gave their time – the girls and men – to come and sing for him. Precisely on the dot of noon we all stood up as they processed silently up the nave with proper solemnity. Then we started with 'The King of Love My Shepherd Is', followed later by Parry's setting of 'Dear Lord and Father of Mankind', with its final protective soft refrain – 'O still small voice of calm'. Our third hymn was the boisterous setting of Robert Bridges' 'All My Hope on God Is Founded' by Herbert Howells – the setting he called 'Michael' in memory of the child *he* lost.

My brother Philip, the Reverend, led the prayers with his usual articulate intelligence, on this occasion generously overcoming his low-church sensibilities to wear unaccustomed vestments. The resident Rector gave an eloquent address from the pulpit, including some of the best Ollie stories, celebrating his joyful spirit but also enumerating the tough challenges he had had to face and adding, 'I can't tell you *why*: bad things just happen.' Lucius read a poem by Christina Rossetti and Alan, Ollie's former keyworker, represented Sunfield with an affectionate funny tribute to their most exhausting pupil. The head, Barry Carpenter, at our request read a poem called 'Welcome to Holland' (with apologies to Edmond's Dutch godfather Kees) which we had first seen pinned on the wall at the Option Institute. The gist of the poem is that having a special needs child is a bit like going on holiday to Italy: you get all excited about the Sistine Chapel and Florence and Giotto and the Mediterranean food and the wine and the dazzling sunshine. At last the big day arrives and you get on the plane; but when you land the other end the steward announces that there has been a change of plan: actually you have arrived in Holland. This is bitterly disappointing, until it dawns on you that, although Holland is not what you signed up for, now you think about it, it has its own, less obvious, charms: it has windmills and tulips and Rembrandts . . .

For me the greatest consolation of that service was listening to the choir singing Fauré's *Cantique de Jean Racine*. It is a well-known piece but we had only stumbled on it recently, by chance, as one of the romantic choral works interspersing Ollie's disc of Gregorian plainsong. Even though it is actually a morning call to prayer, its simple, contemplative, melodic innocence had made it perfect bedtime music. Like Rembrandt's tormented Saul, soothed by David's harp, Ollie seemed, right to the end, to find solace in music, and the *Cantique* had been one of the last sounds he heard as he lay dying. So it seemed the perfect choice for this service. The girls and men had been rehearsing it for a recording and they sang it beautifully, as shafts of light slanted through the south transept, projecting amethyst patterns onto the pale creamy stone behind them.

I wanted it to go on for ever, wanted to remain on this island of peaceful contemplation, delaying the moment when we had to start the rest of our lives. The hardest part was still ahead and for Rosie, the mother, the aching void must have seemed even emptier, the endless daily reminders harder to face. Weeks would pass before we dared to start, gradually, taking down all the elaborate security gates cluttering the staircase. Giving some of Ollie's toys to the children of his helpers, so apt in theory, would in practice prove painfully difficult; the garden, as one neighbour put it so nicely, would be diminished by his absence, the unchewed fennel, flowering eight feet high for the first time, just another reminder of what we had lost.

Of course there would also be laughter – lots of laughter as the repeated tales of Ollie's quirky, provocative, mischievous, weird, batty, creative, enigmatic, exasperating deeds took on a kind of epic, Homeric quality. And we would take increasing delight from the pictures of him which hung on every wall, and his clothes which Edmond now wore. And the sadness? Of course it would never, ever, go away, but as someone wrote in one of the scores of letters we kept, that sadness would eventually transform itself into a kind of familiar, comforting ache.

The choir sang one final pianissimo anthem, 'God Be in My Head'. The Rector gave the blessing from the high altar. There was a pause while Peter King, the director of music, dashed up to the organ loft. Then, lighting up the silence, filling the whole of that glorious effulgent space, the organ thundered out the brilliant, trilling, austere opening chord of Bach's *Fantasia and Fugue in G minor*. I wanted to linger, wanted to wait for one particular sequence of harmonies so improbable, so awesome, so unfathomably sublime that it seems to transcend mere human creation; but already the vergers were opening the west doors, and we had agreed to process out immediately after the choir and clergy, leading the rest of the congregation. So we left our pew, walking briskly down the nave, Rosie looking gorgeous in a black fur hat, Edmond between us in his Sunday-best Norwegian jumper, the three of us solemn, but smiling inwardly with pride: pride for Ollie, the boy who had inspired all these people to come here and give thanks. We walked past them, row after row of faces – more people than I had ever imagined would be here – and then we passed the final row and came out through the great west doors into the bright light.

Select Bibliography

Attwood, A. (1993) *Why Does Chris Do That?* London: National Autistic Society
Excellent beginners' guide to living with an autistic child.

Grandin, T. (1995) *Thinking in Pictures and Other Reports from My Life with Autism*. New York: Bantam Doubleday Dell
One of several books by the well-known autistic academic.

Kaufman, B.N. (1994) *Happiness is a Choice*. New York: First Ballantine Books
The philosophy underpinning the Son-Rise approach.

Kaufman, B.N. (1995) *Son-Rise: The Miracle Continues*. Novato, CA: H.J.Kramer
'Bears' Kaufman's account of the unique approach he and his wife developed to help their son Raun emerge from autism.

Le Breton, M. (1998) *Gluten & Dairy Free Cookbook*. London: Jessica Kingsley

Lewis, L. (1998) *Special Diets for Special Kids*. Arlington, TX: Future Horizons

Lovaas, O.I. (1981) *Teaching Developmentally Disabled Children: The ME Book*. Austin, TX: Pro-ed
The original ABA teaching manual.

McCandless, J. (2002) *Children with Starving Brains: A medical treatment guide for autism spectrum disorder*. Bramble Books
A clinician's guide to biomedical treatments for autistic spectrum disorders.

Maurice, C. (1993) *Let Me Hear Your Voice: A Family's Triumph Over Autism.* New York: Alfred A. Knopf
Parent's compelling account of successful ABA intervention with her autistic children.

Maurice, C., Green, G. and Luce, S. (1996) *Behavioural Intervention for Young Children with Autism: A Manual for Parents and Professionals.* Austin, Tx: Pro-ed.
Updated ABA teaching manual.

Moore, C. (2004) *George and Sam.* London: Viking
Mother's highly praised account of bringing up two autistic boys.

Sacks, O. (1995) *An Anthropologist on Mars: Seven Paradoxical Tales.* New York: Alfred A. Knopf
Includes the famous *New Yorker* article about Sacks' encounter with Temple Grandin.

Seroussi, K. (2000) *Unravelling the Mystery of Autism and Pervasive Developmental Disorder: A Mother's Story of Research and Recovery.* New York: Simon & Schuster
Parent's impressive metabolic detective work.

Shattock, P., Whitely, P. and Savery, D. (2002) *Autism as a Metabolic Disorder: Guidelines for Gluten and Casein-free Dietary Intervention.* Sunderland: Autism Research Institute, University of Sunderland.
Serious science by the British guru of dietary intervention.

Shaw, W. (2002) *Biological Treatments for Autism and PDD.* Kansas: The Great Plains Laboratory
Detailed summary of current research into biological approaches to autism.

Waterhouse, S. (2000) *A Positive Approach to Autism.* London: Jessica Kingsley
An expanded, updated version of the former Stella Carlton's *The Other Side of Autism.* A professional's holistic approach, brimming with open-minded curiosity.

Williams, D. (1992) *Nobody Nowhere*. New York: Times Books
Harrowing account of autistic woman's difficult childhood.

Williams, D. (1994) *Somebody Somewhere*. London: Transworld
The happier sequel by one of the people who has done most
to explain what it feels like to be autistic.

Useful Organisations

The National Autistic Society
393 City Road
London EC1V 1NG
020 7833 2299
http://www.nas.org.uk/

Autism Research Institute
Bernard Rimland, Director
4182 Admas Avenue
San Diego
CA 92116
USA
(1) 619 281 7165
http://www.autismresearchinstitute.com/

Autism Research Unit
School of Health Sciences
University of Sunderland
Sunderland
SR2 7EE
0191 510 8922
http://www.osiris.sunderland.ac.uk/autism/

The Schafer Autism Report
9629 Old Placerville Road
Sacramento
CA 95827
USA
http://www.freewebz.com/Schafer/SARHome.htm

Allergy Induced Autism
11 Larklands
Longthorpe
Peterborough
Cambridgeshire
PE3 6LL
http://www.autismmedical.com

Pfeiffer Treatment Center
4575 Weaver Parkway
Warrenville
IL 60555-403
USA

Treehouse
Treehouse
Woodside Avenue
N10 3JA
http://www.treehouse.org.uk

Gluten and casein-free parents' groups:
gfcfkids@yahoogroups.com
gfcfkidsUK@yahoogroups.com

Peach
(Parents for the Early Intervention in Autism in Children)
The Brackens, London Road
Ascot, Berkshire SL5 8BE
01344 882248
info@peach.org.uk
www.peach.org.uk

The Counseling Center
Auditory Integration Therapy Division
7 Tokeneke Road
Darien CT 06820
USA
(1) 203 655 1091
aithelps@aol.com

Index

THE POWER OF READING

Visit the Random House website and get connected with information on all our books and authors

EXTRACTS from our recently published books and selected backlist titles

COMPETITIONS AND PRIZE DRAWS Win signed books, audiobooks and more

AUTHOR EVENTS Find out which of our authors are on tour and where you can meet them

LATEST NEWS on bestsellers, awards and new publications

MINISITES with exclusive special features dedicated to our authors and their titles

READING GROUPS Reading guides, special features and all the information you need for your reading group

LISTEN to extracts from the latest audiobook publications

WATCH video clips of interviews and readings with our authors

RANDOM HOUSE INFORMATION including advice for writers, job vacancies and all your general queries answered

Come home to Random House

www.randomhouse.co.uk